Promoting
Collaboration in
Primary Mental
Health Care

Promoting Collaboration in Primary Mental Health Care

Edited by

Peter Nolan
Professor of Mental Health Nursing
School of Health Sciences
University of Birmingham

and

Frances Badger
Research Fellow
School of Health Sciences
University of Birmingham

Published in 2002 by:
Nelson Thornes Ltd
Delta Place
27 Bath Road
CHELTENHAM
GL53 7TH
United Kingdom

02 03 04 05 06 / 10 9 8 7 6 5 4 3 2 1

A catalogue record for this book is available from the British Library

ISBN 0 7487 5874 7

Illustrations by Northern Phototypesetting Ltd
Page make-up by Northern Phototypesetting Ltd

Printed and bound in Spain by Graphycems

Contents

LIST OF CONTRIBUTORS

Jon Arcelus is a consultant in child and adolescent psychiatry at Thorneywood Adolescent Unit, Nottingham. His research interests include attention deficit hyperactivity disorder and psychiatric co-morbidity in children and adolescents.

Lynn Ashburner is currently working on a World Bank project in Bulgaria, setting up management courses within the health sector. Previously, she managed MBA programmes and conducted health services-based research into the management of change, reorganisation of health care and collaboration.

Frances Badger is a research fellow in the School of Health Sciences at the University of Birmingham. She has a nursing background, has worked on a number of health and social care studies and has an interest in promoting mental health care within primary care settings.

James Briscoe is a consultant community psychiatrist in North Birmingham. He has a particular interest in developing strong links with primary care practices and organisations and exploring the further potential of primary mental health care.

Paul Craddock has a background in social work and has been a mental health team manager since 1991, working in a number of areas, including forensic work. He is particularly interested in working in any way to improve services for people with severe and enduring mental illness.

Jim Cody has worked as a mental health nurse within the NHS since the mid-1960s and is currently working as a community psychiatric nurse in an inner-city area. His special interest is in caring for people with continuous mental health needs, within a primary care setting.

Diane Cook is Clinical Manager, Eating Disorders Service, with Worcester Community and Mental Health Trust. Previously, she worked in the private sector and as an independent training and professional development consultant. She also has an interest in working with clients suffering from complex PTSD.

Neil Deuchar is a consultant psychiatrist in primary care liaison. Interests include care pathways, primary mental health care, the integration of primary and secondary care and services, and ways of operationalising the National Service Framework in mental health.

Steve Field is acting Regional Postgraduate Dean for the West Midlands, a GP principal in inner-city Birmingham, and Chair of the Implementation Committee for the new UK GP Registrar Scheme. He is committed to developing and supporting the teaching, learning and assessment of communication skills in general practice.

Fiona Gale is a senior primary child mental health worker and Honorary Visiting Fellow in Child and Adolescent Psychiatry at the University of Leicester, and has been involved in education and the development of new roles within CAMHS. Interests include children's perceptions of mental health stigma, primary mental health work, adolescent forensic psychiatry and young people in care.

Tom Harrison is a consultant psychiatrist working in rehabilitation in Birmingham. The holistic approach to severe and enduring mental illness had led him to consider the psychological issues for the general population and he has been working in mental health promotion for the past eight years in the West Midlands region.

Zyl Harvey taught art and worked in a variety of sectors before re-training and working in assisting people with disabilities into employment. Becoming a service user changed her life and opened doors to new roles; writing, presenting and communicating by any means in order to remove the stigma of the 'user' label and to give understanding, courage and hope to fellow travellers and professionals.

Marie Holland has general, mental health nursing and CPN qualifications. She currently works as a primary care-based mental health nurse, enjoying the demands placed upon her skills by the whole variety of mental health problems. Interests include the provision of equitable services to those with severe and enduring mental illness in addition to those with common mental health problems.

Abid Kahn is a consultant in general adult psychiatry in Stafford, working very much within a shared care model with primary care practitioners. He is also responsible for the district-wide intensive care unit and a trainer for the psychiatric training programme. Additional interests include medico-legal work on behalf of patients and with local law firms.

Jennifer Law is a mental health promotion strategist, fostering an entrepreneurial way of promoting mental health, involving the identification of opportunities, and the development and management of radical and innovative projects. Interests include organisational dynamics, entrepreneurism and corporate social responsibility.

Helen Lester has been a GP in inner-city Birmingham for 10 years, is a senior lecturer in primary care and Co-Director of the University of Birmingham Interdisciplinary Centre for Mental Health. Her particular interests relate to primary care provision for people with serious and enduring mental illness.

John Macleod is an epidemiologist at the Department of Primary Care and General Practice at the University of Birmingham and a GP in central Birmingham. His main research activity deals with the explanation and amelioration of health inequalities. He has a long-standing interest in problem drug use, both from a clinical and from an epidemiological perspective.

Julie Marlow is a community mental health nurse for older people working within South Birmingham Mental Health NHS Trust. Although involved in all aspects of mental health care of older people, she has a special interest in dementia care and services provision for people with dementia and their carers.

Peter Nolan is Professor of Mental Health Nursing at the University of Birmingham and has a long-standing interest in the history of mental health services in the UK. His current research interests focus on the emerging primary care services and the characteristics that will distinguish them from services provided in the past. The changing roles of community and primary care nurses are other areas of interest.

Jan R. Oyebode is Course Director for the Clinical Psychology Doctorate at the University of Birmingham, a clinical psychologist with older adults and Acting Director of Psychology, South Birmingham Mental Health NHS Trust. Teaching interests focus on carers' issues and research interests include loss and bereavement, quality of life for people with dementia and adaptation to physical illness.

Peter Spurgeon is Professor of Health Services Management and Director of Management/Organisational Development and Leadership at the Health Services Management Centre, University of Birmingham. His main interests include assessing managerial potential and performance, organisational development and the management of change and organisational culture and risk management.

Tracy Smith is a community mental health nurse for older people within South Birmingham Mental Health NHS Trust. She is involved in all aspects of mental health care for older people, with a special interest in carer and bereavement support and promoting collaboration throughout primary, secondary and tertiary care facilities.

Mary Tyson is a consultant clinical psychologist in the NHS. She has specialised in working with individuals with personality disorder since the mid-1980s, and has a particular interest in attachment styles and their implications for therapeutic outcome.

Panos Vostanis is Professor and Honorary Consultant in Child and Adolescent Psychiatry at the University of Leicester, where he has been involved in the development of multi-agency training programmes in child mental health. His current research addresses the mental health needs of children exposed to trauma and living in adversity, and the evaluation of treatment interventions and service models.

Gillian Wainscott is a consultant psychiatrist working in a regional Mother and Baby Unit in Birmingham and specialising in the care of women with perinatal illnesses. She is keen to optimise women's care through interdisciplinary working and liaison with primary care practitioners.

Derrett Watts trained and worked as a GP, subsequently trained as a psychiatrist and is now a consultant in general and community psychiatry in Stoke. His special interest areas include substance misuse and the influence religion can have for individuals with mental illness.

Tricia Whitehouse is a chartered counselling psychologist, and works in North Birmingham as acting locality lead psychologist within an NHS community mental health team. She also has a small private practice. Particular interests include eating disorders, trauma, personality difficulties and transpersonal psychotherapy.

PREFACE

'Partnership', 'collaboration' and 'participation' are terms frequently used in all aspects of modern life, but especially in health care. Within a political context, they are terms used to incline people to become involved in the democratic process. Community participation is the foundation stone of the new approach to public health. This approach aims to enable communities to have a greater say in the shaping of all aspects of their own health care where, previously, 'top-down' approaches had attempted to improve health through social engineering and the management of the physical environment (Petersen and Lupton, 1996). Participation is now becoming a duty as much as a right, with considerable efforts being made to engage all citizens in the task of creating a healthier and risk-free environment. While definitions of 'partnership', 'collaboration' and 'participation' may vary in their particular emphasis or slant, they all share the notion that individuals have a powerful part to play in the shaping and delivering of health services. Failing to realise this potential will condemn health care to stagnation.

The ideas underpinning partnership, collaboration and participation might be seen as a backlash against ideologies familiar in the 1980s, when competition and the internal market were so much in vogue. Some might see them as representative of a movement to diminish the power and control of the welfare state, by asserting the rights and responsibilities of the individual. Others might interpret them as a desperate attempt to hold together an array of disparate and disconnected health services, which have begun to fragment and have created priorities for themselves other than the needs of clients, patients and their carers. Using terms such as 'partnership', 'collaboration' and 'participation' may be a way of shifting the burden of responsibility on to service users and carers, of indicating that individuals have a duty to take care of their own health and that of others. Or they may be a way of responding to the frequent attacks mounted by critics in recent years, who assert that the NHS has become too cumbersome, an unwieldy and inert bureaucracy unable to respond to individual needs.

Recent government policy has once again stressed that the essence of the modernising agenda is to be found in partnerships between health-service providers and service users, and in collaboration in the planning, provision and evaluation of services. Professionals and the public are reminded that they should be vigilant, to ensure that services are focused on individuals and on helping people maximise their potential. Yet, at the start of the twenty-first century, access to health care is not equitable; 'postcode' lotteries exist; and certain groups are favoured over others, who are equally deserving but who live in an inner-city area, are unemployed or do not have English as a first language, with the result that they cannot claim the services that were intended precisely for them. The Black Report (DHSS, 1980) and *The Health Divide* (Whitehead, 1987) made it clear that, despite an ever-increasing budget for health services, the divide between privileged and non-privileged in terms of access to health care was as wide as ever.

While politicians may run successful campaigns on a platform of reducing such inequities, the gap has persisted for many decades. It may be time to accept that policy in itself will be insufficient to bring about radical change. Collaboration between motivated and innovative individuals may be more effective than a revamp of organisational structures and a focus on education and training have proved to be so far. Even the highest-quality research has not been sufficient in itself. There is more power in committed and creative individuals reflecting on their working practices and on the nature of their interactions with others – their clients and other professionals and agencies – and, in doing so, improving their focus on what is actually happening, where, when and how. By becoming more aware of those factors that determine the outcomes of health care, they have found that collaboration has the 'potential to improve procedures, interpersonal relationships and organisational factors related to power' (Taylor, 2000).

Instead of attempting to improve access for the disadvantaged to health care, and its quality, from the top downwards, it may be time to look at a bottom-up approach. This book endorses such an approach by listening to the accounts of collaboration of a variety of mental health care personnel working in everyday practice with a range of clients – adolescents, young mothers, drug abusers, those with personality disorders and older adults. The book does not seek to engage in yet more debate about how policy can promote collaboration, nor does it claim to present a comprehensive overview of the state of collaboration across all mental health services. Instead, it seeks to describe and understand collaboration from a 'real world' perspective. Direct accounts from frontline workers are richly informative, in contrast to formal reports generated by enquiries, research and audit, which all too frequently nourish the blame culture rather than supporting and encouraging staff.

One of many texts on collaboration, this book makes its contribution by examining the accounts and experiences of practitioners and users. People who have transformed the way they work in order to improve the care of clients, and who have effectively managed relationships between professional groups and agencies, describe how they got started, the difficulties they encountered, the joys, pitfalls and frustrations, and their successes (or otherwise). Few contributors would regard themselves as 'experts', but all are actively engaged in delivering a service and committed to improving it. Some have never written about their work before; others have found writing again about what they do an opportunity for reflection. No 'house style' has been imposed on the writers; instead, they have been encouraged to write using their own voice, and the language with which they are most familiar. The aim is to capture the immediacy and the urgency of their attempts to collaborate. The accounts come from a variety of settings, and each chapter provides a different example of collaboration between different types of users and practitioners. The range of collaborations is limited only by the size of the book; it would be possible to investigate many, many more examples without any duplication.

The accounts are honest and thought-provoking, leading the reader to consider what is it we are hoping to achieve through collaboration, and how can we achieve it. Collaboration is not an end in itself, only a means to an end. If collaboration does not produce positive results for users and practitioners – in terms of easier, more rapid access to resources, more suitable and sensitive service provision, and the satisfaction of a job well done – nothing has been gained by the venture, and the exercise remains a mechanistic response to policy without tangible gain for any of the individuals concerned.

Many justifications are put forward for collaboration in health and social care, but effective collaboration should produce positive results for service users and their carers, which could not be achieved by individuals working on their own. Although collaboration should have benefits for service providers, that is not its main aim. Ideally, good collaboration should benefit everyone – the providers, the service users and their carers.

It would not have been possible to document collaboration in every area of mental health care, so the accounts focus on broad client groups – children and adolescents, older people with depression, and people with serious and enduring mental illnesses. Within mental health services there are many groups with specific needs – for example, people from minority ethnic groups, people with dual diagnosis, people with physical and mental health problems, gay and lesbian clients. We have not devoted chapters specifically to the needs of these groups (there are other texts that are better able to address their specific needs); our aim has been to provide an overview of collaboration. Within the chapters authored by practitioners, certain groups of practitioners feature more prominently than others. This is not intended to imply that other professional groups are not involved in collaboration; it is simply that they do not happen to feature as major players in our sample.

Chapter 1 describes why collaboration stands a better chance of being effective in health care today than at various times in the past. Spurgeon and Field (Chapter 2) set out the policy context within which collaboration needs to be understood and explain why failure to acknowledge the importance of mental health services when Primary Care Trusts are formed will set back progress in mental health care. Ashburner (Chapter 3) discusses the meanings of collaboration, and suggests that confusion about definitions means that many practitioners who are delivering excellent integrated care may be anxious that they are not collaborating in the way that is expected. The insights of a service user as well as a service provider can be found in Harvey's chapter (Chapter 4), which demonstrates how health-service personnel fail to see the full picture. Readers will find this account unusually perceptive, and full of pathos.

The following chapters explore how practitioners set about their work, what they have achieved and what still remains to be done. These contributors do not attempt to make the world conform to theoretical models but instead look to service users to provide confirmation that what is being done is of real benefit to clients and carers. Cook and Whitehouse (Chapter 5) discuss how they have tried to improve services for people with eating disorders. In their work, collaboration between the statutory and private sectors is seen in action. Craddock (Chapter 6) explores the importance of social care and of collaboration between health and social services. He discusses the importance of agreeing management structures and of setting the geographical boundaries for health, social and primary care services. In Chapter 7, Lester, Cody and Deuchar describe how they have worked to make primary care more sensitive and relevant to those with severe and enduring mental health problems. Tyson and Briscoe (Chapter 8) address one of the greatest challenges facing mental health today, that of developing better services for people with personality disorders, a group that has been and continues to be highly misunderstood and stigmatised.

In Chapter 9, Wainscott looks at post-natal mental health and how collaboration can lead to early identification of depression and effective care and treatment. Arcelus, Gale and Vostanis (Chapter 10) discuss children's mental health problems, an area that has been poorly addressed in the past. From the perspective of a single-handed GP who is trying to find ways of collaborating with others, MacLeod (Chapter 11) examines approaches to clients who abuse drugs, while Oyebode's chapter (12) concerns the care of older people, an increasingly large group requiring services.

Kahn, Watts and Holland (Chapter 13) stress the importance of teambuilding and of collaborating with colleagues from other areas of health care in establishing suicide prevention services. In Chapter 14, Marlow and Smith show how nurses have worked closely with primary care to build up a service for older adults. These contributors have also established relationships with a wide range of other service providers whom they can call upon, as needed, to maximise the benefits of collaboration. Law and Harrison (Chapter 15) examine mental health promotion and show readers how they can use their ideas and suggestions to collaborate with others and improve the quality of services.

The concluding chapter brings together the main themes raised by the contributors – the importance of professionals being confident in their own role; having the appropriate skills to carry out the work required; being ready to respect and acknowledge the expertise of others; and being able to build relationships with different professionals and agencies.

The book does not pretend that there is a consensus about the meaning of 'collaboration'. Politicians, policy-makers, managers, clinicians, service providers and people in receipt of services may all define it differently and may have different expectations of it. The book's contributors also interpret collaboration in different ways and set about achieving it using different strategies. None the less, there is unanimous agreement among contributors that collaboration has required them to be very clear about their own roles. They have also learned far more about the roles of others (a positive outcome of collaboration, as lack of understanding of the roles and remit of other professionals and agencies has been a major obstacle to health reform in the past). Casey (1997) observed that individual health-care workers tended to have little understanding of what happened to their clients immediately prior to and following their particular involvement with them. Fragmentation of services, coupled with divisive funding arrangements made it almost impossible for staff to understand the 'bigger picture'.

The aims of the book are, therefore, the following:

- to provide a forum for a variety of practitioners to describe how they have achieved collaboration;

- to explore the variety of individuals' understanding of collaboration in practice;
- to discuss what collaboration means to different individuals;
- to provide an interpretive framework of the necessary conditions in which collaboration flourishes.

All the contributors are committed to improving mental health services in primary care and, while some may not be well known, all of them command the respect of colleagues because of what they have achieved at grass-roots level. The chapters are not meant to be representative of every dimension of mental health care, but instead provide a series of snapshots. Contributors' accounts are especially interesting for the way in which they analyse their own responses to the collaborative venture, as well as describing and seeking to understand the forging of relationships between different health-care personnel and agencies. They can be found practising in very different communities, in rural and urban areas, and in the statutory, voluntary and private sectors. Not all their attempts at collaboration have proved successful and readers will be impressed with the candour of what they have to say.

Readers are encouraged to use the insights and inspiration gained from the contributors' writing in order to improve services in their own working environment, whatever the resources available and the prevailing culture.

Peter Nolan and Frances Badger

REFERENCES

Casey, P.R. (1997) *A Guide to Psychiatry in Primary Care*, Wrightson Biomedical Publishing, Petersfield
DHSS (1980) *Inequalities in Health* (The Black Report), HMSO, London
Petersen, A. and Lupton, D. (1996) *The New Public Health*, Sage Publications, London
Taylor, B.J. (2000) *Reflective Practice: A guide for nurses and midwives*, Open University Press, Buckingham
Whitehead, M. (1987) *The Health Divide: Inequalities in health in the 1980s*, Health Education Council, London

ACKNOWLEDGEMENTS

We are deeply indebted to members of our families for the support and encouragement they generously provided during the gestation of this book. We would especially like to acknowledge the unobtrusive but highly valuable assistance provided by Matthew Badger regarding the tables and figures and to Helen Broadfield for her kindly but firm steering hand.

We would also like to thank the following people and organisations for permissin to reproduce material in this book:

OPCS for Table 2.1 on page 21; The Colston Health Centre for Table 7.1 on page 105; the NHS Centre for Reviews for material Table 13.1 on page 194; J. L. Cox, J. M. Holden and R. Sagovsky for material in appendix II on page 267; and The National Primary Care Research and Development Centre, University of Manchester for material for Appendix III on page 272.

Every effort has been made to contact copyright holders and we apologise if anyone has been overlooked.

PART ONE

THE CONCEPTS OF COLLABORATION

1 IN SEARCH OF COLLABORATION AND PARTNERSHIP

Peter Nolan and Frances Badger

THE NHS VISION

The birth of the NHS, on 5 July 1948, promised a new era in health provision in Britain. It embodied the philosophy that a nation that truly values democratic principles should provide the best possible health care for all its citizens, in order to enable them to contribute to the common good, to achieve personal happiness and to participate fully in the development of a robust national economy. Health care provided free at the point of delivery liberated many from the fear of having to endure illness and suffering, perhaps for an entire lifetime, because of an inability to pay for care and treatment. However, behind the laudable aims and optimistic rhetoric of the NHS there lay another reality. The NHS was, in fact, the child of scarcity, conceived during a period when Britain was recovering from the ravages of war.

The NHS has remained a monument to institutionalised scarcity ever since. It may be that the search for an ultimate solution to the nation's health-care needs is doomed to failure. Perhaps the best that can be achieved is the modification of health-care expectations, which may currently be unrealistic, and an improvement in the mechanisms for deciding who needs care and how it should be provided. Even at the inception of the NHS, it was recognised that a co-ordinated health service, provided by skilled health professionals collaborating with and complementing each other's work, would only partially meet the health-care needs of the nation. Other aspects of social policy – housing, sanitation, diet, working conditions, education, transport and recreational facilities – were known to be equally, if not more, significant. Creating a social context in which people could *remain well*, and lead a fulfilled life, was considered as important as providing appropriate medical and restorative services for them when they became ill. In the early years of the NHS, health-care provision implied co-operation between government departments and the first Minister of Health was also the Minister of Housing, embodying the essential integration of public services (Webster, 1998).

The NHS vision anticipated – and depended upon – greater collaboration between the different health-care services that had come into existence during the nineteenth and early twentieth centuries. The architects of the NHS, Beveridge and Bevan, were aware that services operated independently of one another, and did not share a common culture, or have the same perception of what constituted 'health care' and 'successful outcomes'. The NHS aimed to rehabilitate many of the ideas contained in the Dawson Report of 1920, a far-sighted analysis of health care, the significance of which remained unrecognised at the time. Dawson wanted to bring health services close to where people lived, by building 'health centres' in local communities. These centres would provide a wide range of services for all, from 'the womb to the tomb'. The vision was of a health service focused on the health needs of *communities* rather than on the needs of sick people in hospital. Dawson's view was that hospitals merely provided opportunities for some health-care professionals, principally doctors, to exercise undue power and to monopolise resources. There were many similarities between the philosophy and aspirations of the Dawson Report and the NHS Act of 1946.

By regenerating health services, Beveridge hoped to ensure that people lived in a much better world than the old one. However, within a decade of its inaugur-ation, the NHS was already in financial difficulties. The Guillebaud Report (1956) confirmed that funding the NHS was proving far more costly than had originally been envisaged. The report also implied, with considerable regret, that the NHS had become a national *hospital* service rather a national *health* service, as had been intended.

MEDICAL DOMINATION

Neither Dawson's nor Beveridge's vision of health services was realised. Originally, the NHS was divided into three sections: the hospital sector, managed by regional hospital boards; the primary care sector, staffed by general practitioners (GPs) and dentists who retained their local independence; and the auxiliary sector, including the ambulance service, maternal and infant services, and home helps. These were left under the aegis of local authorities. Power and resources quickly gravitated towards the hospital sector, to the detriment of the community and primary care sectors. Specialist services provided in hospitals exercised ever-increasing influence, not only over the resources of the NHS, but also over its direction. The medical curriculum was totally hospital-based. Student doctors acquired their medical knowledge in hospitals and from hospital-based doctors. Professions allied to medicine, such as physiotherapy, occupational therapy and dietetics, were quick to adopt the medical model of training. Nurse training followed suit and even nurses who aspired to work in the community had first to undergo a hospital-based training. The training of health professionals ignored the fact that many people had (or could have) their health-care needs adequately met in primary care. Even though GPs trained alongside colleagues who went into secondary care, their work in primary care was attributed a lower status and attracted fewer resources.

Not all doctors, however, favoured a medically dominated health-care system, either after the arrival of the NHS or before. The Socialist Medical Association (SMA) formed in 1930 under the presidency of Dr Somerville Hastings, Labour MP for Reading, aimed to make medical services available to all. It encouraged doctors to become active in politics and its first publication, *For a Healthy London*, was taken up by the Labour-dominated London County Council in 1931. The SMA continued to lobby for a national health service throughout the 1930s and 40s. Its various policy statements included *Whither Medicine?* which, as early as 1939, anticipated the basic principles of the NHS. After the publication of the Beveridge Report (1942), the SMA was invited to have regular meetings with the

Minister of Health and by then its membership had reached approximately 1800 doctors. In the 1940s, it sponsored 12 Labour MPs and was thereby able to influence the progress of the NHS Act through Parliament in 1946. In 1981, the SMA renamed itself the Socialist Health Association (SHA), to reflect a new focus on the prevention of illness through the promotion of health.

The history of the SMA is significant because it has always adhered to the founding vision of the NHS, reflecting the concerns of a significant minority of doctors and health-care professionals who have regretted the supremacy of secondary care over primary care services. It has been vigorous in supporting quality health care through effective collaboration between health, social and voluntary services and, above all, through good relationships between health-care personnel and patients.

THE POSITION OF GPs

GPs were initially regarded as being outside the NHS and were left to regulate their own work; many ran their surgery in an individual, often idiosyncratic way. GPs could select the patients they wanted to care for (and refuse those they did not) and decide how to treat them. Their surgeries were like 'cottage industries', all working independently of each other and apparently unaccountable to anyone. In the early days of the NHS, GPs had little access to hospital resources and were not invited to collaborate with the hospitals. Gradually, the significance and potential of their role in health care came to be recognised and they were granted access to hospital diagnostic and pathological facilities (Webster, 1998). Their importance as front-line health-care workers and as 'gatekeepers' for specialist services is now well established.

Approximately 34 000 family doctors currently work in the NHS, providing a comprehensive service to almost the entire population. In addition to medical services, people visiting their GP surgeries can now also expect to find information about and gain access to social care services, health promotion activities, alternative therapies and a range of voluntary service organisations.

PSYCHIATRY, MENTAL HEALTH AND THE NHS

The newly created NHS brought psychiatry, predominantly centred in psychiatric hospitals, under the aegis of health care for the first time. Formerly a part of the Poor Law system, mental health services were to be modernised and the stigma of poverty associated with them was to be removed. Their inclusion in the NHS resulted in an outcome that had not been anticipated. It soon became apparent that approximately three-quarters of NHS beds were occupied by psychiatric patients. The psychiatric hospitals were encouraged to remain independent of the acute sector and were funded to provide their own pathology laboratories, X-ray departments and other investigative and medical facilities. This expansion of services in psychiatric hospitals had the effect of elevating the standing of psychiatry within the NHS, while at the same time isolating it from other NHS services.

A certain naïveté on the part of policy-makers led them to believe that policy alone could reform the mental health system (Rogers and Pilgrim, 2001). Others, such as Martin (1984), recognised that, for change to happen, routines, management styles, and issues of power and status must all be addressed, to enable the infrastructure of care to support real and ongoing improvements in the services provided. Ashford *et al.* (1999) argue that, to be effective and sustained, change must be reflected in policy and the structure of the organisation, and accepted at the level of individual health-care practitioners. This comprehensive approach to change was not applied to psychiatry after the inception of the NHS. While the professional status of psychiatry benefited from being in the NHS, the care of patients continued largely as before. In the early 1960s, the acute NHS hospitals commanded such vast resources that psychiatric hospitals were probably worse off than they had been prior to 1948. Inquiries into the running of psychiatric hospitals revealed that the Poor Law ethos still prevailed. The medicalisation of mental illness was fiercely criticised by Szasz (1960) and others, who objected to the way in which patients' lives were being controlled. He suggested that mental illness was manufactured by psychiatrists (and sometimes by the state) to suit their own ends – professional advancement or control of non-conformist citizens.

From the 1970s onwards, other branches of medicine were criticised. Cochrane (1972) questioned the effectiveness of most medical interventions, while McKeown and Lowe (1976) argued that it was improved standards of living rather than medicine that had been responsible for the decline in the death rate since the middle of the nineteenth century. Illich (1976) argued that, far from curing people, modern medicine actually made some of them more ill. Iatrogenic illness was on the increase and people were becoming dependent on doctors rather than on themselves to deal with minor illnesses and to maintain their health. In the 1981 Reith Lectures, Ian Kennedy condemned modern medicine for its obsession with the disease process rather than concentrating on the needs and welfare of patients.

At the start of the twenty-first century, environmental groups continue this theme, claiming that science and medicine are more harmful than beneficial to health. Disillusionment with traditional medical services is seen in the emergence of self-help and patient advocacy groups, the anti-vivisectionist movement, organisations promoting natural birth and the women's health movement, and in the increasing popularity of complementary and alternative therapies. Litigation on the grounds of medical negligence and malpractice is flourishing.

Today, the new public health philosophy puts the patient at the centre of his or her own health care. Those who seek to challenge and find alternatives to modern medicine have been well supported by Foucault (1991), who argues persuasively that science has been used to explain reality, and to control and standardise it. His socio-political analysis of medicine and how it operates looks at the relationships between ways of knowing, health-care practice and power, and concludes that health-care delivery disempowers the patient.

THE EXTENT OF THE MENTAL HEALTH PROBLEM

Population surveys have revealed that the most common mental health problems are anxiety and/or depression, and alcohol dependence (with anxiety and/or depression). Jenkins (1998) is amongst those who have pointed out that mental health policies have traditionally focused on the care of people with 'severe mental illness' (often taken to mean psychosis), and have neglected the more prevalent forms of mental illness. Bowers (1997) has criticised the use of the term 'minor psychiatric disorder' to refer to these problems because it underplays how distressing, long-lasting and disabling they can be for the people affected. Neither does he find the term 'common mental disorder' much better, being merely a catch-all term for states of emotional distress most frequently seen in general practice.

Leaving aside the terminology, approximately six million people, or a ninth of the total UK population, consult their GP each year about a problem with a mental health component. Indeed, it is now generally accepted that approximately 25–30% of those attending GP surgeries in Britain have a psychological component to their presentation, but only 5–10% are referred to secondary mental health services (Commander *et al.*, 1997). It would be impossible for a greater percentage to be referred since even the wealthiest nations can provide specialist care for only a small proportion of the large number of people with mental health problems (Jenkins, 1998).

Jenkins (1998) suggests the following:

> *... it is no longer tenable to argue that this burden of the common mental disorders should be ignored – the costs of so doing are immense in terms of repeated GP consultation ..., sickness absence ..., labour turnover ..., reduced productivity, impact on families and children and the more difficult to quantify, but nonetheless important concept of the emotional wellbeing of a country and nation. (p. 138)*

The question of how to respond to mental health problems in primary care appears to be a global challenge and not peculiar to Britain or to post-industrial nations. One project of the World Health Organisation (WHO), carried out in 14 countries (including the USA, Japan, the UK, China, Nigeria and India), found well-defined psychological problems to be frequent in all the general health-care settings examined. WHO estimated that the overall rate of such problems among those presenting in primary care was 24%. Depressive and anxiety disorders, and alcohol abuse were the most common (Ustun and Sartorius, 1998).

Shepherd *et al.* (1966) were the first in Britain to suggest that these kinds of mental health problems would be best treated in general practice. They argued that mental health services could be more quickly improved by strengthening the role of the family doctor and the primary care team than by expanding existing psychiatric services. Shepherd and his colleagues found that primary care services were ideally placed to identify early signs of psychological ill health, to initiate treatment and to reduce stigma. Thirty years later, the central role of primary care has been enshrined in the *National Service Framework for Mental Health* (Department of Health, 1999), which summarises the British government's aims and objectives for the NHS in the area of mental health. It lists seven Standards, which relate to mental health promotion, access to services, effective services for people with severe mental illness, caring for carers, and preventing suicide. Standard Two, which concerns primary care, declares:

> *Any service users who contact their primary health care team with a common mental health problem should:*
> - *have their mental health needs identified and assessed;*
> - *be offered effective treatments, including referrals to specialist services for further assessment, treatment and care if they require it. (p. 28)*

Those who design health policies are now clearly opposed to the creation of more professions, preferring the challenge of improving communication and collaboration between existing groups; the challenge has been described as 'everybody's distant relative but nobody's baby' (Department of Health and Social Security, 1983). Communication between primary and secondary services, and even within primary care, has been and remains poor. Psychiatrists and GPs have traditionally had little contact with each other, other than via the occasional letter and even more occasional phone calls (Gask and Croft, 2000).

PLACING MENTAL HEALTH IN PRIMARY CARE

The move away from care in institutions and towards community care has been a feature not only in Britain but throughout the western world. Care of the mentally ill in Britain falls into three periods: the asylum era of the nineteenth century; the emergence of biological psychiatry at the end of the nineteenth century; and the return to the community in the second half of the twentieth century. Shorter (1997) observed that the integration of some aspects of mental health services into primary care was both desirable and inevitable, and part of the process of deinstitutionalisation. Reynolds and Thornicroft (1999) have described landmarks in the process of deinstitutionalisation in the UK:

- the relocation of services from a few, large institutions to smaller, decentralised facilities;
- the publication of strategic and clinical protocols and guidelines;
- the advent of the multidisciplinary team in which professional groups co-operate with each other in treating and caring for users;
- co-operation between NHS services, local authorities and the independent sector to plan and provide an integrated pattern of local services;
- an increasingly influential role for primary care in the purchasing and commissioning of health services;
- the involvement of service users and their carers in shaping services;
- an increased emphasis on risk assessment and improved client management.

Locating mental health care in the primary sector holds out the promise of improved services. Services provided in primary rather than secondary care are much preferred by clients and their carers. In the past, mental health services isolated people from their families and friends (and sometimes abused them). After spending time in a psychiatric institution, it was very difficult for most people to return to their former position in society, due to loss of confidence, loss of social and occupational skills and a reluctance on the part of society to accept them. Some critics have even argued that the driving force behind the asylum system of the mid-nineteenth century was a desire to stigmatise 'anti-social' or 'difficult' individuals, and remove them from society.

There are many lessons to be learned from the experiences of patients discharged from the former mental hospitals. They returned to a society in which community services for the mentally ill were poorly developed, and health and social policies were not in place to support them. Those who were not 'lost to the disorder' were therefore 'lost in the community'. The current emphasis on primary care mental health services is therefore welcome, enabling clients to access services easily and to have their needs met in a non-stigmatising environment.

Attitudes towards mentally ill people have changed, albeit very slowly, in line with a greater awareness of and adherence to human rights. Article 1 of *The Universal Declaration of Human Rights*, adopted by the General Assembly of the United Nations in December 1948, states the following:

All human beings are born free and equal in dignity and rights. They are endowed with reason and conscience and should act towards one another in a spirit of brotherhood.

WHO's policy document *Health for All by the Year 2000* (1985) stated that people in all countries should enjoy a level of health that would allow them to work productively and to participate in the social life of the communities in which they live. In 1990, WHO stated that human beings have the right to a clean and harmonious environment, in which physical, social and aesthetic factors are all recognised as important.

Since the 1990s, UK policy directives have required planners and providers to base services for mentally ill people on humanitarian values, social justice, respect for persons and evidence-based practice. In the voluntary sector, these values have been especially well represented in the work of MIND. Larry Gostin, former Director of MIND, witnessed how mental health services in the United States were transformed as a result of the appeal to individual human rights. Under Gostin's leadership, MIND campaigned on the platform that what is done to and for people should help them to achieve a more fulfilled and meaningful life. The UK Human Rights Act came into effect in October 2000 in the middle of a radical reform of mental health care. The Act should make a significant contribution towards safeguarding the rights of people with mental health problems and their carers, and ensure that they are involved in shaping services that are client-centred and needs-led.

Evidence for the effectiveness of primary mental health care services has been available from the United States for some time. Preskorn (1999) considers it self-evident that services should be provided where people present with their problems. If the primary care physician is not involved in mental health, a vital component of many people's care and treatment will be missing. The multiple advantages to integrating mental health into primary care include the following:

- reduction of stigma;
- cost savings (care is shifted from expensive in-patient settings into office-based family practices); and
- improved quality of care (primary care personnel tend to be more concerned with the functional status of patients than with merely targeting symptoms).

Mental health should not therefore be seen in isolation from other aspects of the person, such as the physical, the social and the spiritual. When people with depression are treated appropriately in primary care, their mental health improves, their relapse rates fall and many are able to devise inexpensive coping mechanisms for themselves that are easy to incorporate into their daily life.

Thornicroft and Tansella (1999) argue that closer collaboration between primary care services and specialist mental health services will help to address the escalating demand for mental health care, which has outstripped the resources of specialist services. High rates of co-morbidity of mental and physical disorders increase the need for individualised care provided by primary care personnel, to avoid gaps in treatment. More enterprising primary care services are already developing links with community self-help and service-user groups and alternative therapists. The aim is to integrate emotionally distressed persons into ordinary social environments by providing them with access to community resources that promote normalisation and demonstrate respect for human rights. Users have stated that they value autonomy, privacy and choice and therefore prefer to live in the community, even though some describe their life as isolated and emotionally bleak (O'Grady, 1996).

A number of specific benefits should arise from closer collaboration between primary care and specialist mental health services:

- earlier detection of mental health problems;
- quicker and easier access to effective treatments, based on sound evidence;
- reduction in variations in the quality of care provided for people with mental health problems;
- improved co-ordination of services;
- increased research into mental health in primary care;
- shared training between primary- and secondary-care personnel;
- greater involvement of mental health professionals in improving mental health in primary care;
- reduced stigma for patients attending specialist mental health services;
- improved management of difficult cases, such as patients with poor adherence to treatment regimes or who require compulsory admission.

(Thornicroft and Tansella, 1999)

Collaboration could have the added advantage of challenging the many myths that abound in many communities about mental illness and inform people that mental illness can happen to anyone. A major aim of such activity should be to encourage the general public not to fear those experiencing mental illness, but to recognise that there are many effective interventions that can assist people to recover. Arboleda-Florez and Saraceno (2001) argue that those who work in mental health services should be aware of the myths and facts about mental illness and should strive to ensure that any advice or education they impart is factually based. Table 1.1 shows some frequently encountered myths and facts about mental illness.

Table 1.1 Some common myths and facts about mental illness

Myths	Facts
Mental and brain disorders only affect adults in rich countries	Everyone is affected – children and adults, rich and poor. The frequency of these disorders is about the same in developed and developing countries
Mental and brain disorders are a figment of the imagination	These are real illnesses that cause suffering and disability
It is impossible to help somebody with a mental or brain disorder	Treatments exist and are effective. Care-givers can be assisted
Mental and brain disorders are brought on by weakness of character	These disorders are caused by biological, psychological and social factors
People with mental illness should be locked up	People with mental illness can function and should not be isolated or restricted

Arboleda-Florez and Saraceno (2001)

THE CHANGING FACE OF PRIMARY CARE

Since the mid-1960s, there has been considerable growth in the number of community nurses and health visitors linked to local GPs, and an increased tendency for GPs to work together in group practices. A new GP contract in 1990 allowed greater flexibility in the categories of attached staff who could be reimbursed, and this resulted in an increase in the number and variety of mental health practitioners working in primary care. At the same time, the rapid reduction in the number of in-patient psychiatric beds meant that the members of the expanded primary care teams were now assuming responsibilities for mental health care far beyond what had been envisaged even a decade earlier.

A survey of general practices in six health districts in England found that 50% had links with a community psychiatric nurse, 21% with a social worker, 17% with a counsellor, 16% with a psychiatrist, and 15% with a clinical psychologist (Thomas and Corney, 1992). Nolan *et al.* (1999) cite figures for the early 1990s researched by Kendrick *et al.* (1993) – 34% of GP practices had links with CPNs, 17% with counsellors, 12% with clinical psychologists, 9% with psychiatrists and 6% with social workers. The types of link varied from liaison, to attachment, to employment. Practices with links with one professional group were likely to have links with others, whilst some similarly sized practices had no links at all. A survey by Usherwood *et al.* (1997) looked at over 500 practices across England and Wales in the mid-1990s. Responses were obtained from 81% of practices, and the researchers found a mean of 0.47 CPNs per practice (nearly all attached to rather than employed by the practice), 0.18 counsellors (all employed), 0.11 psychologists (mostly attached) and 0.10 social workers (also mostly attached). The amount of time spent in the practice averaged five hours a week for an employed counsellor, and seven, four and three hours, respectively, for attached CPNs, social workers and psychologists. Cape and Parham (1998) estimated that around 30% of practices in the UK had dedicated counsellors and found that, in one inner London borough, 35% of the practices surveyed had counsellors based in them. Most of these practices provided a half-day or one day of counselling per week, with a small number providing more time.

Other than GPs, practice nurses represent the largest group of professionals based in general practice with the potential for meeting mental health care needs (Nolan *et al.*, 1999). Practice nurses have been employed by GPs since the early 1960s. By 1977, it was estimated that there were 1,500. This number trebled between 1984 and 1990, and, by 1993, nearly all GP practices had practice nurses attached. Although engaged in administering vaccinations, running diabetic and weight-control clinics, and carrying out routine physical health screenings, their role also includes health education and counselling. They are ideally placed to contribute to mental health care. However, a survey by Nolan and colleagues in the Birmingham Health Authority (1999), and one by Crosland and Kai (1998) in the north-east of England, suggest that practice nurses are very aware of a lack of formal mental health training. The best response to mental health problems in primary care demands an examination of the training and education needs of practice nurses, and of other staff employed by and attached to general practices, and of their role.

Peck and Greatley (1999) reported on a project on primary care and mental health carried out by the King's Fund and the Centre for Mental Health Services Development in three localities in London. They pointed out that advice on how to improve relationships between primary care and secondary care has usually been handed down by experts from secondary care. The way ahead for mental health services now needs to be based upon the views of GPs and their colleagues in primary care. A number of issues need to be considered before any integration of primary care and mental health services:

• Do all mental health problems require the attention of health professionals?
• Which methods of mental health assessment are most appropriate in primary care?
• Is evidence elicited from the management of psychiatric patients in secondary care appropriate for people with mental health problems in primary care?
• Which clients should be referred to secondary mental health services?

PROMOTING COLLABORATION

This book took shape against the background of the General Election of June 2001, when New Labour was re-elected under the leadership of Tony Blair. All the political parties campaigned on a platform of providing quality public services, especially in health care, for the creation and maintenance of a happy and healthy nation. It was as if the Beveridge Plan was being revisited all over again. Much of the health-care rhetoric heard during the election campaign echoed the language of the National Plan and the Dawson Report. Tony Blair argued that the Labour administration elected in 1997 had put in place policies and administrative systems that would enable improved public services; during a second term of office, it pledged to ensure the translation of those policies into practice. The mode of delivery was to be innovative and based on collaboration and partnerships between disciplines, agencies, and individuals. Historically, paternalistic governments in many countries have found reforms relatively easy to encapsulate in policy terms, but notoriously difficult to implement. Governments committed to social reform tend to raise somewhat unrealistic expectations. Innovators frequently forget that change is imposed on an existing reality and that those working within that reality may not always be as committed to change as the policy-makers.

Health-care policy today is inevitably more worldly-wise than it was at the time of the introduction of the NHS. Now it aims to meet health-care needs *within the existing resources*. The NHS Plan (Department of Health, 2000) contains the most recent agenda for health-care reform and its implementation; some of the proposed changes are summarised in Table 1.2. In April 2001, shortly after the publication of the NHS Plan, it was announced that vast swathes of bureaucracy in the form of Regional NHS Executives and Health Authorities would be reduced so that decision-making could move closer to the place where services were provided. The aim was to facilitate more creative and relevant ways of working that could be 'owned' by those engaged in them.

Table 1.2   Requirements of future health services

- Expectations and outcomes of health services must be agreed by all stakeholders.
- Processes must be restructured to focus on outcomes.
- Multi-agency working must reflect an understanding of cultures, values and beliefs.
- Hierarchical layers of management and administration must be replaced by leadership.
- Skills and competencies must be identified through process mapping.
- Appropriate education and training must be commissioned through confederations.
- Training must be evidence-based.
- Workforce numbers must be identified to meet present and future need.
- There must be far more collaboration between services.
- Service users must be at the centre of all health-care provision.

There is considerable variation in the composition of primary care teams, in the skills that individual practitioners possess, and in the extent to which they collaborate. Often, only a few members of the team are collaborating with each other, over a short period of time, on projects that have only short-term funding.

Successful collaboration depends on the personalities of those involved, the working environment, the perceived worth of the job to be done, and the level of job satisfaction enjoyed. Identifying and integrating the best that each partner in the team has to offer is the goal of collaboration. Collaboration aids client involvement in care, energises professional groups, expands professional practice and integrates health-care systems. Collaboration is a high-order activity necessitating trust on the part of the collaborators and a shared belief in what they are doing.

Collaborators also need to have the confidence to accept their limitations. Only when individual practitioners are confident in their own skills, and understand the parameters of their work, can the benefits of collaboration be realised. Being part of a caring, supportive team has a powerful effect on the individuals making up the team. The feeling of belonging, and of being accepted, of being needed for oneself and for one's skills, is confidence and morale boosting within an interactional or communicative process (Burleson *et al.*, 1994). Collaborators must be strong enough to accept challenges and criticisms from colleagues, other professionals, clients and carers, and be prepared to justify what they are doing. Equally, they may have to challenge colleagues about aspects of their work, while at the same time sustaining good working relationships with them.

Recent organisation theory suggests that improved job satisfaction lies more in devising empowering work structures than in attempting to modify the personal attributes of employees. Good educational and career opportunities, managerial support, information and adequate resources lead to a highly motivated and integrated workforce.

CHALLENGES AND OBSTACLES TO COLLABORATION

Promoting collaboration between individuals and agencies – all with different histories, values and ways of working – is more difficult than it may at first appear. A variety of obstacles militate against success, such as territorial claims to specific skills, professional culture and attitudes, social status and class, different codes of practice and ethics, and different rates of remuneration. Attempts to promote collaboration between mental health services and primary care have, in the past, been bedevilled by three obstacles, according to Rogers and Pilgrim (2001):

1 *Conceptual vagueness concerning the precise nature of mental health services and their target audience.* This vagueness made it difficult to link with other services having greater clarity about their objectives.
2 *Lack of influence of health policies, research and education over practice.* This could be attributed to variability in the quality of education and research across the country and lack of interest on the part of clinicians in implementing findings that would benefit the service.
3 *Conservative mental health policies focused on short-term needs.* Most policies have advocated no more than minor adjustments to existing arrangements and failed to bring about real as opposed to imagined change.

Some may be suspicious that the hidden agenda for collaboration is the integration of disciplines and budgets as a means of managing scarce resources. However, Blount (1998), one of the foremost commentators on closer collaboration between mental health and primary care services, sees the initiative as essentially worthwhile, leading to lower service costs, increased patient satisfaction, increased job satisfaction for staff, and growth in understanding of the relationship between mind and body in health and illness. Bringing together the medical, social and voluntary services that promote mental health recovery and mental wellbeing, in order to avoid the separation of 'physical' and 'psychological' in defining people's problems, is the first step towards understanding how they experience those problems.

Some Primary Care Groups (PCGs) and Primary Care Trusts (PCTs) have made significant progress in implementing the changes necessary to transform the culture and organisation of primary care and community health services. However, as Wilkin *et al.* (2001) have remarked, variations in management capacity and in the general support for PCGs mean that the aims set out in the National Plan may take longer than anticipated to achieve. Although PCGs and PCTs have been told that they are 'in the driving seat', because it is they who are in the best position to respond to local needs, the reality does not quite match the rhetoric. There has been a continuous stream of directives and performance targets from central government. Some PCGs have regretted not being able to pursue locally defined agendas and hope that Trust status will enable them to reclaim their autonomy. If the Trusts find themselves as closely managed in terms of performance as PCGs, health professionals are likely to become disillusioned and disengaged. While many enthusiastic staff are currently involved in attempting to improve local services, there is the danger that the demands of managing complex mergers, preparing to assume Trust status, and dealing with the aftermath may divert attention from the real business of raising quality standards, improving access to services, building partnerships and improving health.

There are major challenges to overcome if mental health services are to become more effective and to establish themselves in primary care. In the UK, collaboration implies a radically different approach to health-care delivery from that which prevailed as recently as two decades ago. Then, there was much talk of the 'autonomous practitioner'. The emphasis on confidentiality precluded disclosure of any aspect of the patient's management to other agents or agencies. Such thinking persists today and creates confusion when health carers try to understand how their *Code of Practice* can be aligned with that of other professionals. 'Whose *Code of Practice* do we subscribe to'? is a question frequently encountered in multi-disciplinary team meetings and one that is likely to be heard regularly following the integration of services. Professionals are uncertain how much personal information about clients, families and carers they can give to other colleagues or agencies, especially if clients have requested that the information they give should be treated as confidential.

While GPs and psychiatrists share some common core training, students from other professional groups likely to be involved in primary mental health care have little contact with each other during their training. In addition, the education of practice nurses, district nurses, health visitors and midwives remains largely focused on physical health care, even though it does take increased notice of emotional and psychological responses to ill health. Contact in practice with people enduring substantive mental health problems may, until very recently, have been extremely limited for these groups of practitioners. In particular, the training needs of practice nurses– a group that research has shown is extensively involved in supporting people with mental health problems – remain largely neglected, although there are some signs of improvement.

While a quarter of community mental health nurses also possess a general nursing qualification, the culture of primary care is alien to most of them. Expecting community mental health nurses (CMHNs) to act as a link between primary care and mental health services may place a heavy burden on these nurses. They have to negotiate both cultures, while feeling settled in neither. Tensions may arise for CMHNs who are employed by one service characterised by a hierarchical structure, rules and protocols, rigid management systems and clearly defined career pathways, but who must work in a very different system where management is flattened and ways of working are frequently negotiated. Some of the work that CMHNs may be required to carry out – such as assessments of risk, suicide and mental health status – may be seen by some clients as stigmatising and unnecessary. Yet organisations may require documentary evidence of what has been done for clients during the CMHN's visit.

Blount (1998) warns that simply bringing together health-care providers with different skills and ways of practising will not be sufficient to break down divisions between them that may have existed for decades. Solutions need to be found to a variety of problems, including allocation of space, access to clerical and computing resources, dissemination of information to all members of the team, and the promotion of a shared culture. Other barriers to collaboration will need to be overcome:

- disputes over professional boundaries and responsibilities ('turf wars' and tribalism);
- ideological positions held by different professionals;
- different conceptual models used in the provision of services;
- confusion over terminology used to describe work;
- inequitable access to educational opportunities and resources;
- differences in career progression;
- resistance to change at individual, team and organisational levels;
- staff burn-out and high attrition rates;
- lack of adequate resources;
- lack of effective leadership;
- pressure from central government to see immediate results; and
- perceptions of professional inequality and differences of status.

(Dombeck, 1997)

Additional barriers to interprofessional collaboration include the structural (for example, lines of accountability and pay) and the cultural (for example, stereotypes and status of different professions). There are differences in approach between professional groups, and even different ways of working *within* groups, contrary to the assumption that there is 'a psychological model', 'a nursing model' or 'a medical model'. Disagreement can thus arise over the nature of the problems with which the patient is presenting and the best way of approaching them. Competition inhibits collaboration when professional groups seek to appropriate roles and skills. There is often a reluctance to 'give away' skills, especially to those who are perceived to belong to lower-status groups (Orford, 1993). Some professionals may also opt to keep certain skills in short supply, thus inflating their value. They may only be prepared to teach skills to others in a modified form, usually via courses of just a few days' duration, which permit familiarity but do not confer expertise. Individuals may believe that only they, or the group to which they belong, have the capacity to use certain skills to the full, because they have served a long apprenticeship, undertaken special courses, or possess certain personality traits.

It is worth reflecting that facilitating closer working between primary care and secondary specialised services is the first step towards identifying a model of primary mental health care, which has its own unique aims, strategies and culture. Once this model is in place, crisis mental health services, assertive outreach, home treatment, early intervention in psychosis, welfare, housing, social care and the voluntary sector could all be incorporated into primary mental health services. A coherent primary care philosophy is necessary to ensure that these and other services are not merely 'added on' rather than becoming essential components of the overall service and sharing its values and culture.

A vision of mental health services integrated into primary care is clearly worth pursuing for the sake of those who suffer from mental health problems. There are many ways of understanding and working towards the vision. This book aims to help readers understand how it is being realised in different ways by different practitioners, working in a wide variety of circumstances. What is good for one team may be antipathetic to another, but that does not preclude individuals or teams from knowing what others do. The accounts that follow will enable readers to reflect on ways of working that might best suit their own local circumstances.

REFERENCES

Arboleda-Florez, J. and Saraceno, B. (2001) Mental health and primary care, *Canadian Medical Association Journal*, 3, 1013–1014

Ashford, J., Eccles, M., Bond, S., Hall, L.A. and Bond, J. (1999) Improving health care through professional behaviour change: introducing a framework for identifying behaviour change strategies, *British Journal of Clinical Governance*, 4, 14–23

Beveridge, W. (1942) *Social Insurance and Allied Services*, HMSO cmnd 6404, London

Blount, A.B. (1998) *Integrated Primary Care*, Norton, London

Bowers, L. (1997) Community psychiatric nurse caseloads and the 'worried well': misspent time or vital work? *Journal of Advanced Nursing*, 26, 930–936

Burleson, B., Albrecht, T. and Sarason, I. (1994) *Communication of Social Support*, Sage, London

Cape, J. and Parham, A. (1998) Relationships between practice counselling and referral to outpatient psychiatry and clinical psychology, *British Journal of General Practice*, 48, 1477–1480

Cochrane, A. (1972) *Effectiveness and Efficiency*, Oxford University Press, Oxford

Commander, M.J., Odell, S., Sashidhran, S.P. and Suretees, P.G. (1997) A comparison of the socio-demographic and clinical characteristics of private household and communal establishment residents in a multi-ethnic inner-city area, *Social Psychiatry and Psychiatric Epidemiology*, 7, 421–427

Crosland, A. and Kai, J. (1998) 'They think they can talk to nurses': practice nurses' views of their roles in caring for mental health problems, *British Journal of General Practice*, 48, 1383–1386

Dawson Report (1920), chaired by Lord Dawson of Penn, HMSO, London

Department of Health (1999) *National Service Framework for Mental Health*, Department of Health, London

Department of Health (2000) *The NHS Plan – A Plan for Investment, A Plan for Reform*, The Stationery Office, London

Department of Health and Social Security (1983) *National Health Service Management Inquiry* (usually referred to as The Griffiths Report), HMSO, London

Dombeck, M. (1997) Professional personhood: training, territoriality, and tolerance, *Journal of Interprofessional Care*, 11, 9–21

Foucault, M. (1991) The ethic of care for the self as a practice of freedom. In Bernauer, J. and Rasmussen, D. (eds.) *The Final Foucault*, MIT Press, Cambridge, MA

Gask, L. and Croft, J. (2000) Methods of working with primary care, *Advances in Psychiatric Treatment*, 6, 442–449

Guillebaud Report (1956) *Report of the Committee of Enquiry into the Cost of the National Health Service*, HMSO, London

Illich, I. (1976) *Limits of Medicine: Medical nemesis: the expropriation of health*, Marion Boyers, London

Jenkins, R. (1998) Mental health and primary care – implications for policy, *International Review of Psychiatry*, 10, 158–160

Kendrick, T., Sibbald, B., Addington-Hall, J., Brennerman, D. and Freeling, P. (1993) Distribution of mental health professionals working on site in English and Welsh general practices, *British Medical Journal*, 307, 544–546

Martin, J.P. (1984) *Hospitals in Trouble*, Basil Blackwell, London

McKeown, T. and Lowe, C.R. (1976) *An Introduction to Social Medicine*, Blackwell, Oxford

Ministry of Health (1920) The Dawson Report, HMSO, London

Nolan, P., Murray, E. and Dallender, J. (1999) Practice nurses' perceptions of services for clients with psychological problems in primary care, *International Journal of Nursing Studies*, 36, 97–104

O'Grady, J.C. (1996) Community psychiatry; central policy, local implementation [editorial], *British Journal of Psychiatry*, 169, 259–262

Orford, J. (1993) *Community Psychology*, John Wiley & Sons, Chichester

Peck, E. and Greatley, A. (1999) Developing the mental health agenda for primary care groups, *Managing Community Care*, 7, 3–6

Preskorn, S.H. (1999) *Outpatient Management of Depression*, Professional Communications, Kansas, MI

Reynolds, A. and Thornicroft, G. (1999) *Managing Mental Health Services*, Open University Press, Buckingham

Rogers, A. and Pilgrim, D. (2001) *Mental Health Policy in Britain*, Palgrave, London

Shepherd, M., Cooper, B. and Brown, A.C. (1966) *Psychiatric Illness in General Practice*, Oxford University Press, Oxford

Shorter, E. (1997) *A History of Psychiatry – From the Era of the Asylum to the Age of Prozac*, John Wiley, Chichester

Socialist Medical Association [SMA] (1930) *For a Healthy London*, SMA, London

Socialist Medical Association (1939) *Whither Medicine?*, SMA, London

Szasz, T. (1960) The myth of mental illness, *The American Psychologist*, **15**, 1113–1118

Thomas, R.V. and Corney, R.H. (1992) A survey of links between mental health professionals and general practice in six district health authorities, *British Journal of General Practice*, **42**, 358–361

Thornicroft, G. and Tansella, M. (1999) Co-ordinating Primary Care with Community Mental Health Services. In Tansella, M. and Thornicroft, G. (eds.) *Common Mental Disorders in Primary Care*, Routledge, London, New York

Ustun, T.B. and Sartorius, N. (1998) *Mental Illness in Health Care: An international study*, John Wiley, Chichester

Usherwood, T., Long, S. and Joesbury, H. (1997) *Who works in Primary Health Care Teams in England and Wales?* Department of General Practice, University of Sheffield, Sheffield

Webster, C. (1998) *The National Health Service – A Political History*, Oxford University Press, Oxford

Wilkin, D., Gillam, S. and Smith, K. (2001) Tackling organisational change in the new NHS, *British Medical Journal*, **322**, 1464–1467

World Health Organisation [WHO] (1985) *Health for All by the Year 2000*, WHO, Geneva

World Health Organisation (1990) *Environment and Health*, WHO, Geneva

World Health Organisation (1999) *Making a Difference*, WHO, Geneva

2 MENTAL HEALTH POLICY AND FUTURE DEVELOPMENTS

Peter Spurgeon and Steve Field

*This chapter sets the recent changes in health care within the policy framework and emphasises that, in a period of transition, many health-care personnel will experience uncertainty about their knowledge, expertise and future roles. The authors feel that the argument for locating mental health services in primary care is well made and that this is the best arena in which to treat a great many people with mental health problems, especially those with depression and anxiety. They suggest that psychological approaches could enhance the quality of primary care for all patients, including those whose presenting problem is apparently physical. The work of individual practitioners can be improved through the adoption of procedures to facilitate accurate assessment, and the identification of appropriate interventions to bring about speedy relief from symptoms. The initiation and maintenance of good team practice depends on keeping all personnel up to date and ensuring that the team functions in an integrated manner. Material from this chapter could form the basis for team reviews and audits. (**Editors' note**)*

INTRODUCTION

Mental health services have traditionally been perceived as one of the 'Cinderella' services of the NHS; in terms of resources allocated to ratio of patients treated, this perception is probably not unreasonable. The public still seems to be uneasy about the concept of mental health. The generous response to appeals for money relating to children's services, for example, is not usually replicated as far as mental health is concerned. Public perception is overly influenced by media coverage of more extreme and disturbing cases of mental illness. The reality is that most mental health problems are far less severe, but – and this is also difficult for the public to acknowledge – will affect most families, directly or indirectly.

Despite its somewhat peripheral status in health care overall, the mental health sector has been subject to considerable upheaval in recent years. While the policy of closing large, long-stay institutions was welcome in many respects, funding was insufficient for adequate community-based care to be established as an alternative. This weakness gave rise to some violent episodes, including fatalities; although small in number, these events were highly publicised. The policy shift to care in the community, and the widespread nature of milder forms of mental health conditions, creates in reality an emphasis upon delivery of care in the setting of primary care.

The recently published *NHS Plan* (Department of Health, 2000a) affords some recognition of this situation. There has been an increase in resources, an announcement of the recruitment of a thousand graduate psychologists to help GPs to treat mild forms of depression, and the appointment of 50 early-intervention teams in the next three years, to help support those suffering from early onset psychosis and schizophrenia. Such investment in primary care is vital. As Verhaat *et al.* (2000) have shown, unless GPs feel they have the capacity and support to care for mental health patients, they will inappropriately refer relatively mild conditions to already swamped secondary services.

CARE IN GENERAL PRACTICE

Mental health problems are very common and primary care teams provide most of the help that people need (Goldberg and Huxley, 1992). In a typical working day, a GP can expect to see a significant psychological component in many consultations. Up to 40% of patients attending their GP for any reason have a mental health problem (Goldberg, 1991); in 20–25% of patients a mental health problem will be the sole reason for consultation. The most common mental health problems are anxiety and depression. In an average practice of 10 000 patients, 1000 would consult with a 'minor' mental health problem each year; there would also be 50 patients with 'severe' depression, 20 parasuicides and one successful suicide (Fry, 1993). Table 2.1 shows a breakdown of the kind of mental health problems that would be expected in a general practice dealing with 18,000 patients.

Table 2.1 Population and estimated general practice prevalence of mental disorders

Diagnosis	Weekly prevalence per 1000 adults aged 16–64	Number of patients aged 16–64 on a GP list of 18 000 patients
Mixed anxiety and depression	77	87
Generalised anxiety	31	36
Depressive episode	21	24
All phobias	11	13
Obsessive compulsive disorder	12	14
Panic disorder	8	9
All neuroses	160	182
Functional psychosis	4	5

OPCS Survey of Psychiatric Morbidity Report 1 (1995)

It is well established that GPs miss 30–50% of presentations of depression (Goldberg and Bridges, 1987). Many GPs also lack confidence in managing mental health issues (Kendrick *et al.*, 1995), perhaps a reflection of the fact that only 30% of them have held a postgraduate psychiatric post (Kerwick *et al.*, 1997) and only 2% of practice nurses have undergone formal mental health training (Crosland and Kai, 1998). In two recently published papers, Cape *et al.* (2000a, b) examined the evidence for the contribution and value of GPs' psychological management of common emotional problems. Although evidence is relatively scarce, and method-ologies are questionable on occasions, there is encouraging evidence that, with relatively little training, GPs can have a significant positive impact upon such patients – when they have the time and technique to offer help. Indeed, it is known that many patients suffering from various forms of depression only visit their GP once and appear to recover with little help.

Bashir *et al.* (2000) also report that the use of a facilitator had a positive impact upon GPs in terms of their capacity to recognise symptoms of mental health problems. In the cases that do have their illnesses diagnosed, the quality of care and the clinical outcomes are variable (Meltzer *et al.*, 1995; Nichol *et al.*, 1995). There is little evidence of specific practice policies for the care of the long-term mentally ill (Kendrick *et al.*, 1991); referral to secondary care can also be complicated by referral to an inappropriate secondary-care team member (Strathdee *et al.*, 1990; Scott *et al.*, 1994) and by significant non-attendance rates (Gournay and Brooking, 1995).

GPs, working increasingly as part of a primary care team, have taken on much of the load of mental health care that has resulted from the closing of mental hospitals and the reduction of psychiatric beds. The role of the GP and the primary health-care team has, however, been unclear, and the lack of participation in planning community care has been a cause for concern (Groves, 1990). In order to cope, the primary health-care teams have expanded in numbers, often with the addition of counsellors, but the work has been absorbed without any additional education and training for either the individuals or for the teams. The additional responsibilities far exceed those predicted a decade ago (Goldberg and Gournay, 1997). Bower and Sibbald (2000) report that the presence of on-site mental health workers, such as counsellors, has had little direct impact upon the clinical behaviour of GPs. None the less, the growth of counselling in general practice has been very rapid over the past two decades.

THE OFFSET COST RATIONALE

The potential cost-saving contribution of counselling provision in a primary care setting is thought to be considerable. It can save the more expensive time of the GP, as well as saving offset costs – patients receiving early mental health support have been found to utilise health services overall to a far lesser degree (Spurgeon and Barwell, 2000).

In an early US study, Goldberg *et al.* (1970) compared service utilisation 12 months after patients were referred to an outpatient mental health programme with the 12 months prior to referral. In the year after referral there was a 14% reduction in the number of patients seen for non-psychiatric purposes and another 16% reduction for tests and procedures. In another study in the USA, Mumford *et al.* (1984) analysed health insurance claims over the period 1974 to 1978, in order to review 58 studies of the effectiveness of outpatient psychotherapy. Using a variety of outcome measures, the results indicated reductions in in-patient and outpatient medical-care utilisation of 10–33%. The evidence demonstrated that psychotherapy had the greatest impact on hospital in-patient utilisation and its associated costs.

Broadly, there appear to be at least two reasons why access to psychotherapy or counselling may reduce health-care utilisation and associated medical costs. First, it may be that those patients with emotional distress present with physical or somatic problems in an attempt to seek medical intervention for relief. From this perspective it may well be the case that a great deal of medical intervention is inappropriate, as long as the real underlying emotional distress of the presenting patient is ignored. Under these conditions the patient is likely to return for treatment as the symptoms continue to evolve and, despite the best efforts of the doctor, the underlying emotional issues remain. Health-care utilisation and associated costs will continue to escalate and the patient will gain little relief from his or her contact with health services.

It is clear that at least half of all visits to GPs do not result in a clear medical diagnosis. Psychotherapy or counselling under these conditions is able to reduce the emotional distress that drives medical utilisation. In a parallel way, medical problems may trigger emotional reactions, which, in turn, may heighten a patient's susceptibility to other forms of emotional or physical distress. There is some evidence to suggest that counselling can have a beneficial effect in major disease areas such as diabetes, asthma and CHD.

Table 2.2 shows the reasons why patients were referred for counselling over a three-month period to seven practice-based counsellors (Wiles, 1993).

Table 2.2 Reasons for referring for counselling

	% of patients
Depression, anxiety, panic attacks	28.3
Marital/relationship problems	21.7
Sexual abuse	11.7
Anger, violence, suicidal feelings, self-harm	11.7
Depression after distressing event (such as miscarriage)	10.0
Bereavement	8.3
Not coping	8.3

A second reason why psychotherapy or counselling may have positive cost offsets is related to the interplay between the medical and the psychological state of a patient. Existing medical conditions may be exacerbated by emotional distress and, furthermore, emotional distress may complicate the treatment process, resulting in higher utilisation and costs. In a similar way, medical conditions may be associated with negative emotional components, which complicate treatment if left unaddressed.

AN INTEGRATED APPROACH

Traditionally there has been a separation between primary and secondary care for patients with mental illness (Goldberg and Jackson, 1992). Communication has usually been only by letter (Williams and Wallace, 1974; Pullen and Yellowlees, 1985). Poor communication only increased the divide between primary and secondary care, but the recent development of community mental health services has led to an expansion of specialist services in the community setting, with a subsequent improvement in communication. GPs have found the new services more responsive to the needs of their patients (Strathdee, 1988); referral practices have also changed, with rates of referral increasing. Consultation liaison models, community out-reach and on-site mental health professionals in primary care have not, however, led to any significant improvement in clinical outcomes, cost effectiveness or patient satisfaction (Gask et al., 1997; Bower and Sibbald, 2000).

It is generally accepted that good quality mental health care results from an effective partnership between health services, the social services, the voluntary services and the service users. However, the concept of partnership and shared care remains contentious, even within the medical profession. There has been no consensus on the distribution of responsibilities between GPs and specialists (Royal College of General Practitioners, 1993). The attitude of inner-city GPs also appears to differ from that of their suburban colleagues; both groups favour shared care with specialists, but those working in the inner cities significantly less than their suburban colleagues. Inner-city GPs are also less inclined to organise overall care. This is despite inner-city GPs being *more* likely to be exposed to patients with serious mental health illness (Brown et al., 1999).

A truly integrated approach must unify medical and mental health care and therefore remove the dichotomy of 'physical' and 'mental' in defining problems presented by patients. Integrated primary care combines medical and mental health services, for a fuller approach to the spectrum of problems and complaints that a patient may present with in primary care (Blount, 1998). The aim is for patients to feel that they have presented to the appropriate person and in the appropriate place.

In the context of the provision of mental health services, integrated primary care means the bringing together of physical and mental health care in the setting of primary care. It therefore avoids the split of 'physical' from 'mental' presenting complaints, resulting in a more holistic approach to patient care.

Until recently there has been a separation between primary and secondary care for patients with mental illness, but an effective partnership between all the parties is vital to good-quality mental health care. There are many other points of access to health and social care: for example, the Samaritans, MIND, the National Schizophrenia Fellowship and the developing NHS Direct all provide valuable services. Patients, users and carers need a more transparent, co-ordinated and user-friendly service – this is how integrated primary care should be.

All services should ideally be located on one site, to facilitate formal and informal communication between team members. Team members will need to develop a shared vision of what the integrated team is seeking to achieve and how it is going to achieve it. The exact design of how the integrated team works will develop over time and each team will have its own particular characteristics, which will depend on local circumstances. The environment should be supportive; frequent team meetings are essential to provide the opportunity to discuss cases and to enable the development of trust, interdependency, mutual accountability, and respect for each other's skills.

There is evidence that integrated primary care is cost-effective in terms of the benefits that arise from optimising both physical and mental health care outcomes (Friedman *et al.*, 1995). The impact on health and economic outcomes comes from an improvement in the immediate health of patients who consult with acute concerns such as stress-related physical conditions, and in the longer-term health of patients with recurrent and chronic conditions. Significantly, untreated depressed patients use two to three times the annual medical services of the equivalent non-depressed patients (Simon *et al.*, 1995). Integrated care, leading to improved detection and treatment of depression in the local community, will result in savings in both health and social care, as well as wider-ranging economic benefits.

Effective integrated care involves all members of the primary health-care team learning and working together. An important first step in the development of integrated care is the move to jointly held medical records, with an eventual shift towards patients holding their own. Integrated primary care should be seen as a remedy to problems identified by the stakeholders. Policies should develop in partnership with all members of the new teams and the patients and carers. Integration means a partnership with patients and carers, enabling them to gain a better understanding of their problem and its management. Local self-help groups also have an important part to play in the integrated primary care system. Embedded in the National Service Framework for Mental Health (Department of Health, 1999) is the acknowledgement that systematic changes will be called for if a service sensitive to the needs of the local communities is to emerge. In order for that to happen, historic thinking about mental health care provision will need to be challenged.

THE PRIMARY CARE GROUP/PRIMARY CARE TRUST LEVEL

The development of Primary Care Groups (PCGs) and, from them, Primary Care Trusts (PCTs) should allow for a more integrated approach to planning all health services for local communities. The local model for providing mental health care may vary depending on circumstances, but an increasing number of PCTs will gain responsibility for all mental services, including specialists, community mental health care teams, local day and in-patient care. This is surely the right direction for all PCTs to take, moving towards a model that can deliver fully integrated care that responds to the needs of local populations.

The National Service Framework (NSF) acknowledges that achieving such services will take some time, and provides a strategy that should act as a means of attaining this vision. It emphasises three key aims:

1 Safe services – to protect the public and provide effective care for those with mental illness at the time they need it.
2 Sound services – to ensure that patients and service users have access to the full range of services that they need.
3 Supportive services – working with patients and service users, their families and carers to build healthy communities.

The role of PCTs

Among the Standards set, two are aimed specifically at PCGs/PCTs. PCGs/PCTs must aim not only to implement the parts of the NSF that are relevant to them but also to influence the local NHS Trusts, health and local authorities to deliver on their areas of responsibility.

The key areas for PCTs are reflected in Standards Two and Three.

Standard Two: Any service user who contacts their primary care team with a common mental health problem should:

- have their health needs identified and addressed;
- be offered effective treatments, including referral to specialist services for further assessment, treatment and care if they require it.

Standard Three: Any individual with a common mental health problem should:

- be able to make contact around the clock with the local services necessary to meet their needs and receive adequate care;
- be able to use NHS Direct, as it develops, for first-level advice and referral on to specialist help-lines or to local services.

PCG/Ts will need to build capacity to manage common mental health problems and manage referral pathways to specialists as well as working with patients, their carers and self-help groups. Their performance will be assessed by a number of local milestones and national targets, which include reductions in the rate of suicide, adherence to prescribing guidelines, experiences of users and carers and access to specialist services.

PCG/Ts will need to exhibit local leadership to deliver the objectives laid down in the NSF. They will need to engage with the key local individuals, groups and agencies, and produce a coherent plan of action supported by their health authority and regional mental health implementation teams.

Achieving the aims of the NSF

The aims of the NSF for Mental Health (Department of Health, 1999) are ambitious and they can only be achieved with an integrated approach based firmly in primary care. To achieve these aims, additional resources have been made available, but the change will also require leadership and a fundamental change in the workforce. Work will also be needed to ensure that patients become more empowered in terms of choices and opportunities and mental health promotion.

The first step will be for each PCG/T to work with the local specialist mental health services to assess mental health needs of their local community. The aim of this should be to inform local delivery plans in accordance with those set out in the NSF. A whole systems approach is required, taking in diagnostic models, service delivery arrangements, pathways of care and national and local policy on setting service level agreements for mental health care. It is important for all stakeholders to be engaged in planning the local arrangements, including health and social services staff, but also local voluntary services, users and carers. A sense of shared vision and partnership is vital to underpin the development of an integrated care system.

The local scoping exercise will throw up many demands, both needs and wants. There will be variation in local capacities and capabilities, which will lead to variations across the country in the speed of moving to an integrated system of primary care. However, this should not detract from the long-term vision.

THE PRACTICE LEVEL: THE PRIMARY HEALTH CARE TEAM

The first step should be for each PCG/T to work with the local specialist mental health services to develop resources for each practice to assess the mental health needs of its local community. The primary health care team should work with the local community, to develop skills and competencies to manage common problems, and agree referral arrangements for assessment and treatment. The development of NHS Direct should give patients and carers another access point, complementing existing national help-lines.

The skills of the primary health care team would initially be enhanced by on-site access to specialist knowledge provided by psychiatrists, community mental health nurses, social workers and other therapists. The traditional primary-secondary interface would be gradually replaced by an integrated system, which, as it matures, would lead to the local mental health services being embedded into the primary care services, until they become seamless. Patients with mental health problems who would otherwise have made an appointment to see their GP could be offered an alternative assessment within the primary care setting by another appropriately skilled member of the integrated primary health care team. This could be a community mental health nurse or a practice nurse who has acquired additional mental health skills.

The future may also see a new type of health-care worker in primary care – a behavioural health consultant, acting as part of the primary health-care team. This development has already been seen to provide added value in the United States (Stroshal, 1998). The behavioural health consultant might see the patient alone, or the patient and referring practitioner together. The aim of the consultation is to target the psychosocial concerns of the patient and to increase the impact of the medical and psychosocial interventions of the doctor or nurse. This new role could help improve compliance with treatment plans for patients whose psychosocial concerns are often not addressed, for example, patients with diabetes, asthma or heart disease. The behavioural health consultant may be an entirely new form of health worker; alternatively, the role might evolve from that of the community mental health nurse. The role of the specialist psychiatric doctor or nurse would complement the behavioural health consultant but would be reserved for more chronic psychological problems.

WHO guidelines

The World Health Organisation (WHO, 2000) has produced guidelines on the management of mental illness. It has also proposed practical steps that can be implemented in a practice, which could act as a foundation on which to build an integrated primary care team.

Practice organisation

- A practice policy for receptionists' responses when faced with a patient who is very agitated or anxious.
- Some longer slots booked in surgeries to allow for people with emotional problems.
- Routine follow-up appointments for people prescribed antidepressants, with a doctor or another member of the team.
- Encouraging patients with chronic mental disorders to see the same team member at each visit.
- A register of patients with severe or chronic mental illness to ensure regular follow-up and monitoring.
- Reviews of the 'mental health workload' of each partner. If it falls disproportionately on one or a small number of partners, it is advisable to consider ways of relieving the pressure; alternatively, there could be a plan to acknowledge and support the specialisation of the partner(s) as part of the way the team operates.

Information and support for patients

- Information leaflets or audiotapes for people suffering mental ill health.
- Information readily available to patients and all members of the practice team about community or voluntary groups who can help patients suffering mental ill health.

Skills within the primary care team

- Reviews of the skills of all members of the team – doctors, health visitor, practice nurse, counsellor, district nurse, and school nurse. What kind of problems/patients is each competent to deal with? Are all members of the team aware of the skills of others within the team?
- Checking the training and support needs of practice nurses or others who are involved in certain activities, such as giving depot injections or monitoring of lithium.
- Ensuring that the primary mental health skills within the team are periodically updated in such areas as: structured problem-solving; activity planning, especially in depression; teaching controlled breathing, relaxation techniques in anxiety states and panic attacks; motivational interviewing in alcohol and drug misuse; supporting graded exposure to feared situations in anxiety, and particularly with phobias; encouraging more appropriate thinking (cognitive skills) in depression and anxiety; re-attribution of symptoms from physical to emotional causes; asking about suicidal intentions; managing self-harming behaviours.
- Serious consideration of clinical supervision, peer or external, for team members who take on a significant counselling or mental health workload.

Liaison with community mental health and substance abuse services
- Regular, face-to-face meetings with the relevant person from the community mental health team(s) that serve the practice.
- Arrangements to 'share' people with a severe mental illness and those with substance abuse.
- Displaying the contact details of the key worker for each person with a severe mental illness prominently on the patient notes.

Psychological therapies
- Reviewing the access, via secondary care or non-statutory agencies, to cognitive, behavioural, family or other psychological therapies.

Stress management for the primary care team
- Meeting with members of the practice team to consider how you might provide support for each other to minimise your own stress.
- Liaison with the PCG to consider some form of regular psychological support system for health professionals.

WORKFORCE, EDUCATION AND TRAINING ISSUES

Workforce planning has not been a strength of the NHS. In 1999, the House of Commons Health Select Committee recommended that there should be a major review of this issue. The resulting consultation document *A Health Service of all the Talents: Developing the NHS workforce* (Department of Health, 2000b) signposted a new system that will lead to an improvement of processes, which should, in turn, lead to better needs assessment and planning at all levels within the NHS. The new system, which also draws together the medical and non-medical training levies, should improve the flexibility of basic and post-basic training programmes (including undergraduate and postgraduate medical training) and aid the development of more interprofessional training opportunities.

It is vital that work is undertaken to establish the current position of staff working in primary care, including those involved in mental health. The profile should include GPs, psychiatrists, psychologists, nurses, social services, counsellors, therapists, carers and workers in the voluntary sector. This will enable the NHS to commission training programmes to produce a new workforce with the appropriate knowledge, skills and attitudes to deliver integrated primary health care, reflecting the priorities set out in the NSF. The new workforce will need to represent the community that it serves; it is, therefore, important that work is done to attract and then retain people from the ethnic minorities into the primary care workforce.

All education and training in the future should be evidence-based and emphasise the importance of interprofessional learning and working. If the integrated primary care system is to work, all health professionals must gain experience in integrated settings during their training. Ideally, this would be in both the under-graduate and postgraduate phases of training.

Historically, the training of doctors, nurses and other allied professionals in the UK has been uni-professional, with very little contact between professional groups. There are, however, examples of good practice in interprofessional learning in primary care; one such example is the University of Birmingham's community mental health programme (Barnes *et al.*, 2000), a postgraduate programme of interprofessional education in community mental health. The programme is part-time, with teaching concentrating on psychosocial interventions using an inter-professional focus. It was planned and delivered in partnership with a number of stakeholders, including service users. Its participants are nurses, occupational therapists, social workers, psychologists, psychiatrists and development workers.

The programme was also evaluated in partnership with stakeholders, and this evaluation of the programme demonstrated the positive effects of that partnership with service users, and of interprofessional education. The benefit is evident in the course design, its evaluation and in the learning outcomes. And it appears to go beyond the direct contribution of users to course content. It seems that a 'saliency effect' has been created, too, so that professionals accommodate to a user perspective in their tasks.

There are many other examples of good practice that promote and support interprofessional education for mental health. They include the *Calipso* CD-ROM training package from the University of Leeds (Williams *et al.*, 2000), the *Teamwork* training pack (Bleach, 1996), and PRiMHE (Primary Care Mental Health Education, www.primhe.org). The latter is an initiative that aims to bring together health professionals who are active in primary mental health care, to provide a nationally co-ordinated programme of mental health education. It provides an online discussion forum for teachers, researchers and PCG leaders. It also produces a journal, training materials and arranges educational meetings. The Unit for Mental Health Education in Primary Care of the Royal College of General Practitioners organises excellent courses for people wishing to teach mental health skills to primary care teams in their local area. The Sainsbury Centre for Mental Health is also active in promoting integrated care and in producing educational packages and courses. There are many other resources available across the UK; the challenge is to make people aware of them and to disseminate good practice throughout the NHS, in order to develop the workforce quickly.

New and existing staff will need help and support with their continuing profes-sional development; all staff should have personal development plans (PDPs). Support and mentoring from educationally competent colleagues is essential in order to help the learner to identify learning needs, and to plan learning. The GP tutor network is an excellent model, which is developing to meet the needs of GPs and other primary care staff to support the development of PDPs, life-long learning and reflective-practice skills. In many PCGs, nurse tutors and practice manager tutors are also working in tandem with their GP tutor colleagues (Field, 1998). Investment in teambuilding and in leadership courses will be needed to support the development of integrated primary care. Leadership and management skills will also be needed.

None of this will happen without the commitment of government to commit substantial resources to achieve its aims. They have promised a substantial investment; they now must deliver.

CONCLUSION: KEY DEVELOPMENT AREAS

A number of key development areas will provide the focus of activity over the next couple of years:

- Agreed protocols between primary and specialist services for the management of depression (including post-natal), anxiety, schizophrenia, drug and alcohol dependence and those requiring psychological therapies.
- Linkages to the local health improvement programmes (HImPs) to promote mental health and combat discrimination and social exclusion of people with mental health problems.
- Frequent reviews of the workforce to ensure that teams have the necessary numbers, and individuals have the appropriate knowledge, skills and attitudes to provide appropriate care to users and support to carers.
- CPD programmes to support staff development, which include mental health subjects and issues. These should be informed by mechanisms to review the practice's prescribing of benzodiazepines, antidepressants and antipsychotic medications.
- Systems in place to ensure that service users have appropriate care plans.
- Systems to measure the experience of service users and carers.

The reader will now have a better understanding of the scope and direction of current health care reforms. The agenda is huge and will not be achieved in the short term. It is understandable that many professionals find coping with change on such a scale demanding and that attrition rates are very high in the present climate. Perhaps the most important point made by this chapter is that health-care providers must respond to a new ideology, in which patients will no longer be viewed as passive, but rather as active, informed and empowered participants in their own care and treatment. The authors feel that the new emphasis on health as opposed to illness could lead to the emergence of a different kind of health-care provider, the 'behavioural health specialist'. This specialist will carry out health assessments and work closely with local communities in health promotion. Practitioners working in the reformed health services, which may absorb many of the alternative therapies, will require high-quality continuous education and training. (Editors' summary)

REFERENCES

Barnes, D., Carpenter, J. and Bailey, D. I. (2000) Partnerships with service users in interprofessional education for community mental health: a case study, *Journal of Interprofessional Care*, 14(2), 189–200

Bashir, K., Blizard, B., Bosanquet, A., Mann, A., and Jenkins, R. (2000) The evaluation of a mental health facilitator in general practice: effects on recognition, management, and outcome of mental illness, *British Journal of General Practice*, 50, 626–629

Bleach, A. (1996) *Teamwork: A training resource pack for the review and development of mental health teams*, Pavilion, Brighton

Blount, A.B. (1998) *Integrated Primary Care*, Norton, New York

Bower, P. and Sibbald, B. (2000) Systematic review of the effect of onsite mental health professionals on the clinical behaviour of general practitioners, *British Medical Journal*, 320, 614–617

Brown J.S.L., Weich S., Downes-Grainger E. and Goldberg D. (1999) Attitudes of inner-city GPs to shared care for psychiatric patients in the community, *British Journal of General Practice* 49, 643–644

Cape, J., Barker, C., Buszewicz, M. and Pistrang, N. (2000a) General practitioner psychological management of common emotional problems, (i) Definitions and literature review, *British Journal of General Practice*, 50, 313–318

Cape, J., Barker, C., Buszewicz, M. and Pistrang, N. (2000b) General practitioner psychological management of common emotional problems, (ii) A research agenda for the development of evidence-based practice, *British Journal of General Practice*, 50, 396–400

Crosland, A. and Kai, J. (1998) 'They think they can talk to nurses': practice nurses' views of their roles in caring for mental health problems, *British Journal of General Practice*, 48, 1383–1386

Department of Health (1999) *National Service Framework for Mental Health*, Department of Health, London

Department of Health (2000a) *The NHS Plan: A Plan For Investment, A Plan For Reform*, The Stationery Office, London

Department of Health (2000b) *A Health Service of all the Talents: Developing the NHS workforce, consultation document on the review of workforce planning*, Department of Health, London

Field, S.J. (1998) Continuing professional development in primary care, *Medical Education*, 32, 564–566

Friedman, R., Sobel, D., Myers, P., Caudill, M. and Benson, H. (1995) Behavioural medicine, clinical health psychology and cost offset, *Health Psychology*, 14, 509–518

Fry, J. (1993) *General Practice: The facts*, Radcliffe Medical Press, Oxford

Gask, L., Sibbald, B. and Creed, F. (1997) Evaluating models of working at the interface between mental health services and primary care, *British Journal of Psychiatry*, 170, 6–11

Goldberg, D. (1991) Filters to care – a model. In Jenkins, R., Griffiths, S. (eds.) *Indicators for Mental Health in the Population*, HMSO, London

Goldberg, D. and Bridges, K. (1987) Screening for psychiatric illness in general practice: the general practitioner versus the screening questionnaire, *Journal of the Royal College of General Practitioners*, 37,15–18

Goldberg, D. and Gournay, K. (1997) The general practitioner, the psychiatrist and the burden of mental health care, Maudsley discussion paper 1, The Institute of Psychiatry, London

Goldberg, D. and Huxley, P. (1992) *Common Mental Disorders: A biosocial model*, Routledge, London

Goldberg, D. and Jackson, G. (1992) Interface between primary care and specialist mental health care, *British Journal of General Practice*, 42, 267–267

Goldberg, I.D., Krantz, G. and Locke, B.Z. (1970) Effects of a short-term outpatient psychiatric therapy benefit on the utilisation of medical services in a prepaid group practice medical programme, *Medical Care*, 9(5), 419–428

Gournay, K. and Brooking, J. (1995) The community psychiatric nurse in primary care: an economic analysis, *Journal of Advanced Nursing*, 22, 769–778

Groves, T. (1990) After the asylum, *British Medical Journal*, 300, 1128–1130.

Kendrick, T., Sibbald, B., Burns, T. and Freeling, P. (1991) Role of general practitioners in the care of long-term mentally ill patients, *British Medical Journal*, 30, 508–510

Kendrick, T., Burns, T. and Freeling, P. (1995) A randomised controlled trial of teaching general practitioners to carry out structured assessments of their long-term mentally ill patients, *British Medical Journal*, 311, 93–98

Kerwick, S., Jones, R., Mann, A. and Goldberg, D. (1997) Mental health care training priorities in general practice, *British Journal of General Practice*, 47, 225–227

Meltzer, H., Gill, B., Petticrew, M. and Hinds, K. (1995) Physical complaints, service use and treatment of adults with psychiatric disorders, *OPCS Surveys of Psychiatric Morbidity in Great Britain Report 5*, HMSO, London

Mumford, E., Schlesinger, H., Glass, G., Patrick, C. and Cuerdon, T. (1984) A new look at evidence about reduced cost of medical utilisation following mental health treatment, *American Journal of Psychiatry*, 141, 1145–1158

Nichol, M.B., Stimmel, G.L. and Lange, S.C. (1995) Factors predicting the use of multiple psychotropic medications, *Journal of Clinical Psychiatry*, 56, 50–66

OPCS (1995) *Survey of Psychiatric Morbidity Report 1*, HMSO, London

Pullen, I. and Yellowlees, A.J. (1985) Is communication improving between general practitioners and psychiatrists? *British Medical Journal*, 290, 31–33

Royal College of General Practitioners (1993) Report of a joint college working group Shared care of patients with mental health problems (Occasional Paper 60), Royal College of General Practitioners, London

Scott, J., McCluskey, S. and Smith, L. (1994) Three months in the life of a community mental health team, *Psychiatric Bulletin*, 18, 615–617

Simon, G., Von Korff, M. and Barlow, W. (1995) Health care costs of primary care patients with recognised depression, *Archives of General Psychiatry*, 52, 850–856

Spurgeon, P. and Barwell, F. (2000) Personal responsibility, empowerment and medical utilisation: theoretical framework for considering counselling and offset costs, *European Journal of Psychotherapy, Counselling and Health*, 3(2), 229–244

Strathdee, G. (1988) Psychiatrists in primary care: the general practitioner's viewpoint, *Family Practice*, 5, 111–115

Strathdee, G., Brown, R.M.A. and Doig, R.J. (1990) Psychiatric clinics in primary care, *Social Pschiatry & Psychiatric Epidemiology*, 25, 95–100

Stroshal, K. (1998) Integrating behavioural health and primary care. In Blount, A.B. (1998) *Integrated Primary Care*, Norton, New York

Verhaat, P.F.M., Van De Lisdonk, E.H., Bor, J.H.R. and Hutschemaekers, G.J.M. (2000) GPs' referral to mental health care during the past 25 years, *British Journal of General Practice*, 50, 307–308

Wiles, R. (1993) Counselling in general practice, Institute for Health Policy Studies research paper, University of Southampton, Southampton

Williams, P. and Wallace, B.B. (1974) General practitioners and psychiatrists – do they communicate? *British Medical Journal*, 1, 505

Williams, C., Cottrell, D. and Harkin, P. (2000) *Calipso* [CD-ROM training package], University of Leeds, Leeds

World Health Organisation (2000) *WHO Guide to Mental Health in Primary Care*, Royal Society of Medicine Press, London

3 THE CONCEPT OF COLLABORATION IN PRIMARY CARE

Lynn Ashburner

This chapter takes us to the heart of the book, with the author's reminder that policy has to be incorporated into a pre-existing world of health care. She discusses the various conceptual and practical interpretations of the term 'collaboration' and argues that there is a significant gap between the rhetoric of policy documents and the reality of collaborative teamworking. The effectiveness of primary care nursing depends on the extent to which nurses feel integrated into the care team and the scope of practice that they are allowed to undertake. There is a need to move away from an ad hoc approach to team formation and to recognise that leadership, management, resources and support are essential if collaboration is to be effective and sustainable. Individuals need to be clear about their skills, their roles and how their work relates to that of others. Once established, collaboration requires constant vigilance, as collapse or fragmentation can easily occur. The importance of good supportive management and leadership cannot be over-emphasised, if grass roots practice is to be consistent with policy rather than merely a rehash of what it has always been. (Editors' note)

INTRODUCTION

This chapter takes an overview of the concept of collaboration. It examines what it may mean in a health service context and looks specifically at the role of the primary health care team, with reference to the role of the community psychiatric nurse (CPN). It will draw upon research carried out for the West Midlands NHS Executive (Ashburner *et al.*, 1998), which focused on the West Midlands Region and explored the organisation of primary care nursing, with a particular emphasis on education and training issues. The remit for this research was to establish what was *actually* happening in primary care across the region, as opposed to what was *claimed*. In the course of doing this work the role of primary care teams was also examined.

Given the emphasis within recent policy directives on promoting partnership and collaboration, it is important to explore and understand the 'gap' between a broadly welcomed policy initiative and the reality of making collaboration actually happen at the service delivery level. When people talk about 'primary care teams', 'partnership' or 'collaboration', there is often confusion about what exactly they mean. The differences in conception may be significant. This can cause problems not just in basic communications, but also in the clarity of the management and organisational role in planning and establishing the most appropriate form of collaboration for the delivery of health care.

Whether the term used is 'collaboration', 'partnership', or 'primary care team', none of these can represent a panacea for current ills, or a blueprint for the future. None of the terms is precise enough, nor is there sufficient research on the effectiveness of different forms of collaboration for clear guidelines, or any concept of 'best practice', to emerge. One of the dangers of establishing some models over others, often under the guise of 'best practice', is to suggest that solutions can be imported or imposed in that way. The chief weakness is that such ready-made solutions cannot be context-sensitive. There is an increasing need, notably within the organisation of primary care, for collaboration to go beyond the health service, to include such agencies as social services, voluntary organisations, education, housing and, in some instances, the private sector.

This chapter explores what is meant by 'collaboration', then considers the health-sector context and looks at the data from the study. A short section looks at what the conditions for effective collaboration might be and concludes by raising the specific issues that relate to primary care. The objective is to facilitate those involved in collaborative ventures in developing the model of collaboration that is most appropriate for a particular context.

WHAT DO WE MEAN BY COLLABORATION?

The purpose of collaboration is to create mutual benefit, to enhance capacity and to achieve ends that would not otherwise be possible. Collaboration is not only the objective but also the means to a desired end. However, because it is something of a 'buzz word', it needs to be understood in all its facets – both its strengths and its weaknesses. This will help to avoid its random application to any and all forms of contact between different groups, agencies or organisations.

There is an implication that the way that health care is organised needs to be changed, but health-care organisation has always required collaboration, so what is different now from the way that the NHS has always operated? There have always been inter-relationships between different groups; overlaps between health and social services; and indeed some community psychiatric nurses have always worked alongside district nurses, practice nurses, midwives and health visitors within primary care. However, much of this has emerged from patterns of individual practice and much has occurred along informal lines. This type of informal collaboration is not necessarily 'inferior' to more formal forms but informal arrangements can lead, with regard to outcomes, to gaps, possible failure if key parties move away, or uncertainty when problems arise.

Collaboration implies a level of formality and it has different bases. There may be a need for collaboration at the strategic planning level, at the organisational level or at the practical level with service delivery. The focus of the collaboration may be on different combinations of parties or groups at each of these levels and even on different aspects of health care. This suggests that a proliferation of collaborative ventures will lead to increasing complexity in the number and type of relationships for individual staff. Unlike conventional organisations, primary care has never been dominated by linear, hierarchical structures, with clear lines of authority and responsibility, so an increase in the extent of networked forms of organisation will not involve a significant change but a development of what is familiar.

An attempt to define what collaboration might mean in practice can be done by categorising it according to different dimensions:

- the *level* across organisations, etc. at which the collaboration takes place, and its *purpose*;
- the *parties* to the collaboration and its *boundary*;
- the *context*: the history and organisational variables such as *culture*, power, etc., which affect the collaboration and its effectiveness;
- *co-ordination*: whether via hierarchy and rules; by market forces/self-interest or by more egalitarian means based on trust: issue of *authority*;
- *formality*: the level of formality or *permanence* of the arrangement – how loose and flexible?

It may be useful in understanding the differences in degree from informal to formal arrangements to use the concept of a continuum, with organisational 'autonomy' at one end and 'merger' at the other. Looking at different definitions, the loosest forms of collaboration are networks, followed by co-operation, then collaboration, then formal partnerships and finally mergers, which result in total integration. The terms might be defined as follows:

- *Network* is used to cover many forms of relationship, both formal and informal, individual and organisational, and either between or within organisations. Networks are characterised by their focus on sharing information or managing; a focus on a common interest, or the early stages of a more formal arrangement; and they can also exist alongside other forms and facilitate the process of collaboration.
- *Co-operation* suggests the sharing of resources, tasks, processes or services. Again, this may be formal or informal. Co-operation between organisations may be short-term, focused on a specific objective and can remain marginal to the main organisational design.
- *Collaboration* implies a more formalised form of sharing for a process, which may be more extensive or longer-term. Collaboration can become organisationally established and, most importantly, will have an impact upon the host organisation's processes, power structures and design. Issues of power and culture across the organisations or groups are important, given that the individuals active in the collaboration carry the status of their organisations into the process. Individuals will also carry their respective hierarchical positions within their own organisation to the collaboration.
- *Partnership* implies a further development towards permanence or legal recognition, with an implied equality in the relationship. It also suggests a move towards a widespread level of collaboration within the totality of the host organisations, with the possibility of greater levels of ambiguity since the focus

is less likely to be on specific tasks and processes. For example, there may be a partnership initiative at a strategic level but with little impact, in the short term, at the grass roots. More complete or mature partnerships may result in *mergers*.

This analysis shows that the concept of 'collaboration' is the one that most closely reflects the requirements of sharing and co-ordination within primary care. The different organisations and groups remain autonomous, but at many levels individuals need to enter into formal or semi-formal arrangements, with regard to the sharing of resources, the co-ordination of effort and processes, in the management and delivery of services. The potential benefits for primary care are that collaboration optimises health outcomes and the use of resources, avoids duplication and brings better-quality solutions. The implications for each party organisation are that it facilitates participation and learning within a multi-disciplinary approach. However, it can also increase the level of complexity in management lines of responsibility, with fewer clear structures; the collaboration becomes very dependent upon strong channels of communication.

Collaboration between organisations can be of benefit by opening up access to more sources of information, skills and knowledge and reducing uncertainty. However, it can also weaken conventional structures and power bases, as new power bases are established and the focus moves towards more formal types of collaboration. In organisational terms, as well as being policy-led, the development of greater levels of collaboration makes sense. This is particularly so, given the diversity and pluralism that characterise public-sector services, the context of continual change and the need for flexible and responsive structures that can meet variable demands.

However beneficial, desirable or appropriate collaborative working is, it does bring additional problems and can put extra pressure on organisations and individuals. Setting up and maintaining collaborative structures and processes can be time-consuming, and there is a danger that the focus can shift to the process away from the purpose. Sustainability is a particular problem, which means that ongoing attention needs to be paid to communications and co-ordination. Participants and leaders need different skills to work and manage in this way, since there will be a mix of different expectations about the methods of work, the objectives, and the benefits of the collaboration. There will be a need to co-ordinate people from different organisational cultures, with different procedures, practices and even language. This also raises important questions about issues of accountability. If collaborative teams work across conventional organisational structures, where does accountability lie? Where individual professions retain their individual accountabilities for their own practice, how does this fit in with overall accountability for the shared process? These are important questions that need to be addressed within the contexts in which they arise.

Managerially, there is a requirement to manage a process that may not be directly within the manager's control, and this puts the emphasis on the calibre of relationships rather than on formal hierarchical power. This has implications for the managerial role. The manager needs to consider the following:

- placing an emphasis on managing via negotiation rather than authority;
- recruiting and training for suitably skilled staff;
- developing trust;
- giving a lead on common strategic direction;
- assessing the performance of the collaboration against objectives;
- building a supportive internal culture; and
- retaining an overview of the processes, and how they relate to the larger organisation.

At the early stages there is a need to be able to assess the capacity and readiness of the organisations and individuals to collaborate and to understand how other parts of the organisation may be indirectly affected. In a primary care sector where overstretched resources for education and development are inevitably directed first at clinical needs, these nevertheless remain important issues with regard to the future development of individual staff and the service.

THE HEALTH-SECTOR CONTEXT

To focus on collaboration brings the whole rationale for the organisation of healthcare delivery into the spotlight. Ideally it is not enough to begin with what happens at present as a given and then seek to optimise the level of co-operation and collaboration, but to use the opportunity to reflect on other fundamental questions of organisation. There are issues of how health needs are defined, prioritised and grouped; where these services should be based and which organisation should provide them; and which health-care professionals should provide which aspect of the care. In all the varying ways of organising, there will be a need for a range of forms of collaboration with regard to both the organisational context and the delivery of care itself. In primary care, especially, there is a very complex network of roles and organisations – across different organisations within or between the primary care sector and secondary, and between the groups of professionals themselves, as they organise their work and deal with individual cases. The development of Primary Care Groups (PCGs) and Primary Care Trusts (PCTs) could well lead to greater emphasis in the future on the integration of nursing roles, as well as on the integration between different parts of the NHS, social services, voluntary groups and other agencies. This may be seen by some as an opportunity and by others as a threat.

Relevant research

The potential for collaboration across the whole of primary care and between health and social services is extensive. This chapter focuses primarily on the role of primary care nurses and the concept of the primary care team, utilising data from a recent study designed to supplement an earlier research project carried out for West Midlands NHSE R&D Directorate on the role of nurse practitioners (Ashburner *et al.*, 1997). The research sought data from all health authorities across the region and carried out more detailed case studies in three, which had different geographical and demographic characteristics. (Though they contained a wide range of contexts, they cannot be regarded as representative.) Within each of these authorities, three general practices with differing profiles were selected for in-depth interviews. Practice profiles were diverse and ranged from single-handed practices and rural practices to multiple partnerships and urban and inner-city settings. Within this sample of nine general practices all clinical staff employed by the practices, or attached to them, were interviewed; in large practices, only a sample of GPs were included. Interviews were also held in all Community Trusts related to the practices.

The interviews focused on four areas:

1 primary care nursing roles;
2 the integration of those roles;
3 inter-organisational relationships; and
4 training and development issues.

The focus for current collaborative work in the area of primary care teams centres on individual general practices. It must be emphasised that this does not encompass the totality of primary care. This emphasis may change as PCGs develop, and collaborative ventures broaden across groups of GPs and into the wider community. Current literature therefore reflects the situation to date in the discussion of the organisation of primary care and the GP role. The preliminary findings of a study by Kendall (1996) suggest enormous differences in the ways in which general practices are organised and also in the responsiveness of GPs to considerations of strategic management and corporate approaches. It is GPs who remain in control of the development of primary care. Lazenbatt's (1997) study of the nursing contribution to targeting health and social need in Northern Ireland indicated that, under the right conditions, nurses can promote integration of services, interdisciplinary and collaborative intra-professional relations, to provide innovative health-care services. The advent of PCGs has increased the power of the GP over the organisation of primary care and it is as yet unclear how much the nursing role in the management of primary care has been enhanced or diminished. Given the numerical predominance of GPs on PCG boards, the latter remains a strong possibility. Ashburner and Birch (1999) suggest that a multidisciplinary approach and collaboration are integral to nursing development in primary care, but there is a question about how far major changes will be achievable without the support of the medical profession, who have more limited experience of multi-disciplinary working.

Nursing roles

The West Midlands NHSE study took place within the wider context of the debate on the development and extension of nursing roles. The concept of collaboration reflects a concern for general practices about how they can use their resources in more creative and efficient ways. As Wilkin and Butler (1996), and Kendall (1996) indicate, solutions to GP workload may involve the introduction of extended and expanded nursing services. Wilkin and Butler have tried to identify a direction and process for collaborative partnerships and have sought ways of evaluating primary and community care initiatives. Nursing roles, especially, are evolving in response to several issues:

- the effects of policy changes;
- advances in knowledge on treatments and disease;
- the changing needs of clinical colleagues, especially doctors;
- the greater levels of collaboration between nurses in primary care; and
- the need to collaborate more formally with external agencies and organisations such as social services.

With the emergence of clinical nurse specialist roles, community psychiatric nurses (CPNs) or community mental health nurses (CMHNs) are taking on new responsibilities. They can provide specialist expertise to support care of patients. The CPNs in the study described the orientation of their work broadly as the assessment of the mental health of an individual within a family and social context, and the provision of a range of therapeutic strategies for individuals with a variety of problems. Commenting on what these nurses do, Hannigan (1999) describes their work as involving the following:

- the provision of clinically effective interventions;
- a closer attention to meeting the needs of people experiencing severe and long-term mental health problems;
- meeting the needs of mental health patients in a primary care setting;
- collaboration with workers from other agencies and disciplines; and
- the development of active partnerships with mental health service users.

Current changes to the way that mental health services are delivered will necessarily have an impact upon how primary care teams are formed and how they develop. The study was carried out prior to many of the more recent changes and therefore focused more on the organising principles of primary care nursing rather than the specifics. Nolan *et al.* (1999) note that, as a consequence of the White Paper *The New NHS – Modern and Dependable* (Department of Health, 1997), the influence of primary care both in the commissioning and the provision of mental health services is likely to increase. They observe, however, that by far the largest professional group currently involved in mental health in primary care are practice nurses, many of whom feel unprepared for this type of work. They identify lack of access to appropriate educational support and poor inter-professional relationships with mental health personnel as the main contributory factors.

Differences between practice nurses and community nurses

The West Midlands study noted several important differences between practice nurses and community nurses (which include CPNs, district nurses and health visitors) in working practice – that is, in the type of work that they do and their range and level of skills. Whereas community nurses have an established range of clinical skills, with skill levels related to grades, the skill levels of practice nurses were extremely variable, and much wider. Their work was focused on supplementing the work of the GP, rather than on a wider nursing role in the community. Notably, the practice nurse is employed directly by the GP, while community nurses work with autonomy, within a general contract. The study concluded that the differences between these nursing roles reflected and fulfilled specific health care needs, and there was little evidence of the roles converging. There was also little opportunity for practice nurses and CPNs to meet in the normal course of their work. Not all CPNs were seen as part of the core primary care team; many would be attached to several such teams and it was frequently inconvenient to attend all meetings.

There was no uniform pattern of community psychiatric nurse involvement in primary care teams. Some included CPNs, but many did not; in others, prior to the mental health reorganisation, they were seen as temporary members. Nolan and Badger (1998) presented similar findings from their study, which aimed to improve the knowledge of mental health care in primary care settings, and to improve collaboration between practice nurses and CPNs. An initial conclusion of this work found that, unless special initiatives are undertaken, there is often little or no contact between CPNs and practice nurses. Such findings, across studies, show that moves towards teamworking and integrated care are not only seen as long overdue but are also needed to ensure that other key workers such as CPNs are not excluded.

However, CPNs are more likely to be part of a community mental health team than they are to be part of a primary care team and this is largely due to their historical roots. CPNs began their work in the community but have increasingly become involved with work more directly in primary care. GP referrals have increased in volume and broadened in nature. Nationally, there is a very mixed picture. Some areas that previously encouraged CPNs to enter primary care settings, and raise their profile with GPs, are now rethinking this policy. Fundholding influenced the emphasis of service specifications for CPNs and there was a large volume of referrals for minor mental health needs. As a consequence, CPNs developed allegiances with colleagues in primary care other than their historic partners in the community mental health team. Crucially, these CPNs were managed within the primary care sector rather than within the mental health directorate. Some mental health trusts may have wanted to regain control over such nurses and redirect their work towards the target patient group of the community mental health teams. Critically, this would mean giving up, for example, the preventative work in which they had become involved, and their newly formed links with other nursing groups within primary care.

There is a need for a clear strategic view of mental health service delivery. When it is based around community mental health teams, there is a retention of separation, and a resistance to integration. In the new scenario, CPNs accustomed to working with autonomy with their own client group, within or in relation to a primary care team, would have to work as part of a mental health team and lose some of that autonomy. Their work with the less mentally ill, and the skills developed in doing this, could be lost.

According to the study (Ashburner *et al.*, 1997), district nurses and health visitors have similar fears about becoming employed by GPs. In addition, the dominance of PCGs by GPs is an important issue. In part, this is the reason why so many practice nurses are now involved in the care of those with minor mental health problems, possibly putting greater pressure on them and other members of the primary care team.

The CPNs in the study described their work as being involved with the provision of acute care in the community and included work with the seriously mentally ill. None saw themselves as fully part of the primary health care team. Despite a long history working in the community, the CPNs' level of visibility with other community nurses and among practice nurses is even lower than that of other groups of community nurses. Some had made a specific effort to become more involved. One CPN interviewed was an F grade, who did mental health assessments of patients; most of them were then taken on by her for treatment, although there was also a psychologist and counsellor attached to the practice. It was only in the most severe cases that the patient was passed on to the secondary psychiatric team. In this respect, this CPN was self-sufficient and seldom needed to relate to other nurses in the team. She described much of the work as short-term intervention, on a one-to-one basis, counselling and stress management. Patients were seen both at the surgery and in their home.

Another CPN was part of a project that was seeking to integrate primary and secondary care of patients and improve communications as part of a Care Programme Approach. She felt that this had provided a useful opportunity to explore what changes might be possible but was concerned that, once the project finished, the changes might not be sustained.

The arrival of PCGs and the development of a looser network of primary care 'teams' or collaborations across several general practices, offered an opportunity to address many of these issues. Retaining different nursing roles ensures a level of expertise within defined clinical areas, so there seems little prospect of an 'integrated' primary care nursing role becoming established. In fact, as each group of nurses developed and extended their roles, there was a clear indication that 'integration' should mean not the integration of nursing roles across different groups, but the integration of the total effort of the primary care team. This is the real focus for collaboration. Within such collaboration, each practitioner has a specific set of skills and varying degrees of autonomy.

COLLABORATIVE WORKING IN PRIMARY CARE

Defining the term 'team'

Primary care encompasses community care, as well as care focused on the general practice. Yerrel and Reed (1997) suggest that even the notion of primary care teams, which cover both community care services and general practice, does not describe how primary care currently operates. They emphasise that teams are having to be made. The same goes for collaborations.

There has been a focus on encouraging teamworking in primary care for a number of years. With a certain amount of experience gained so far, and the new push for increased collaboration, there now needs to be careful consideration of the context. We need to consider exactly what is meant by the word 'team', what the team is for and thus what sort of team is needed.

A number of particular issues within primary care can make teambuilding problematic:

- the beginnings of organisational fragmentation of primary care;
- generalists and specialists beginning to work in the same vicinity;
- different professional groups having their own standards of practice;
- differing geographical and organisational locations, which limit the scope for those making the effort to create effective teams.

The concept of a 'team' suggests a fairly tight-knit group working to a common objective. It may, therefore, be more appropriate to refer to 'collaborative working'. Teams may have been formulated for purposes other than collaboration – because people share the same building, for accounting purposes, or because of some short-term motive.

Barriers to effective teamworking

Before exploring the development of collaborative working there is a need to understand the main problems that have troubled teams operating within primary care.

Some innovative practices have put in place high-profile developments, working towards an 'integrated team' approach, which were defined in relation to that practice's needs. However, the West Midlands study (*see* page 34) found that there was no widespread development of primary care 'teams', or clarity over how these should be defined. Individual team members had different expectations of what the team was for, who should be part of it and on what basis. Such a lack of consensus or understanding could cause unnecessary confusion or conflict, but in reality it generally meant that the team operated more in name than in function. In one practice, described by the Nursing Development Manager at the Health Authority as 'leading edge', the health visitor described the team thus:

> *'I think it depends on what you see as a team. I would say we are really just working together. I would not say that we were working as a team. And I think that what is going on is that we all work alongside each other, we all ask each other questions but everybody seems to be very protective of their own little area and isn't that keen to share.'*

Even in practices that felt themselves to be progressive, the GPs were described as not being fully part of the team. There were issues about how much information GPs shared with other staff, and how practice meeting decisions were made. Some GPs said that they conferred with practice nurses over the development of new services, while others did not. Some nurses felt they could make some contribution to decision-making over practice development, but many could not. Even where teamworking was described as 'best practice', there was a question over the extent to which GPs were really a part of the team. From the community nurses' perspective, there was little in the way of collaborative decision-making – community interface – across the general practice, either over the direction in which services might develop, or over specific issues of patient care.

In most cases, therefore, when practices talk about teams, they mean local primary care *nursing* teams. For a collaborative model to become established there would need to be a widening of the basis of such groups.

Events such as teambuilding 'away days' had been held in some practices, but participants often questioned the outcomes. In some cases, GPs would not attend; even when GPs had attended, there was sometimes no subsequent change in behaviour.

Although most teams were practice-based, one or two met across practices, but this was usually in cases where GPs ran more than one surgery. This has implications for the form that the team took and who was included. The most usual core team comprised practice nurses, district nurses, health visitors and nursing auxiliaries. Others had health-care assistants, nursery nurses and nurse visitors to the elderly, while a few larger teams also included midwives, nurse practitioners, CPNs, counsellors and school nurses. The problem for this latter group was that their patient group usually covered several practices and attending several team meetings was described by some as putting an unnecessary strain on an already heavy work schedule. CPNs in particular found themselves more isolated from the possibility of being invited to team meetings; when asked about potential members, most 'core' members did not mention CPNs. There were also comments about what membership of the team meant, and this often excluded occasional or part-time members.

The study identified other barriers to effective teamworking. Most nursing teams did not have a nurse manager or leader, as such. In many, the unofficial co-ordinator had been self-nominated out of a desire to help the group function. Whoever took on the role did so on top of their other duties. In one practice with four GPs, one GP said that the team was not large enough to warrant the allocation of such duties, although he did see the potential advantages in having a nurse manager role. Questions were raised – given the number of different nursing groups involved in the team, where would the managerial role lie? Despite being directly employed by the GP, the practice nurses were not always seen as the most senior members of the team. One health visitor felt that the team leader should be a community nurse, because they would find it easier to challenge the GPs, should it ever be necessary. Resources for the development of nursing teams were limited. Just one Community Trust had appointed a Nursing Teams Co-ordinator to facilitate and co-ordinate the development of integrated and autonomous nursing teams.

More central to the issue of the different nursing groups working together is the fact that each professional group defined its own areas of practice and professional standards. This also meant that different groups had different employers and this meant different systems for accessing training, etc. There are also issues of how much actual scope there is for individuals to interact, share and communicate within a team. There was seldom a common physical location at which the team could be said to be based, to ensure that those on duty were likely to cross paths with others. Then the location of much of the work in the community and different shift patterns meant that many team members never saw other team members. This placed very real problems on communication and co-ordination. Interaction between team members was problematic for all teams studied. Given that each professional is accountable for their own practice, this does not enable the establishment of a culture of mutual reliance.

These findings are broadly substantiated by other literature on the development of primary health care teams. Gregson *et al.* (1992) noted that all primary health care teams had problems in common. They found that, of those who had patients in common, there was active collaboration between only a quarter of GPs and district nurses and between one in ten GPs and health visitors. Similarly, an Audit Commission report (1993) on patients' experiences found that GPs failed to co-ordinate properly with community nurses and that patients received conflicting advice from different health professionals.

West and Poulton (1997) explored the extent of teamworking in primary care and compared this with the way other multidisciplinary teams functioned. The study covered 68 primary care teams, 20 community mental health teams, 24 from an oil company, 27 NHS management teams, and 40 social service teams. The outcome measures were the levels of team participation, support for innovation, task orientation, and clarity of and commitment to team objectives. The primary care teams scored significantly lower than other teams on all team-functioning factors, except task orientation. The most effective teams were based around more specific objectives, such as financial targets, and part of their performance benefit was that people preferred to work with others rather than on their own. The conclusion of the study was that a restructuring of the organisation of primary care is required if primary care teams are to develop clear shared objectives, to facilitate a co-ordinated approach to the delivery of care. Such problems do not exist to the same extent in profession-specific groups, such as teams of district nurses or mental health teams. It may therefore be more useful to think about different groups of workers in different forms of collaboration rather than assuming all will form effective teams. All need to recognise the principles for good collaboration.

The benefits of teamworking on the production of goods and services are generally accepted, but perhaps primary care does not need to change in order to be able to sustain the same sort of 'effective' teams. In fact, such teams may not be the most effective form of collaboration, given the way that primary care is organised and delivered. There may be an assumption that a primary care team is just like all other multi-professional teams, where the most important characteristic is the sharing of a single objective. That objective could be identified as the provision of optimum health care for a defined population, but, in reality, the more specific objectives of each individual on the team might be only marginally connected to the objectives of others, given the different clinical areas. The level of inter-connection between individuals on any 'team' varies according to each individual objective, task or issue. The objectives of the primary care team tend to be more disparate, so it cannot easily be compared with other forms of team. In nurse education, for example, Atkins and Walsh (1997) counsel against pushing too hard for collaboration, stressing that a nurse's development is based upon his or her ability to develop as an individual, respecting professional autonomy.

Given the working context – multiple employers, different forms of work organisation and varied levels of support – is it feasible to create such traditional team-based groups? According to a traditional view of what 'effective teamworking' might be, many of the teams would not be seen as effective. The concept of 'collaborative working' rather than that of 'teams' enables the establishment of a different kind of group, looser in form and with a variable membership. Among the nurses interviewed, there was no shortage of individuals working to improve the effectiveness of their teams, and effective collaboration was emerging where nurses actively worked together to co-ordinate their work. Whereas close forms of teamwork were often envisaged by the core group of nurses in a practice, few groups had moved from very loose coalitions of professionals working independently – a move away from the idea of a formal team.

What was actually happening was a much looser form of collaboration, which, because it was not recognised as the required form, was not being developed in a way that would optimise its advantages. What was needed was a recognition of the different forms that collaborative working could take and, within these, people, processes and structures that facilitated communication and sharing of information, across the boundaries of different locations, professional groups and organisations.

ESTABLISHING EFFECTIVE COLLABORATION

The creation of PCGs and PCTs offers an opportunity to address some of the factors that may be limiting the development of more effective organisational forms. Periods of significant change bring with them the greatest opportunity to introduce other types of change.

Current literature and study findings suggest that several key factors lead to effective collaboration. The following factors need to be openly discussed within the group:

- A shared understanding of the objectives and how best to achieve them – given the need for individual and professional objectives, it is important that the superordinate objective is couched in terms that all individuals can sign up to. Agreement on objectives may be easier than agreement on how best they are to be achieved. There is a need to understand how objectives within the collaboration relate to individual organisational objectives.
- A definition of 'membership' – is it all on the same basis or at different levels? Is it fixed or flexible, etc? Are all the stakeholders represented at the right level and contribution?
- A clarification of roles, rules, procedures, accountabilities, and the modes of co-operation within the group – the processes that will be shared and those that will

remain discrete should be specified. There is a need to recognise people's expectations of others.

- The critical role of leadership – this demands a range of skills, including vision, facilitation and adaptability.
- The necessity for communications between parties to be clear and open, to avoid misunderstandings – when people are geographically separate, there should be even more emphasis on effective communication. It is vital to be able to ensure that the requisite information is sent and received, and there may be a need for a separate role to oversee this.
- There must be a willingness to participate in all parties, and a development of trust.
- A shared culture is required, or an understanding of each others' organisation culture or structure, if there are differences.
- An understanding that co-empowerment ensures that people feel enabled to contribute in a way that is commensurate with their role – there may be a need to acknowledge any inequalities and to respect differences, to ensure that no single party dominates, etc. Not all parties will necessarily be of equal status or have equal access to resources, power, etc.
- The identification and resolution of potential conflicts of interest, within the group or between the group and outside – if differences arise there is a need to focus on the added value brought by being in collaboration.
- Different modes of individual support may be needed to ensure participation and shared decision-making.
- Maintenance – there needs to be some stability of membership to ensure that shared understandings are maintained. Effort is required to maintain collaborative working, especially when new parties enter.
- Realism – all things are not possible, actual constraints need to be acknowledged, and different problems will emerge as the group evolves and matures.

There is a need for change at the level of the individual and not just in the form of new organisational initiatives. As PCGs and PCTs become established, there is increased collaboration between health and social services. Exworthy and Peckham (1999) show that initial efforts to increase coterminosity to promote collaboration were insufficient to resolve deep-rooted inter-agency issues. Another study by Hiscock and Pearson (1999), drawing on data from four sites, actually suggests that, as policy guidance urges close collaboration and joint working between health and social services, the long-established cultural and professional gaps are widening and deteriorating. This is largely due to each group's preoccupation with changes within their own organisation. The very real problem is that too great a level of organisational turbulence results in too little time for ensuring that the changes are brought in and established in the most effective way.

Glen (1999) suggests that effective collaboration depends upon establishing understanding that respects differences in values and beliefs. There will be differences in response to the multiplicity of patient/user needs. A US study on collaborative practice (Stapleton, 1998) showed how the development of collaborative relationships required much time and effort, with significant attitudinal, institutional and behavioural barriers to overcome. As collaboration occurs between individuals, each one must understand the concept of collaboration as it operates in each context, and be committed to investing the time and energy required to develop relationships and overcome barriers.

CONCLUSION

In the organisation of primary health care, the concept of 'collaboration' is more appropriate than that of the 'team', since it allows for greater flexibility in form, types of relationships and membership. There is an opportunity for the emergence of many new forms of collaborative working, as long as workers are not constrained by pre-conceived ideas of what these should or should not look like. It is vital to recognise the need for specific skills to work effectively in a collaborative culture. The emphasis needs to be on shared objectives and on co-ordination and this requires appropriate forms of leadership and communication.

Who should have the power and control? Should collaborative ventures be focused on general practice or managed by GPs? What is more certain is that GPs need to be part of collaboration, and cannot be allowed to remain apart. If any single group is dominant within a PCG, there is a risk that other professional groups may have problems ensuring an equal voice, retaining share of resources, or even (with regard to community nurses) their professional autonomy.

Representatives of the different professions need to remain accountable as individuals, even when they are part of a co-ordinated whole. They should all have an equal opportunity to participate. Any collaboration must include all stakeholders, and involve an understanding of who are the beneficiaries of that collaboration.

There is a significant gap between rhetoric and reality with regard to the development of teamworking and collaboration. The efficiency and effectiveness of each primary care nursing role depends upon the way that it is integrated into the overall provision of care. There is a need to move away from the ad hoc and voluntary nature of these developments and their leadership towards a recognition that collaboration can only be effective and sustainable if there are sufficient resources, along with management effort and support.

Studies have shown a commitment to collaborative working, but this can only be achieved if individuals are clear about their position with regard to their own practice, and how it relates to the work of others. Considerable management time and resources will be needed in order to enable the emergence of the necessary shared understanding, ensure the right levels of training and support, and develop the necessary processes and structures to ensure effective communications.

Prior to the introduction of PCGs there were no real drivers for change. Now, policy directives have introduced additional impetus. Government policy sets the broad future agenda for primary care. The role of PCGs is now well established but the precise way that different nursing roles will be co-ordinated, both between each other and within the wider context of the primary health sector, is less clear. This relates especially to the delivery of mental health care. It is the responsibility of management to ensure that such large-scale change processes are supported and co-ordinated so that grass-roots practice is consistent with policy, and is more than the simple relabelling of existing organisational forms.

Issues around professional territories in primary care and distribution of power need to be resolved if they are not to be taken forward into new systems of working and prevent a favourable environment for teambuilding and shared culture to emerge. Nurses, one of the largest groups in health care, experience particular difficulties in feeling part of a team, and in accessing appropriate training and education. They may be disenfranchised in the new system if their needs are not identified, addressed and monitored. If primary care is overburdened with professional disciplines and different kinds of personnel, there is a danger that it will fragment, or that more energy will be expended in changing the system than in providing the service. Ways of working will have to be negotiated, and systems must be set in place for discussing and resolving issues. All members of the team should feel a sense of belonging, and of being needed and valued. (Editors' summary)

REFERENCES

Ashburner, L. and Birch, K. (1999) Professional control issues between medicine and nursing in primary care. In Mark, A. and Dopson, S. (eds.) *Organisational Behaviour in Health Care: The research agenda*, Macmillan, Basingstoke

Ashburner, L., Birch, K., Latimer, J. and Scrivens, E. (1997) *Nurse Practitioners in Primary Care: The extent of research and practice*, CHPM, University of Keele, Keele

Ashburner, L., Latimer, J. and Quy, S. (1998) *Primary Care Professional Education Development* [project report], CHPM, University of Keele, Keele

Atkins, J.M. and Walsh, R.S. (1997) Developing shared learning in multi-professional health care education: for whose benefit? *Nurse Education Today*, 17(4), 319–324

Audit Commission (1993) *Practices Make Perfect: The role of the family health services authority*, HMSO, London

Department of Health (1997) *The New NHS – Modern and Dependable*, HMSO, London

Exworthy, M. and Peckham, S. (1999) Collaboration between health and social care: coterminosity in the 'new' NHS, *Health and Social Care in the Community*, 17(3), 229–232

Glen, S. (1999) Educating for interprofessional collaboration: teaching and values, *Nursing Ethics*, 6(3) 202–213

Gregson, B., Cartlidge, A. and Bond, S. (1992) Interprofessional collaboration in primary health care organisations, Occasional Paper 52, Royal College of General Practitioners, London

Hannigan, B. (1999) Specialist practice in community mental health nursing, *Nurse Education Today*, 19(6), 509–516

Hiscock, J. and Pearson, M. (1999) Looking inwards, looking outwards: dismantling the 'Berlin Wall' between health and social services? *Social Policy and Administration*, 33(2), 150–163

Kendall, S. (1996) *General Medical Practice Workload Study Phase II: The facilitation of practice development within primary health care teams*, Buckinghamshire College with the Royal College of Nursing. Information supplied by authors, research funded by Welsh Office

Lazenbatt, A. (1997) Targeting health and social need: the contribution of nurses, midwives, and health visitors, *Health and Well-being into the Next Millennium*, Department of Health and Social Services, Belfast

Nolan, P. and Badger, F. (1998) Practice nurses and CPNs: bridging the gap, *West Midlands Journal of Primary Care*, **4**, 60–62

Nolan, P., Murray, E. and Dallender, J. (1999) Practice nurses' perceptions of services for clients with psychological problems in primary care, *International Journal of Nursing Studies*, **36**(2), 97–104

Stapleton, S.R. (1998) Teambuilding – making collaborative practice work, *Journal of Nurse-Midwifery*, **43**(1), 12–18

West, M. and Poulton, B. (1997) A failure of function: teamwork in primary health care, *Journal of Interprofessional Care*, **11**(2)

Wilkin, D. and Butler, T. (1996) *Commissioning Primary Care from Provider Organisations: A development and research programme*, National Primary Care Development Centre, University of Manchester, Manchester

Yerrel, P. and Reed, A. (1997) The anachronism of policy for nursing in general practice: conceptualising a way forward, *Nursing Times Research*, **2**(4), 245–257

PART TWO

COLLABORATION IN AREAS OF PRIMARY MENTAL HEALTH CARE

4 EFFECTIVE COLLABORATION WITH USERS

Zyl Harvey

This chapter provides an unique perspective on collaboration within primary mental health care. The author suffered from depression, which eventually led to her early retirement. Owing to personal experience as a primary health care provider, she had certain expectations when she became a service user who needed the intervention and support of professionals. This chapter provides important insights into a 'journey through depression', and suggests how respecting users' desires to contribute to their own recovery is a vital aspect of managing depression, the most common of the 'common mental health problems'. Collaboration and the development of trust between users and practitioners are crucial in promoting recovery. The author reminds practitioners of the amount that voluntary organisations can contribute and suggests that their services should be utilised more and integrated into primary care provision. (Editors' note)

THE CONTEXT OF HEALTH CARE

For the last quarter of my working life I was employed by the social services department of a large local authority, assisting service users into employment, and providing them with ongoing assistance and support. I worked with people with a range of disabilities: physical, sensory and learning disabilities. For the purposes of this chapter, however, I will draw on my experiences with mental health services. One perspective is based on the collaborative aspects of my work; the other is entirely personal. When I unexpectedly became a mental health service user myself, I found a marked lack of what I had most looked forward to – collaborative opportunities.

On the positive side, my experience as professional turned user has given me the opportunity to truly appreciate the potential of collaboration – both as an aim and as a response to the development of a sense of purpose. My only regret is that I was forced into early retirement; with the insight provided by my own first-hand experience, I could have been so much more effective in my work.

DEFINITIONS

For me, the term 'users' means people who have had, or are currently receiving treatment within the mental health primary care system. My use of the term 'professionals' covers a wide range of workers, from the psychiatric team and the staff who supervise work and rehabilitation, to volunteers who work for recognised organisations, which train those volunteers to implement their policies.

Whatever their status, the common factor among these professionals is that they are almost always restricted by working practices. They are a cause of irritation and frustration to some, but for others they provide welcome boundaries.

By definition, 'collaboration' is a two-way process. It is not confined to professionals and users, or may not even be truly present between them. Indeed, it can be at its most useful when taking place between a user and another person, in any situation *other* than in conjunction with a professional. It is dependent only on the extent of willingness and trust between those involved, which enables them to communicate with a marked degree of equality. It contains many challenges, but has no limits.

BACKGROUND

In the part of the Midlands where I was employed, from the mid-1980s onwards changes in mental health-care provision led to the closure of residential units attached to hospitals. Many long-term residents became the responsibility of local government, passing into the care of social services departments. Pressure on existing services led to a re-examination of the potential of some of the existing service users; those who were able were encouraged to leave the shelter of day centres and enter the world of work.

This was a national trend. Successful ventures had already been undertaken in Birmingham and York, and elsewhere, in conjunction with the employment service. Using the local authority in an agency role, financial support was available for participating employers. Initially, the main target group comprised people with learning disabilities, but the success of the policy prompted rapid expansion into other areas of disability, including mental health, that is, people who were or had been receiving psychiatric treatment.

I had had no formal training in mental health care. My counselling qualification, together with years of experience in various posts requiring well-developed communication skills, including teaching, youth training and liaison with employers, was deemed adequate by the local authority. This, coupled with my personal enthusiasm and eagerness to learn as much as I could from the extra training made available to me, led me into work that proved to be totally absorbing, yet alternately frustrating and rewarding.

I embarked on a sharp learning curve, working closely with the employment service, as well as many local authority personnel departments. I gained practical experience in day care units run by the social services, and built up contacts within the health service with occupational therapists and management teams, as well as working closely with other local authority departments and the employment service. I also became a volunteer with my local branch of MIND.

Within the social services system I found that day centres for people with physical, sensory or learning disabilities appeared to have a mainly static population. Attendance at many of the day centres provided access to other, free services – everything from dental care to further education or training. Work was not generally seen as a viable option; indeed, it was viewed by some with suspicion.

If service users went into employment, access to these other services would be withdrawn, and would become their own responsibility.

In mental health care, however, there was an impression of movement, and because many of the service users had experienced employment, work was frequently mentioned as an ultimate goal. Service users had frequently progressed from hospitalisation into residential care, followed by a period of supervised independent living care. After that, transfer to day centre care and socialisation was merged with occupational and/or educational training.

Historically, there was no sense of urgency. Users would emerge from health care into social services care, knowing that if they did not manage to reach the ultimate stages of independence they could fall back into the earlier parts of the system. Few managed to exit permanently, and those who did found for the most part that they had had to adapt to the pace of the system, rather than the system adjusting to their rate of individual recovery.

The users of the mental health services, in particular, came out of complete dependency on professional care in hospital or residential care, where most decisions were made for them, or, at most, a limited choice was offered. A stage of co-operative, supervised care in a residential setting followed, during which users were 'steered' into what the professionals thought was best for them, or what it was possible to offer. This lasted until they were 'well enough' to cope with average daily living experiences; in other words, when they did not require an undue amount of supervision, and knew how to access help in an emergency.

For both users and professional carers it was so easy to perpetuate co-operation; risks were more easily avoided when the professional made the decisions and the user co-operated. Indeed, this stage was welcomed by many users who had not yet reached a level of confidence that would allow them to take their final steps into complete independence. On the other hand, for some users there was a sense of irritation when independence was delayed and they were held back in a situation where their frustrations made them feel anything but co-operative.

WHERE DOES COLLABORATION COME INTO IT?

At the final stage, a limited amount of collaboration was deemed appropriate, permitted or encouraged, but the service appeared to stop at the point at which the user was deemed 'well enough'. Often, the user was left feeling 'What now?', but there was no structured opportunity for supervised progress after that. My role was to provide the opportunity for work experience, leading into supported employment. It was an attempt to answer the 'What now?' question and this was the point at which I felt true collaboration could start.

As the service's vocabulary adjusted to new experiences, the old terms of 'success' and 'failure' were replaced by 'change'. From my past experience of working with school leavers, I knew that the most successful work would be based on a foundation of mutual trust, and I took as much time as necessary to establish this. Then the user and I together explored the elements of entering or re-entering work: preparation and training, obtaining work, monitoring progress. We reviewed aims and adjusted to changes as they happened. The work looked into many areas of the user's life. Helping to remove barriers to fulfilment, assisting when times were tough, sharing the joys of achievement – the tasks were as varied as the individual. For some, the barriers were based on association with past experience; for others, it was their relatives or carers on whom they were dependent who had fears that had to be overcome.

When I was first employed in this type of work there were few boundaries. The results proved the value of this, with many examples of service users achieving more than they thought possible. Carers and relatives were given support and reassurance as *they* adjusted to the new circumstances, and the users learned that other agencies also could and would be prepared to provide the partnership of collaboration.

I learnt that a sense of purpose is crucial, not least for those who are in danger of losing it, or for those who may be helped to avoid an escalation of their need for care. Later, as I floundered through the onset of my own depression, I began to understand more of the circumstances of the user. I had only been able to empathise with others as they struggled with it, but now it became a reality for me.

THE IMPORTANCE OF THE SENSE OF SELF

I represent what is, unfortunately and disturbingly, an apparently growing number of professionals involved in some aspect of mental health services who have become users themselves. Some soldier on, propped up by medication and the goodwill of colleagues; others leave the service, gladly or reluctantly, perhaps never recovering sufficiently to return, or grasping any opportunity to take an alternative career route.

In 1997, I became one of an increasing number who experience 'burn-out', manifested in my case as depression. When I became a user of the system, I experienced for myself the delays, lack of continuity and inaccuracies that I had seen lead to frustration in others. As I struggled to keep working, trying to make use of the support systems that were available, yet not able to believe their impartiality, I found I was not exempt from the prejudices I had fought on others' behalf. As they had done, I felt isolated and defeated. I slid into the depression and out of the world of employment into the world of users.

As a full-time service user, uncertain of whether I would ever return to any type of employment again, I encountered different attitudes – some helpful, others less so. Struggling to retain remnants of the person I once was, as a benchmark for the person I might again become, I found how painful it can be when the memories do not match the present abilities. I could remember that I had often produced detailed written reports, but it was a memory that seemed unreal, at a time when my concentration span was no more than five minutes.

However, I could also remember aspects of the service with which I had worked. I could remember the passivity and the co-operation, and I was determined that my own route of treatment would not end at that point of 'good enough' or 'well enough'. I longed to be valued and respected as an individual, to have my willingness to recover tested to the maximum – in other words, I looked forward to the extra element of collaboration, and hung on to the belief that eventually I would reach that point.

The way I saw the system operating, after the period when the user has been dependent on others making the decisions, and the following period when recovery or progress is measured on a scale of co-operation and agreement, collaboration is a demonstration of the user's individuality being recognised. Emerging from the fog of loss of all the elements that make life what it is – control, willpower, personality, choice, aims and significance – the user reaches a point at which collaboration can start. At this stage, the user's sense of self can be nurtured through the period of change that leads to where they want to be.

That had been my theory and the basis of successful practice when I was at work. I found my own experience confirmed it, as I longed for signs that my individuality as a person, rather than a 'case', was being recognised. But that sense of self is elusive (I had not realised just how elusive until it disappeared for some months). I did not feel it was there, even with my GP and the community psychiatric nurse, and certainly not with the psychiatrist. I did not feel that my individuality was starting to surface until about halfway through the one-to-one counselling sessions, almost 12 months after my diagnosis. I could rationalise it and say that this was probably more indicative of my personal state than of a general situation. However, I had noticed in my working life that, when a user had realised that they were being treated with genuine concern as an individual, it proved to be a turning point. Their response and subsequent rate of progress had often been remarkable.

LIMITATIONS OF THE SYSTEM

Primary care provides a raft of various services, from the GP to the psychiatric service, and an assessment leading to different levels of care and treatment. Monitoring and review of progress leads eventually, as the user regains independence, to the setting up of rehabilitation, until a satisfactory level of mental wellbeing is achieved. At its best it provides a seamless route to recovery. Unfortunately, the best is not always available, due to unavoidable limitations, and casualties return to the system.

Within primary care services the most common major limitations are of continuity and consistency. Inevitably, staff change at treatment units, or may be absent at crucial times. Goalposts are moved by the system, and senior management may impose changes in a successful structure, which render it ineffective by comparison.

For example, my area of service was at its most successful when it started, with 50 people having been found employment in five years. A decision was made at the highest level to separate elements of the tasks and to increase staff, reasoning that, by implication, the number of successful outcomes would increase. But instead of duplicating the successful model whereby all staff knew all aspects of the work, and accompanied a service user from start to finish, the new method of separating the elements of the work restricted staff, and caused unrest. This caused problems for management, so another method was set up, whereby staff circulated within the elements of the service, to broaden their experience.

The result was that the service suffered from fragmentation and lack of continuity between staff and users. Users had to adapt to frequent changes of staff at a point at which they could have been using all their energies to build up a basis for productive collaboration. Their individuality suffered. What had been a service geared to providing support for individual work experience became merely the provision of a limited range of training programmes.

MY PERSONAL EXPERIENCE

Because of my age (58 at diagnosis) and an ongoing physical condition, assumptions were made by the health service professionals that I would have to take early retirement; indeed, this was eventually confirmed by my employers. I had no alternative but to agree, even though I had hoped for several more years of working life. The implications of retirement, of course, were that I would not even be given access to the type of rehabilitation service of which I had been part. I had little idea of what, if anything, would be available for someone in my position.

People of working age could be seen as potential 'positive outcomes' if they went through rehabilitation, and entered some form of work or work experience. They attracted funding to the system. I was outside that particular system, so I could be offered nothing more than medication and regular contact with my GP, supplemented by contact with the CPN, and eventual access to a limited number of counselling sessions. I realised that whatever I could remember of my working life might stand me in good stead as I steered myself through various routes to what I hoped would be recovery. I trusted that I would eventually reach and recognise the stage of 'What now?', and hoped for appropriate support.

Even though I had seen the struggle when I was working with people making the effort to reach this stage, I was not fully prepared for my own experience. The main uncertainty was about the validity of my aims – could I even get halfway towards being the person I had been? On days when I seemed to have lost the tenuous threads linking 'Who I had been' with 'Who I might eventually be', it was a major effort. Other people's beliefs in me seemed well-intentioned but unrealistic – goals were fantasy, not possibility.

Eventually, the tiny milestones I was determined to note each day (washing myself, dressing, answering the phone when it rang) became more consistent. I began to assemble the pieces and construct my new persona, rather than a poor replica of the previous one. It has proved to be an ongoing process, but one that received a boost when true collaboration started, within the counselling sessions. The completion of these sessions, spread over several months, marked my discharge from mental health care.

Since then I have actively and increasingly sought opportunities for collaboration in various capacities, as many people do. It has brought me most satisfaction in new areas of 'work'. By giving me a sense of purpose it has redressed the balance of my life. Small difficulties have begun to take their rightful place. I am no longer overwhelmed by commitments. I identify and make choices, and am therefore more in control of the way my life is proceeding.

ANSWERING THE 'WHAT NOW?' QUESTION

Finding a route

Because collaboration is not as readily available via the primary care mental health system as it is outside, users often have to find their own route to something that answers the 'What now?'. It may be returning to, or entering new employment; it may be finding something worthwhile through contacts with other users; or it may be seizing the opportunity to embark upon a new phase of life. There are many examples of informal collaboration – from self-help groups starting in someone's home to users becoming volunteer workers or contributors to supportive charities, according to their interests and abilities.

Some examples

CASE STUDY **THE NEEDS OF SERVICE USERS**

One user with a background in public relations set up a seminar to focus on the needs of service users in general. It was attended by local health officials and government representatives, and had a major effect on the morale of users and primary care staff, who felt they had the ear of the health department, and the opportunity to influence local and national decision-making.

One GP wished to set up a record of local resources, and invited two of his patients to work together to achieve this. They both benefited from the purposefulness of the task, and found the added bonus of a mutually supportive friendship.

In a town rich in access to 'alternative' and 'complementary' therapies, certain yoga and t'ai chi groups are recommended by a local CPN, as they are known to welcome and successfully integrate users.

Choices of different levels of involvement within one organisation are helpful, as the following example shows.

CASE STUDY **LEVELS OF INVOLVEMENT**

One national organisation not only offers information via its website and a help line, staffed by trained users, but also broadens into contributory and collaborative areas, such as pen friendships, options to contribute to clinical research, and local group meetings. Members' contributions to a quarterly magazine demonstrate a depth of fellow feeling and empathy, while at the same time a request for positive and encouraging tales of recovery can produce a wealth of useful techniques.

It is not always necessary for the user's background to be revealed; indeed, when the user is accepted in a new situation on his or her own merit, this can mark a different and highly valued stage of recovery.

CASE STUDY   PROMOTING SELF-ESTEEM

One user attended a class for people interested in improving their writing skills, and became involved with other projects as a result, finding a purpose in compiling a family history. Although initially it was suggested as a therapeutic exercise, the user was accepted on his own merit, which greatly improved his self-esteem.

Another user who regularly contributes to a music appreciation group knows that he is invited to do this solely on his merits as a knowledgeable person.

A lifetime user who had been part of an ongoing caseload for an overworked social worker unexpectedly found more immediate, unconditional and practical help at hand from visiting evangelists. As he became more self-sufficient he eventually began to repay their support by training and becoming part of their mission.

The common factor in all of the above examples appears to be that someone, whether a professional, a friend or a member of a volunteer group is seen to believe in that individual. Use is made of the user's interests or skills; this in turn develops the user's sense of purpose, going hand in hand with building confidence, and generally restoring self-esteem. In some of these examples it happened so effortlessly that without professional analysis it would continue without acknowledgement.

Success is not guaranteed when the user accepts the ideas of professionals, in a spirit of co-operation; what might seem to be a worthy idea from the professional point of view sometimes provides little or no motivation for users. Similarly, success cannot be guaranteed with collaborative ventures, however akin they are to the user's sense of purpose. Even when this happens, if it has been handled in a supportive non-critical way, non-achievement can be a valuable learning experience. I had 'false starts' as well as successes, but these were discussed within the counselling context, or with supportive friends, and I saw the 'moving on' as part of the process as a whole.

PRIMARY CARE, THEN...?

I carried one particular memory clearly through my own turmoil – I knew I had to regain a sense of purpose, particularly with the daily routine of employment taken away from me. I knew also that my personal situation meant that I would have to rely largely upon my own resourcefulness, such as it was.

As I emerged from months of dependency, which had been punctuated by periods of varyingly enthusiastic or reluctant co-operation, I drew heavily on a supportive network of friends. One chapter of my life was drawing to a close, but what was a new chapter going to offer me? The absence of any recognized continuation service for someone who was going to be retired from work became apparent. The system's aim seemed to be that I should be enabled to retreat quietly into old age, grateful for the treatment I had received, and hoping that I would never need to return to the service.

Fortunately, my GP was monitoring my progress with interest. He could see that I was determined to achieve more than avoiding another descent into depression, and encouraged my attempts at self-rehabilitation. Slowly re-educating my attention span, I spent my time reading and writing. I tried picking up threads of previous activities, but new experiences, such as pottery classes and learning to develop two hours of concentration at a time, proved to be more successful. A small writer's group was also useful, as the discipline offset the random nature of my bursts of cathartic rambling.

These activities served to occupy the months between being assessed and embarking on the psychological counselling with which my GP practice was engaged at the time. In the interim I was also allocated to a CPN at the local mental health unit, and given the choice of sessions there or at home. I received some very necessary practical support and guidance during this period of enforced exile from a working life. It also proved to be useful groundwork in preparation for the counselling sessions.

The counselling I received via the primary care service proved to be the beginning of truly collaborative working. In the first session, I was asked to provide a 'family tree' of significant people in my life, to bring on my return. This was language I could understand and to which I could respond. From one session to the next, sifting through my fractured thought processes as the counselling progressed over a number of months, a sense of purpose was increasingly brought back into my life. Then, inevitably, I reached the 'What now?' point.

Support groups were discussed with the counsellor, but we concluded that they were not the answer for me, as I was probably too accustomed to providing support for others. (Later, when I did feel the time might be right to make enquiries, I found there was a geographical connection with my previous employment – another consideration the professional has to take into account.)

A professional guide has to be ultra-sensitive to the user's needs and capabilities. Knowing what other support is available, both locally and nationally, and the nature of that contact, can make a significant difference to a recovery and rehabilitation programme, if offered at the right time. Making this information available is as much the responsibility of the organisations, as of the primary care services, if the aim of outside support groups is to provide an alternative route. In the direct or indirect settings they provide, away from the structure of primary health care, they may offer a choice of methods of developing that all-important sense of purpose, and ability to collaborate.

THE CURRENT SITUATION

Indisputably, a great deal of stigma still persists about mental health in general, and at all levels. In my working life, I fought it on behalf of others; it remains there today, for me to fight again, this time as a user. Information would undoubtedly help. Although it is available, there is scope for more contact to be made, and for liaison to be improved between the general public and the primary care services. The question is not only how to do it, but where is the common ground for it to happen?

One answer would appear to be related to the organisations that act as a halfway stage between the mental health services and the user no longer needing any contact with any services. This is precisely the point at which collaboration can be most effective. Although voluntary organisations may assist people to prepare for and get back into work, or provide opportunities for contributing to voluntary work themselves, and sheltered workshops are provided at some day centres, producing goods and raising money for funding, these are not for everyone. Other opportunities need to be identified, and the more organisations can be drawn into providing alternatives for all users, and benefiting from what the users have to offer in return, the more effective will be the message to society in general.

By identifying the gaps that currently exist, it is possible to start looking at how existing services can be improved. The two main gaps highlighted by my experience were the sparse provision for the age group I was approaching, and the total lack of provision for professional casualties. It did mean that I avoided being pigeonholed, which was important for me, but it should surely be available as an option. Attempts are being made by some professions to provide contact groups, but ignorance remains about mental health in general, and at all levels. The user who attempts to regain or retain a working foothold may be treated with suspicion or even outright hostility. They may never regain their previous status and their working life is likely to end prematurely, even though they may still have much to give.

A great deal of help and support can be achieved by the availability of information. It may not be sufficient to point out where information may be obtained, or even to pass on the leaflets. Part of the professional's role is to check the outcome. Was it available? Has it been of use? There is also a responsibility to ensure that information is comprehensive, accurate and up to date.

Physical and practical accessibility is of prime importance, as mental ill health does not preclude physical disabilities; indeed, such physical disabilities may even make the user more prone to mental health problems. Not all premises are easily accessible and, although this should not lead to delays, it sometimes does. Flexibility is essential, to accommodate the varying health of users. Do units continue to start their working day at a time when the 'medication hangover' is still active? Are meetings arranged before noon, when an option for a later time would be welcomed? Are services available in the evenings?

THE IDEAL

My own experiences led to two main discoveries – the lack of effective and wide-ranging information about voluntary groups and organisations, and the problems encountered by professionals where services available to users are unacceptable, either because of their geographical position and/or because of the personnel involved.

The information issue is in the hands of the organisations themselves, together with primary care, but much more could be done with efficient liaison. I discovered accidentally that one organisation at least gives opportunities for members to contribute to professional research, as well as being a rich source of user information and peer-group support. Modern technology makes it possible for a database to be made available to all primary care services.

The second difficulty was more personal, but it prevented me from joining an active local group. Attempts to set up another group in an adjacent area proved futile, so I now have little direct contact with fellow users. However, I find I can use various means of communication to provide insights and support for users, and also for professionals in training. A whole new opportunity opens when this route is pursued and organisations involved in professional training are receptive to offers of liaison, although this usually appears to be a result of networking, rather than contact through formal channels.

As I recovered some of my skills, I approached a local university in search of interest for a particular project. Although the project did not become operational, I made contact with a School of Health Sciences, and I have become a member of its training resources, using my personal experiences of depression in talking to and teaching future mental health and general nurses. Undergraduates have time and inclination to listen, discuss aspects of treatment and ask questions. The aim is for them to acquire a better understanding of depression, and become more aware of contributory factors and the impact depression may have on all aspects of life. My own experiences, once the object of therapeutic interventions and the clinical gaze, are now a source of reflection and enlightenment for others. Being able to help others to understand and provide insights into what depression is and how it affects people is an endless source of satisfaction for me. Hopefully, my personal insights gained in this way may offset some of the divisions between users and professionals of the future.

The value of my small contribution leads me to believe that effective and efficient liaison between primary care and other organisations could be achieved by tapping the rich source of capability among users who are willing and ready to collaborate. By offering this as an option to members, voluntary organisations would be responsible for assessing the suitability of applicants, obtaining GP approval, and any other safety checks deemed necessary. With the co-operation of the primary care services and the volunteer sector, it should be a relatively easy matter to organise training and provide contacts for these liaison workers, working in geographical and service areas of their choice.

Information about the voluntary organisation's functions would be provided, for example, to professionals within the health authority, at GP practice meetings, mental health day centre staff meetings, or local authority mental health units. Users, carers and the public in general would be able to access the information in different places, from day centre user groups to local interest groups unconnected with any of the services. A whole field of opportunity is opened up when this route is pursued.

The colleges and universities where future professionals train might be receptive to offers of liaison. This does sometimes happen already, but it is usually the result of an accidental meeting, or by way of individual personal interest. If contact is made in this way, there is scope for requesting use of the facilities of the college or university.

The social benefits of, for example, a regular gathering open to all, including deliverers of the professional services, but with a non-medical focus, might be a useful preventive measure. Isolation, particularly intellectual isolation, is recognised as one of the major causes of depression. Such a gathering might be a bold step for professionals, but it could be quite enlightening.

I believe it is possible to encourage society as a whole to take responsibility for collaboration. It involves identifying and rewarding examples of effective work, facilitating and encouraging existing and new initiatives, and making use of the richest resource – the experience of users. It will need courage from users and particularly from professionals, who will be required to emerge from the safety of their professionalism, step over their self-defined limitations, and enter an arena of genuine humanitarianism. Those who can measure up to the challenge have everything to gain and nothing to lose.

This personal account of a provider of services becoming a user is candid and thought-provoking. The author reflects on how services should ensure that users are aware of the care and treatment options available to them, and encouraged to find their own path through recovery. Health-care reform must go beyond the mere restructuring of services; it must ensure that the needs of users are identified by drawing on the experiences of people who have thought about how services have affected them, both positively and negatively. The author notes that health-care practitioners may feel secure within their own professional boundaries and be reluctant to move beyond them, making it impossible to move services forward. Trust between colleagues is essential before boundaries can be broken down and this chapter brings home to readers the importance of caring for their own mental health, and the mental health of their colleagues. (Editors' summary)

5 FOOD FOR THOUGHT: TOWARDS IMPROVING SERVICES FOR PEOPLE WITH EATING DISORDERS

Diane Cook and Tricia Whitehouse

As well as having to endure censure from others who perceive eating disorders as self-inflicted, people with these conditions are also prey to multiple physical illnesses. Eating disorders are complex and multi-faceted, as this chapter makes clear, and interventions may be lengthy and equally complex. The authors are persuasive in their view that the key to improvements in the services offered to people with eating disorders is good teamwork, and having appropriate services available at the right time. Collaboration between clinicians and clients, between different professional groups, between primary and secondary services, and the involvement of social services as well as agencies within the voluntary and private sectors, enable clients to receive services that are sensitive to their social, psychological and physical needs. Creating an environment in which these clients can be supported depends on professionals who are good communicators, secure in themselves and able to give and receive honest feedback. The authors, who are skilled clinicians, provide valuable insights into how to set up, manage and sustain services for people with eating disorders. (Editors' note)

INTRODUCTION

What are eating disorders?

Eating disorders are emotional disorders, which find expression in focusing on food consumption and over-concern with body size and shape. They represent a means of coping with stress within a social environment that overvalues appearance and promotes a morbidly thin ideal, particularly for women. However, because of the effects of starvation and compensatory behaviours such as vomiting, laxative/diuretic abuse and over-exercising, this way of coping results in high levels of morbidity and mortality. If untreated, eating disorders may result in a wide range of bio-psycho-social morbidity, including severe malnutrition, amenorrhoea, osteoporosis, electrolyte imbalances, heart, kidney and liver damage, social isolation, depression, self-harm, suicide and death.

Eating disorders usually start during adolescence and, in the absence of prompt, appropriate treatment, the earlier the onset the more likely the individual will suffer from some degree of irreversible physical and psychological damage and impaired social functioning. Eating disorders have the highest incidence of morbidity and mortality among psychiatric/psychological conditions, including schizophrenia and depression. Preventive measures, early recognition and early intervention are crucial in order to promote speedy recovery and minimise the long-term physical, psychological and social effects that can arise in moderate and severe eating disorders.

Eating disorders constitute a major problem in our society and present a consid-erable challenge to health care service providers. Research findings indicate that eating disorders are increasing. They continue to affect primarily young women, but the incidence of disorders in children, males, older women and psychiatric patients is increasing.

Why has the problem been neglected?

The identification, treatment and management of eating disorders are not core components within the training programmes of mental health professionals. At best, students will receive one or more teaching sessions introducing them to eating disorders. Any deeper understanding of the problem derived from evidence-based practice remains both patchy and inadequate. As a result there is very little awareness of the causes and effects of eating disorders and even less knowledge about appropriate treatment. This is especially worrying in relation to primary care services, as early recognition and treatment are crucial if the incidence of severe and chronic disorders is to be minimised.

Eating-disordered patients may be perceived as difficult, manipulative and controlling people, motivated by vanity or relatively minor emotional difficulties. Staff involved in their care, who may have little understanding of the physical, psychological/psychiatric and social effects of the disorders, may see them as self-inflicted conditions with a relatively simple solution. They may believe that sufferers can just eat their way out of trouble. In reality, eating disorders are often severe, complex and enduring mental illnesses, which are prone to relapse and chronicity.

The other major problem is that the treatment of severe, chronic eating disorders may be long-term and expensive, and is often considered to be an inefficient use of limited resources. There is a huge disparity in attitude towards eating-disordered clients who relapse repeatedly and towards those with other major psychiatric illnesses. A decision not to treat an eating-disordered patient may be rationalised by the patient's inability to recover fully from previous treatment. Sometimes, treatment may be delayed until the patient has deterior-ated to a life-threatening degree. In contrast, if a patient suffering from manic-depressive psychosis or schizophrenia shows signs of relapse, a strategy of early intervention, to prevent or minimise the consequences of relapse, is considered essential. Few clinicians would refuse to provide appropriate, possibly very intensive, care to a relapsing schizophrenic on the grounds that he has been treated for one or more such episodes in the past and has not stayed well as a result of that treatment. Such an attitude, however, is commonplace towards eating-disordered patients.

To compound the situation, there are few specialist practitioners and even fewer comprehensive specialist services to provide appropriate treatment. The Eating Disorders Association has stated, and clinical experience confirms, that inappropriate treatment, in terms of content and/or duration, may be counter-productive.

Why does the problem warrant more attention?

Eating disorders are an expression of, and themselves create, a deep well of misery, dysfunction and disability for sufferers, and, often, for those who are close to them. In addition to pre-existing aetiological factors, the long-term effects of starvation include personality changes, relationship breakdown, loss of employment/education, social isolation and, often, psychiatric co-morbidity such as depression, self-harm, alcoholism, obsessional-compulsive disorders, and even psychotic episodes. Many women with chronic eating disorders who have children may have their parenting ability compromised as a result of associated physical and psychological illness and the effects of unresolved psychological conflict on family and social relationships. Furthermore, there is a significant risk of intergenerational transmission of eating-disordered attitudes and behaviours.

In spite of the costs involved in treating people with eating disorders, the long-term physical consequences of inadequate, or no treatment, such as osteoporosis, heart, liver and kidney disorders, mean that treatment should be more cost-effective in the long run, particularly if the disorder is diagnosed early. Maintenance and follow-up can be long-term, but are relatively inexpensive and essential to prevent relapse and further deterioration.

What follows is an account of how someone with an eating disorder accessed care, how she was treated and who was involved in her treatment. The importance of multidisciplinary and multi-agency working, and of good communication, is evident throughout.

CASE STUDY JAN

Jan, a single white woman aged 21 was referred to the Eating Disorders Service (EDS) by her GP. She had a history of three episodes of anorexia nervosa at ages 13, 16 and 18, precipitated by stress relating to the physical and emotional upheavals of adolescence and exam pressures. Episode 1 started by her avoiding lunch at school; she was also observed walking round and round the school grounds on her own. A teacher expressed her concerns to Jan's mother, who contacted their GP. Jan was referred to an adolescent service where she was admitted for a brief period, re-nourished and discharged back to the care of her GP. At follow-up she had maintained her discharge weight and had begun to menstruate. She was still very slender and her body-image dissatisfaction was marked, but it was not felt that further intervention was necessary. Indeed, it was believed that it might disrupt her education and social development.

At 16, exam pressures led to bouts of comfort eating and some weight gain, which prompted episodes of compensatory vomiting and laxative abuse. Jan also joined her local gym and attended aerobic classes three times a week. She began to focus her life almost entirely around studying, bingeing, vomiting and exercising. Her mother, noticing that Jan seemed quite low in mood and was isolating herself, tried to encourage her to cut down on her studying and contact her friends. Jan became verbally abusive and tearful at what she perceived as her mother's interference in her life and distressed that her mother had not noticed her lack of friends.

Jan began a strict diet and lost weight rapidly over the next few weeks. She was taken back to the GP, very much against her will, and referred to adult mental health services. Following assessment, which focused on her relatively recent weight loss, she was offered dietary advice and short-term cognitive behavioural counselling, combined with education about the effects of starvation. Jan did not disclose that she had been bingeing, vomiting and purging for some months. She regained weight to within the normal range and utilised the counselling she was offered to help manage her anxieties about the forthcoming exams. She gained 10 GCSEs, achieving high grades.

A similar situation developed around A-levels, though this time Jan self-referred. She had begun to have palpitations and dizziness after vomiting and had fainted following a particularly strenuous workout at the gym, which she now attended five or six times a week. She also experienced 'lost time' where she could not remember what had happened. On this occasion, Jan disclosed to her GP the extent of her bingeing, vomiting, laxative abuse and over-exercising. What had previously been considered as relatively minor anorexic episodes were revealed as a serious, entrenched and enduring eating disorder. Jan, although of acceptable weight, was not menstruating regularly. The severity of her symptoms indicated a need for specialist treatment and Jan was referred to an Eating Disorders Service (EDS). However, due to limited resources, there was a minimum six-week waiting list for assessment and a further delay before treatment could be offered. Jan was re-referred to her local community mental health team (CMHT) for support in the interim.

When the GP referral was received by the CMHT, Jan was referred for assessment to a psychologist who had a special interest in eating disorders. (Details of Jan's assessment plan can be seen in Table 5.1.) Following this assessment, the psychologist wrote to the consultant psychiatrist, requesting a psychiatric assessment and monitoring of Jan's medication. She also wrote to Jan's GP, requesting that he monitor Jan's physical health, and arrange for various laboratory investigations to be carried out on a regular basis (see Table 5.2 for a summary of these). The dietician was contacted and asked to review Jan's weight, calculate her body mass index (BMI), and negotiate the beginning of re-nourishment.

Jan was placed on the waiting list for the next anxiety management group. Her case was presented to the team, with a request for a community mental health nurse (CMHN) key worker to be allocated, to offer Jan support between sessions. At this time the CMHN assigned to Jan's surgery was overwhelmed with other demands and had no capacity to take on another complex client. The psychologist took on the role of key worker, in addition to that of therapist; it was not an ideal situation, but one that is often a reality in the community.

Since Jan's previous referral, the Trust had been fortunate enough to obtain the services of a dietician trained in cognitive behavioural therapy (CBT) for the treatment of eating disorders. Dieticians are not generally qualified in CBT and many have no specialist knowledge of eating disorders, or other mental health issues, so Jan was very fortunate to receive this support. Working closely with the dietician, the psychologist was able to explore Jan's history of eating problems and was able to focus on the factors that predisposed her to resort to such an extreme coping mechanism. Because of time constraints, it was not possible to explore each of these factors fully, but Jan was fortunate to receive support from the clinicians who had worked with her previously. She appeared to cope well with help from the local team and, when an appointment with the specialist service became available, she did not feel the need to attend. Jan successfully completed her A-levels and gained a place at university, thereby moving out of the catchment area of the specialist service.

Jan next presented to her GP two and a half years later, having been advised by a counsellor at her university to take a year out and seek treatment for her eating difficulties and depression before returning for her final year. She complained of feeling very low and apathetic and described a similar array of signs and symptoms as at age 18. In addition, her weight had dropped significantly and she had not menstruated for over 18 months. An urgent referral to the CMHT was made and Jan saw the psychologist with whom she had worked previously. The assessment procedure was as before, with many of the relevant details being taken from her notes. Jan was clearly in need of immediate in-patient treatment, and the NHS specialist EDS was contacted. There were no available beds and the team were advised that there was a minimum three-month waiting list. However, the consultant psychiatrist attached to the unit agreed to assess Jan, while the psychologist attempted to obtain an extra-contractual referral (ECR) to a private-sector specialist unit, which had beds available immediately. On the recommendation of the psychiatrist, Jan qualified for admission to the specialist unit. This process took four weeks, during which she continued to deteriorate, despite regular sessions with the psychologist. Once the ECR was confirmed, Jan attended for assessment by the private-sector EDS team, who felt that in-patient care was indicated. She was offered admission the following day.

This picture of repeated episodes, increasing in severity, is one frequently seen in the history of people with eating disorders. Jan was very fortunate to live in an area where there was a specialist unit and a GP who was aware of these types of problem.

REFERRAL AND ASSESSMENT

In the NHS

The referral of people with eating disorders to appropriate services can vary. In some instances, referral may be to the team where a decision is made to allocate a client to a particular clinician/s, who will be able to provide the most appropriate care and treatment. Alternatively, the referral may be to a consultant psychiatrist, who may then refer on to another clinician. Referrals from primary care usually come via the GP.

As can be seen from the case study, a number of people became involved in Jan's assessment and care. These included:

- a consultant psychiatrist, responsible for Jan's medication and psychiatric overview;
- a psychologist, responsible for Jan's psychotherapy and acting as key worker;
- a GP, responsible for overseeing Jan's physical health;
- a dietician, responsible for monitoring Jan's weight and re-nourishment.

In the private sector

In the private-sector facility referred to in the case study, referrals are either to the consultant psychiatrist or to the specialist team. Referrals come from multiple sources, including self-referral (rare), GPs, consultant psychiatrists, other senior clinicians within the NHS, and from other services dealing with eating disorders. The assessment is carried out by a minimum of two members of the team and should include all items in Table 5.1 and Table 5.2.

Table 5.1 Assessment

	Community (NHS)	In-patient (private)
Detailed personal history, including: • reason for referral; • family structure and roles; • relationships; • occupation, work, study, etc.; • use of leisure time; • previous treatment and how perceived; • other agencies involved, past and present; • self-perception; • hopes and fears for the future; • expectation of treatment.	•	•
Eating disorder pathology and body image assessment	•	•
Mental state examination, including assessment of other self-injurious behaviours, past and present	•	•
Routine physical examination	•	•
Weight and calculation of BMI	•	•
Laboratory investigations (see Table 5.2 opposite)	•	•
ECG		•
Bone scan		•
Pelvic ultrasound for early adolescent onset		•
Other physical investigations as necessary	•	•
Co-morbidity	•	•

Table 5.2   Laboratory investigations

	Anorexia nervosa	Bulimia nervosa
Full blood count	•	•
Urea and electrolytes	•	•
Calcium	•	•
Magnesium	•	•
Phosphate	•	•
Serum proteins	•	
Liver function tests	•	
ECG	•	•
Glucose	•	
Thyroid function tests	•	
Vitamin B12, folate	•	
Erythrocyte transketolase (thiamin)	•	
Bone markers	•	

The assessment process

The assessment process focuses on the individual needs of each patient. It is a comprehensive and ongoing process that facilitates a flexible response, in terms of monitoring and treatment provision, to the patient's changing needs over time. The initial assessment will begin at the patient's interview with the consultant and, if admission is necessary, will be completed following admission.

Jan's assessment revealed a BMI of 14.2 (normal range 20–25; a BMI of 17.5 and below is a positive diagnostic criterion for anorexia nervosa). Her potassium levels were also low, primarily due to frequent vomiting and abuse of laxatives. Liver function and thyroid tests were both abnormal. A bone scan revealed signs of osteoporosis and her ECG showed minor irregularities. She had restricted fluids in addition to food and was somewhat dehydrated. Her blood pressure was very low and she often felt dizzy. Her concentration and short-term memory were poor.

ADMISSION AND INTRODUCTION TO THE TEAM

Eating Disorders Service Co-ordinator

Following admission Jan was introduced to the Eating Disorders Service Co-ordinator, who spent two hours with her giving her written and verbal information about the service and the treatment regime, including the re-nourishing process. This time is regarded as necessary in order to build trusting relationships and to ensure that the client knows what to expect and the extent to which they are expected to be involved in their own treatment. The co-ordinator liaised closely with the dietician and worked with Jan to formulate an initial menu plan, taking into account her dislikes. Jan is a vegetarian and also avoids milk and vegetarian cheese because she feels she is sensitive to them. The co-ordinator, aware that Jan may be avoiding certain foods because of their fat and/or calorie content, rather than because she is sensitive to them, made a mental note to discuss this with the team, and with Jan when she was a little more settled. Allergy testing was considered.

It was the responsibility of the co-ordinator to introduce Jan to the nurse manager and to the staff nurse who was allocated as her 'named nurse'. Jan was then introduced to the other patients and staff. During her induction, Jan was given a great deal of information and met a number of people. It was unlikely that she would remember everything and the staff understood that reinforcement of what she had been given would be necessary. Time spent with the co-ordinator is of central importance to the induction process; that person provides an informative, supportive relationship for patients throughout their treatment. Whatever Jan remembers or forgets, she needs to feel that she has been treated with kindness, consideration and respect. This is perhaps the most important part of her introduction to the service and to those who will be caring for her.

The co-ordinator's role is to ensure that the administrative components of the service run smoothly, from funding issues to arranging clinical meetings. She deals with enquiries about the service, and provides information and support to relatives and carers. She liaises with finance, admissions and catering within the hospital and with primary care workers and others in the community. She works closely with the nurse manager and nursing staff and participates in service development. In addition to her role as co-ordinator of the service, she works in partnership with the dietician to provide support around food, from menu-planning to helping patients manage their anxieties over daily eating and weight gain. She also weighs the patients regularly and keeps records of their progress.

THE TREATMENT REGIME

Reviewing Jan's treatment provides an opportunity to examine the various roles of those involved in her care and treatment.

Consultant psychiatrist

The consultant is a key person in Jan's management, with medical responsibility for the service. He is involved in the assessment process, both initial and ongoing, and attends to the overall medical and psychological needs of the patients. He works closely with the patient and the team in formulating, delivering and reviewing treatment interventions, through regular formal and informal meetings. He writes regular progress reports to referral and funding agencies and plays a crucial role in securing adequate time and funding to treat patients effectively.

Many of the patients are tertiary referrals with multiple pathologies, who require lengthy and patient work on various aspects of their life. The consultant liaises with health authorities, primary care teams and other agencies involved in providing care, to enable effective and appropriate treatment to be given during admission and following discharge back to the local teams. He works closely with the team to agree a discharge process and is involved in formulating care plans to help meet ongoing treatment and follow-up needs.

Nurse manager and nursing staff

The role of the nurse manager is varied and demanding. She is ultimately respon- sible for the day-to-day running of the treatment programme and deployment of staff, in addition to participating in the clinical work of the service. She works closely with the whole team, including liaising daily with the consultant and super- vising sessional therapists. She represents the team at management meetings. Like the co-ordinator, she provides day-to-day support, information and guidance to patients, colleagues, relatives and carers.

Nursing staff are involved in patient care from admission to follow-up. In addition to providing specific therapeutic interventions, they create the clinical and administrative framework within which the care package as a whole is provided. Nurses liaise with all members of the team and all departments within the hospital, from the housekeepers to finance, and play a significant role in shaping the patient-centred culture of the service.

The nursing staff had a vital role to play in Jan's treatment. Her named nurse was responsible for overseeing her treatment programme and had regular discus- sions with her about her progress, fears and concerns. She helped Jan to identify strengths and formulate aims and objectives for her treatment, and helped identify needs relating to discharge. Nursing staff were there to support her during and after mealtimes, when she couldn't sleep at night and when she needed support to resist the urge to self-harm. They were at the end of the telephone line for support and advice during weekend leave. Jan's relationship with each of them, and their relationships and communication with each other, were pivotal to the success of Jan's treatment overall. Feeling understood and being able to learn to trust others to care for her in a respectful, honest and consistent fashion were prerequisites for Jan participating in her various treatment sessions, rather than just attending them.

Dietician

For Jan, the most important initial considerations were to rehydrate and begin to re-nourish her, while providing practical and emotional support. Because she had been eating and drinking very little prior to admission it was important to do this gradually, to avoid overwhelming her digestive and circulatory systems. She was seen by the dietician and a bodystat was done.

The bodystat, or bioelectrical impedance analysis (BIA), has been used with many client groups as a non-intrusive way of measuring body composition. Feedback includes the percentage proportion of fat to lean, water level and the calorific value required by the individual to maintain weight. Although there is a margin of error in the use of the BIA, as there is in any measure of body compos- ition, provided it is used correctly and consistently with the patient, under the same conditions over a period of time, it can be relied upon to demonstrate changes in body composition.

Patients are more willing to accept re-nourishment when they have access to their bodystat results. These results can show that appropriate management of re-nourishment leads to weight increase that is spread across both lean and fat tissue, rather than just fat. They also indicate that rapid, secretive exercise, without adequate intake of carbohydrate, causes a reduction in lean tissue rather than fat.

The dietician calculated the calories needed to increase Jan's weight and then, together, they formulated an eating programme that would allow her to gain two to three pounds a week. This plan was communicated to the co-ordinator who would help Jan manage her food on a day-to-day basis.

Because Jan felt unable to face the amount of food necessary to establish weight gain, it was agreed that she would, initially, be allowed to supplement her intake with high-calorie drinks. The ultimate aim of re-nourishment is a normal intake of food sufficient to maintain a healthy weight and functioning, in response to appetite and in line with normal social behaviour. However, in the treatment of eating disorders, food is essentially medicine, and the intake of sufficient calories and nutrients to restore health is of prime importance.

At very low weight, and where starvation behaviours are evident, it may be necessary to allow lots of time for mealtimes. Obsessive rituals around food, such as cutting food up into small pieces and chewing endlessly, are starvation behaviours, not just an avoidance of eating (although they may be this too). Also, where digestion is impaired through starvation, this behaviour may be helpful in extracting the maximum nourishment from food. Such rituals may resolve, and should at least partially resolve, when the physiological state of starvation is reversed, as the patient begins to eat regularly and gain weight. When this happens, it is helpful to permit the patient to leave the table and to be escorted to a supervised area away from the dining room as soon as their meal is eaten. It is unnecessarily stressful to expect everyone to sit at the table until the last person has finished; increased stress will further exacerbate symptoms and behaviours related to eating disorders.

If rituals around food do not resolve following re-nourishment, this will be addressed within the therapeutic programme at a number of levels. In addition to individual work with patients, the dietician also provides nutritional education in a group setting, which Jan attended. In the group, Jan learned that the re-nourishing programme was not just about weight gain, but also about maintaining both physical and psychological health, and that the idea of food as medicine was important to her recovery. She discovered that, to aid her recovery, food has to be:

- individually prescribed;
- observed to be taken;
- taken regularly; and
- regularly reviewed and adjusted.

And that the functions of food as medicine were many, including:

- to maintain life;
- to reverse/minimise the immediate and long-term effects of starvation;
- to resolve starvation behaviours;

- to help manage the urge to binge and vomit;
- to re-learn hunger and satiety signals;
- to stimulate metabolism; and
- to facilitate other treatments.

Adequate nutrition is essential in order to ameliorate the physical, psychological and behavioural elements of eating disorders, which arise from, or are intensified by starvation, vomiting and purging. This is necessary to facilitate the exploration of underlying causes, identification of ongoing problems and treatment aimed at resolving them.

The dietician is involved throughout treatment, from admission to discharge. Her role requires her to provide information and training to staff and she has regular contact with all members of the clinical team. She liaises closely with catering staff in order to ensure that they understand the need for strict portion control and appropriate provision of menu choices. She also provides guidance on the provision of special diets for vegetarians, ethnic minorities and those with other special dietary needs. The role of the dietician is thus pivotal to the survival and wellbeing of the patient, and also to the success of all other interventions.

Occupational therapist

A central feature of the OT's role is to undertake a task analysis, which identifies the patient's needs in terms of their activities and cognitions. Individual treatment packages are then developed, in collaboration with the patient, to develop the skills that will meet these needs at a practical level. A major problem for Jan in terms of her social functioning was that, having left her friends behind when she moved house and school, she had not been able to build new friendships and was very isolated. Her life had revolved around studying, exercise, dieting, bingeing and vomiting. Also, her self-esteem was very low and she had little confidence in herself. She struggled in the treatment groups because she did not believe that she had anything of importance to say and felt that people looked down on her.

Assertiveness training and social skills groups helped Jan to build confidence. Experiential and creative work enabled her to express herself in a variety of ways, and then to find the words to describe what she was feeling. She improved her ability to interact with others within the treatment programme and was then encouraged to use her new skills to begin to solve the problem of not having friends.

Jan worked on a one-to-one basis with an OT to identify goals relating to social-ising and building friendships. Accompanied by the OT initially, Jan began going to the cinema, the bowling alley and to various other social and recreational activities. At first she was very self-conscious, but she was able to bring her feelings back to her individual and group work for discussion and support. Doing more gave Jan more to talk about with others and so she felt less boring, more confident about being included, and more able to express her thoughts and feelings to others. Even better, she began to meet new people and made some friends, so reducing her reliance on the OT for company.

Jan began to enjoy being able to socialise, but confided that she particularly missed two friends from primary school to whom she had been close since nursery days. Although they had contacted her after she moved, she had been too low to reply and had lost touch. With support, Jan wrote to both and was delighted when, some weeks later, the three of them had a reunion at the hospital. Jan also received OT support for menu-planning, budgeting, shopping and cooking. These, and attendance at the breakfast club, helped her to begin to take responsibility for her own meals and portion sizes, and to believe that she could eat healthily without putting on too much weight.

When Jan was ready to return to university, the OT staff helped her to find accommodation and kept in regular contact with her, including visiting her, until she had settled in.

OT staff are involved in patient care from assessment through to discharge and follow-up. The skills and competencies Jan built with their help were utilised in all of her treatment settings and, just as importantly, in her return to university and a life outside hospital. OT staff liaise closely with all members of the team, their work has a direct impact on the work of others and, in turn, is informed by that of fellow clinicians.

Psychotherapist

All patients are assessed for psychotherapy, which usually commences at the time when the person enters the service. Depending on the patient's cognitive functioning and physical state (which varies widely from individual to individual), contact with the therapist may be purely supportive initially. This is important in helping to create the therapeutic alliance that facilitates further work when this becomes possible.

Because her eating difficulties arose in response to managing stress and emotional problems, Jan was offered individual psychotherapy. Although she found the process very difficult at times, she was eventually able to link her perfectionist 'people-pleasing' behaviour and low self-esteem to events during her childhood, in particular the death of her younger sister when Jan was seven. This had left her parents emotionally unavailable to her, locked into their own distress. Her mother had become depressed and withdrawn, caring physically for Jan but unable to do any more, while her father buried his grief beneath a mountain of work and began to drink excessively. When drunk, he had been unpredictable and, although previously a gentle man, he had become increasingly physically violent towards both Jan and her mother. As a result, her parents' relationship had broken down and they had divorced shortly before Jan moved to secondary school. Her parents' divorce had necessitated a house move, so Jan found herself in a new school in a new area, without any of the friends who had been her main support until then.

As Jan's experience illustrates, the causative, precipitative and maintaining factors of eating disorders include trauma and deficits in care, which are increasingly recognised as resulting in post-traumatic stress disorder (PTSD). This results in a lack, or disruption, of the ability to recognise and differentiate affective and physical states, and in chronically raised stress hormones. With regard to eating disorders, the treatment model takes into account that the physiological response to unmanageable stress reinforces psychological patterning and interferes with the opportunity for new learning as the individual develops. Increasing bodily sensations at adolescence, combined with emotional upheaval and physical changes, threaten the ability of vulnerable individuals to contain conflict arising from past and present experiences and overload their ability to recognise, differentiate and manage internal states. Diet and exercise may be seen as a way to boost self-esteem and to create a sense of being in control; in this way, a pathway to an eating disorder opens up.

In severe cases, eating disorders may represent personality development that is powerfully shaped by deficits in self-regulation. In such a situation, the relationship with food is used to represent and/or deny unmet needs and conflict, and to preserve a sense of being in control, without needs and wants and free of negative feelings, thoughts and actions.

In order to work with eating-disordered clients/patients, the therapist must have an awareness of the following:

- the origins and effects of deficits in self-regulation;
- the consequences of starvation and compensatory behaviours on physical, psychological and social wellbeing;
- family and the wider social context; and
- the function of self-harm behaviours as a regulatory mechanism.

Psychotherapists working with eating disorders may need to work at different levels according to the changing needs – and levels of awareness – of their clients. They should be able to work in an integrative way, utilising a number of treatment modes, while maintaining a framework of aims and objectives relating to the patient's needs. They must also have a firm commitment to multidisciplinary working and to value input from other clinicians, including, where necessary, the prescription of psychotropic medication. It is a common misperception that, if the underlying issues are attended to, the eating disorder will vanish, and that neither food nor the medical model of treatment is the real answer. However, established moderate to severe eating disorders create the physiological and psychological conditions for their own maintenance, and all aspects of these disorders need to be addressed simultaneously.

Ideally, therapists should avoid being either opaque or over-enthusiastic and should be accepting, open, friendly and calmly responsive. They should aim for an elaboration of meaning based on the reconstruction and understanding of the effects of past and present experiences. Abstract interpretation and an opaque or over-directive approach will hinder the elaboration of chaotic internal states into meaningful sensations, feelings and memories.

Initially, Jan's psychotherapy focused on cognitive management of her day-to-day difficulties around eating and only when she was able to think more constructively about these was she able to move to more exploratory work on 'making sense, making links'.

In the treatment of eating disorders, psychotherapy aims to do the following:

- provide support and build a trusting relationship;
- facilitate management of current thoughts, feelings and behaviours;
- develop more appropriate ways of coping;
- identify and resolve underlying issues;
- reduce, and eventually overcome self-harm behaviours;
- improve interpersonal functioning; and
- facilitate personal development, maturation and individuation.

Psychotherapy will become part of the treatment programme as soon as the patient's physical and cognitive functioning permit, and usually continues until discharge from the service. The psychotherapist attends team meetings and has regular contact with colleagues on a formal and informal basis. Family therapy may be considered, especially in the case of younger patients who expect to return to live in the parental home after discharge from in-patient care. Family therapy will usually commence when the patient has made therapeutic gains, in terms of insight, self-awareness and interpersonal behaviour, within individual therapy. Family therapy is undertaken by a therapist other than the patient's individual therapist.

The therapist's input will mediate, to some extent, the expectations of progress in other areas. For instance, when Jan was confronting particularly difficult issues in her therapy, her weight remained static for some weeks, but she was making progress psychologically and, providing she did not *lose* weight, the situation was felt to be acceptable in the short term. This necessitated reports and information concerning the rationale for Jan's clinical management at this juncture, from the consultant to referral and funding agencies, in order to safeguard Jan's ongoing treatment.

Similarly, when Jan was over-exercising and vomiting, her physical condition deteriorated and she was unable to participate effectively in her psychotherapy until her physical state was stabilised. The therapist, aware of the reasons for Jan's apparent lack of engagement and progress, was content to continue in a more supportive role in the mean time. Without good communication within the team, these situations would have been managed less effectively, and Jan's overall progress may have been jeopardised.

Body-image therapist

Diagnostic criteria of eating disorders, body-image distortion and dissatisfaction are often severe and entrenched. At low weight, body-image distortion may be of delusional severity and may be accompanied by equally delusional thoughts around the handling and consumption of food. Where anxiety is expressed as bodily disgust, physical pain, postural distortions and a restricted range of movement (often in spite of frantic over-exercising), and where there is a need to have fun and actually enjoy the physical body, specific body-image work is necessary.

Body-image work may be provided by OT or nursing staff, or by a body-image therapist. Massage is provided only by the body-image therapist, who is a qualified and experienced aromatherapist, reflexologist and counsellor.

As with all who suffer from eating disorders, Jan's relationship with her body was negative and confused. She had received little physical comfort as a child, and her father's beatings resulted in a powerful connection between high levels of anxiety and physical pain. As a child she could only relax at home immediately following one of her father's outbursts, when there would be a period of calm before the next storm began to build up. Since her early teens she had associated being in control of her thoughts and feelings with self-punishment and food deprivation. Her body brought her no pleasure and she regarded herself not only as fat, but also as physically repulsive. When distressed and unable to contain her feelings through starving, bingeing, vomiting and laxative abuse, she would resort to banging and bruising herself, and occasionally burning her skin with a cigarette.

Jan's self-harm behaviours enabled her to dissociate from what she perceived as unmanageable distress. However, self-harm, once established, can become an increasingly habitual way of dealing with anxiety, and obstructs the development of more constructive ways of coping. Jan would, of course, explore the reasons for her self-harm in psychotherapy, but while this process was under way, it was important to identify and better manage thoughts and behaviours arising from her distorted perception of her body. Initially, body-image distortion may be severe and unvarying in intensity. As treatment progresses, the patient may feel worse (or better) about his or her body than at other times; later still, with increasing self-awareness derived from therapeutic work, the patient will recognise that his or her body image varies according to personal level of comfort or anxiety.

Body-image work is tailored to the physical condition of patients, and includes the following:

- massage;
- body-mapping and other exercises in size estimation;
- discussions about media images of women and men;
- shopping for clothes;
- line dancing;
- personal space exercises;
- swimming;
- team games;
- cognitive techniques to challenge distorted perceptions; or
- cognitive techniques to manage the effects of distorted perceptions.

Massage usually begins with a hand, foot or shoulder massage, and progresses to full body massage only if the patient is in agreement, and is comfortable with it. Massage has a number of uses with eating-disordered patients:

- It improves circulation and muscle tone where exercise is undesirable due to low weight.
- It assists with relieving the symptoms of tension and anxiety.
- It has proved invaluable in patients who have suffered sexual or physical abuse, providing an opportunity to distinguish between good and bad touch, helping

them to regain control over their body so that they can learn to say 'no' to unwanted attention.
- It allows patients to perceive the size and shape of their body through touch, often a very different experience from when they look in the mirror.

Body-mapping, choosing and trying on clothes and other size-estimation exercises confront patients with their misperceptions in a very concrete way, while cognitive techniques provide a means to manage the thoughts and behaviours arising from body-image distortion and dissatisfaction. Swimming, team sports, outings and other recreational or sporting activities allow the patients to regain some confidence in their body – and may even be enjoyable! Physical tension and rigidity, along with shallow breathing, create a physiological state that induces and maintains anxiety and even panic attacks. Movement, which involves rotation of the body, helps to release this physical rigidity and necessitates deeper breathing, releasing physical and emotional tension.

Near the end of her in-patient stay, Jan found herself laughing helplessly during line dancing, as legs and arms all went the wrong way and people bumped into each other. The concentration needed to get the steps right and keep in time with the music, and with others, resulted, for a while, in a complete lack of concern with what she looked like. She was completely absorbed in a physical activity, the purpose of which was not weight loss but fun, in a way that, perhaps, she had not experienced since before the death of her sister. Although Jan's body-image distortion and dissatisfaction did not resolve completely during treatment, they were much improved and she was more able to link how she felt about her body with how she was feeling at any particular time. She also developed a number of coping strategies to avoid her anxiety escalating to the point of self-harm (either eating disorder behaviours or self-injury) under stress.

SUPPORT FOR RELATIVES AND CARERS

Support for relatives, carers and friends is an essential component of service provision, without which some interventions may be less effective. Jan's mother, not fully recovered from the loss of her child and the breakdown of her marriage, felt overwhelmed and guilty about Jan's admission to hospital. She attended the family support group, which is facilitated by a psychotherapist, and the relatives group, which was set up by the nursing staff to provide information about eating disorders and practical advice on how best to help. In addition to this, following a meeting between herself, the consultant and the nurse manager, it was felt appropriate to offer her a number of supportive one-to-one sessions with a therapist (not the same one as Jan), to allow her to express her own feelings and concerns within a safe environment. In the event, she found them so helpful that she opted to enter psychotherapy on her own account. Jan was relieved that her mother now had some support, and felt less responsible for her and more able to plan ahead. Their relationship, though still difficult at times, improved because they both felt more able and willing to communicate with each other on issues that had previously been unmentionable.

Jan and her mother had very little contact with Jan's father. After much hesitation, Jan contacted him and he visited. Their meeting, unfortunately, was not successful, as it was difficult for him to see her eating disorder as anything but attention-seeking, manipulative behaviour, used to control others. He quickly became angry, which frightened Jan, and she decided that she did not want to see him again until she was stronger. However, in spite of her own troubles, Jan was able to see how her father's behaviour related to his own pain and loss, so she wrote to him, expressing the hope that they could keep in touch by letter, even though things were difficult at the time. Jan needed a great deal of support in this, as did her mother. There is no guarantee that her relationship with her father can be healed but, after much soul-searching, she had felt it important to leave the door open a little. In the event, Jan was saddened that her father was unable to move closer to her, but she also accepted that she did not have the power to make everything OK for everyone.

THE IMPLICATIONS OF JAN'S EXPERIENCE

A number of points in the management of Jan need to be highlighted. She was fortunate to be treated in the community by clinicians with experience of eating disorders who, when she became very ill, referred her to an established specialist service with an integrated model of treatment. However, service provision for people with eating disorders varies considerably and is usually far from ideal.

To begin with, there is no generally recognised model of best practice for the treatment of eating disorders, especially those with complex aetiology and who may have, or be at risk of developing, severe, chronic conditions. Many interventions have been found to be helpful in the treatment of eating disorders, but there is little guidance on treatment combinations and sequencing. Evidence-based research identifies cognitive behavioural therapy and interpersonal psychotherapy as the treatments of choice for bulimia nervosa while family therapy and individual psychotherapy are recommended for anorexics. However, most research is undertaken with outpatients who have mild to moderate and relatively uncomplicated eating disorders, and who receive stand-alone interventions. Although this may be sufficient and effective for many patients, it will not be appropriate for the more severe conditions.

Where there is no designated service, or where the service consists of a single interested clinician, it is practically impossible to elaborate an appropriate multidisciplinary response, which takes into account both the nature of eating disorders and the individual needs of the patient. In these circumstances, stand-alone treatments, such as a bulimia group, or individual counselling, may be all that can be offered. Even more problematic, the majority of clinicians treating eating-disordered patients as part of a generic caseload, may not be aware of the physiologically determined effects of starvation and trauma, or the need for ongoing, comprehensive medical monitoring. Jan, for instance, at the age of 21, was found to have a relatively minor degree of osteoporosis, which is an irreversible effect of starvation sufficient to suppress menstruation. Some clients, referred to a specialist service for the first time in their late teens, 20s and 30s, have moderate to severe osteoporosis because they were not regularly monitored, and not treated until their disorder became life-threatening.

Even where there are experienced and knowledgeable clinicians, the treatment of more severe eating disorders, requiring intensive day care or hospitalisation, poses many dilemmas. To begin with, day-care facilities are few and far between. They may not be offered by a specialist service, let alone a generic community service. And in-patient beds may be impossible to find, or there may be long waiting lists for both assessment and treatment. This means that the re-nourishing process is left entirely to the patient, who may or may not have good advice, but will be unsupported and unsupervised in any efforts to eat. As a consequence, an essential part of the patient's treatment needs will not be met and the rest of the treatment programme will be undermined at best, and effectively sabotaged at worst.

In cases such as Jan's, where there is under-nourishment severe enough to demand hospitalisation, but no beds available, decisions about alternative care must be made. Such decisions are extremely difficult and should not be the responsibility of any one member of the team. Enquiries need to be made to all possible sources of support and an informed decision made by all those involved in the client's care. This can often be difficult to organise, with interested parties being scattered over many sites, sometimes miles apart. Yet, in order to provide good care, it is important that regular meetings take place between all involved professionals, both with and without the patient present.

Clearly, the major problem faced by clinicians working with eating-disordered patients is the dearth of services. Although the Eating Disorders Association lists over 170 NHS services as providing treatment for eating disorders, many have limitations:

- Many have no specialist service or clinician, but occasionally receive referrals of eating-disordered patients.
- Some have a single clinician (nurse, doctor, psychologist, dietician or OT) who has a special interest in eating disorders and receives referrals. Most carry a generic caseload, though some provide a specific service. Of these services, none have beds attached, and offer outpatient care only. If the clinician leaves, the service may come to an end.
- A few are specialist services, which are able to provide outpatient care. Not all have specialist beds (although some do) or access to general psychiatry beds. Some, but not all, are able to offer day care.

The information provided by the EDA cannot be regarded as completely accurate, as service provision fluctuates and not all provisions will be reported to the association. Nevertheless, it is clear that the treatment of eating disorders is seriously under-resourced.

ACCESSING BEST SERVICES AND CROSSING SECTOR BOUNDARIES

Many of the specialist services providing a comprehensive treatment package for those suffering severe eating disorders are in the private sector. However, the picture of the relationship between public- and private-sector provision is not clear. The problems have been both political and administrative, and their effects on patient care have often been of great concern.

To begin with, there is a huge misconception that all private treatment is more expensive than comparable NHS care. This was not the case with the service described in the case study. Health authorities referring to such a service will be surprised to find that treatment costs compare, often favourably, with the NHS. However, in spite of comparable costing structures and a general lack of specialist services, the culture militates against referral to private-sector services. Until recently, this opposition was backed by government pronouncements, guidelines and policies.

One problematic issue resulting from the reluctance to use private-sector services is the lack of a secure referral and treatment process. Referral may be delayed far beyond the boundaries of safety, almost until no other option can be found (as in Jan's case). Or, in severe, chronic but relatively stable disorders, patients may be superficially monitored, rather than actively treated, while their long-term physical and mental health is increasingly, and irreversibly, damaged. In rare cases, individuals have been admitted to a private-sector service, settled in and made progress, and have then been unceremoniously transferred to an NHS service because a bed has become available or the authority concerned has refused to spend more money in the private sector (even though total costs will not be very much affected). This is not good practice, either clinically or administratively. It is disruptive and distressing for patients and staff, and does nothing to foster productive communication and respect between clinicians in both sectors.

In spite of this kind of situation, good relationships can be, and are, built between the NHS and the private sector. Working closely to promote continuity and consistency of care for patients, and attending training offered by the special-interest groups of both sectors, leads inevitably to an exchange of information, a sharing of expertise and a sense of being colleagues with shared interests and concerns.

There is an urgent need for closer formal and informal links between the NHS and the private sector, mutually agreed pricing strategies and high-quality treatment programmes developed by the two sectors in co-operation with each other.

THE IDEAL SERVICE

What can we learn about improving services for people with eating disorders? The ideal service does not, and may never, exist, although there are a number of examples of good practice to emulate. While it may not be possible, or necessary, to build such services in every locality, a realistic aim would be the provision of local day-care services, where specialist clinicians could provide the following:

- medical monitoring (by a GP, or a general specialist psychiatrist);
- dietary advice, counselling and re-nourishment planning (provided by a dietician, nurse, OT, or other professional with appropriate skills);
- supervision and support at mealtimes (by a nurse, OT, or nursing assistant with in-service training and experience relating to eating disorders);

- body-image therapy (provided by a physiotherapist, nurse, OT, or psychologist);
- psychotherapy (provided by a suitably qualified/experienced professional, preferably with a core specialism in mental health, such as a nurse, psychologist, doctor, or OT).

Ideally, the above roles should be carried out by different individuals, but where this is not possible it is better that clinicians have a dual role than a vital component of treatment is omitted.

A service providing the above interventions will address all of the symptoms and behaviours of eating-disordered individuals described in the diagnostic criteria; the psychotherapy will address underlying issues. Teams of specialist clinicians working within local day-care services should be able to manage most eating disorder referrals, being able to offer more intensive day care to those with more serious disorders. More importantly, the existence of local, intensive day-care provision will facilitate early discharge and continuity of care for the minority of patients who continue to require in-patient care on a regular or occasional basis. It is also important to have links with rehabilitation services, social work departments, housing associations, and so on, to facilitate the management of practical issues that arise during and following treatment.

REVIEWING EATING DISORDER SERVICES

There are a number of important issues to take into consideration when reviewing existing services or when initiating new ones.

Creating an 'eating disorder-aware' culture

This is vitally important in primary care, which is often the first point of contact for patients and their families. This can be achieved through the following activities:

- developing collaborative working relationships with specialist services, including sharing information and undertaking joint assessment and treatment initiatives;
- education and training in eating disorders for all mental health professionals;
- provision of clinical supervision by specialist practitioners for all staff working with eating-disordered clients;
- research initiatives to provide data relating to current incidence and prevalence, patients unable to access appropriate services, links between untreated/partially treated eating disorders and a range of diseases, compared with their incidence in the general population.

The creation of an 'eating disorders-aware' culture has the following benefits:

- It facilitates early recognition and intervention.
- It ensures continuity of care between specialist services and the wider mental health team.
- It facilitates prompt re-referral to specialist services if necessary.

The need for early detection

Early detection is dependent on the creation of an 'eating disorders-aware' culture, and is essential for the following:

- to treat mild to moderate disorders efficiently and effectively;
- to minimise the potential for patients to develop severe, chronic disorders;
- to maximise wellbeing for those suffering with severe, chronic disorders; and
- to provide appropriate information and support to relatives and carers.

Hostel accommodation

There is a desperate shortage of appropriate hostel accommodation for those who are ready to leave hospital or intensive day care, for whom returning home would be counterproductive, but who are not yet ready to live completely independently. Well-managed hostel accommodation would provide a bridge to independent living that would enhance the possibility of a better level of recovery for many patients.

ORGANISATIONAL AND TEAM MANAGEMENT OBJECTIVES

Increased awareness and clinical skills are not, of themselves, sufficient to improve the treatment of those suffering from eating disorders. Organisational and team management objectives, based on a range of reliable local and national data, are of crucial importance. At present there may be no formal aims, objectives and strategies in place, in many services, for the treatment of eating disorders. If this were the situation with other major psychiatric illnesses, mental health services would not be able to function. Yet the treatment of a common, severe, enduring and mentally and physically damaging mental illness is frequently not included, or even considered, as part of mainstream services. This must change.

> This chapter highlights the complex nature of eating disorders and the way they manifest themselves. The authors show how Jan had been wrestling for many years with problems and how professionals either failed to detect symptoms or to see that the same condition can have an effect at different periods of a life. The chapter introduces a new perspective on collaboration – that is, collaboration with the private sector, which is likely to increase over the coming years. Perhaps the greatest sources of Jan's problems were a lack of appropriately trained personnel, of services and of collaborative mechanisms between the public and private sectors. A great many professionals were involved in Jan's care, but the authors justify this on the grounds of having the appropriate expertise, and enough people to reinforce the patient's progress. The authors highlight the fact that clinical staff have many other responsibilities in addition to the direct care of the patient, including keeping records up to date, ensuring finances are in order and ensuring relevant personnel are involved and informed.
>
> Perhaps the keenest insight provided in this chapter is how the culture of an organisation can affect what people do and how they relate to each other and to

others outside the organisation. Merely possessing clinical skills is not sufficient. It is far more important to have the right kind of attitude, to respect others and to have a desire to do the best for the client. Significantly, the authors raise the question of what can be provided for clients with eating disorders, in the absence of specialist services. All health professionals should be aware of the social, psychological and medical consequences of untreated eating disorders. (Editors' summary)

RECOMMENDED READING

Brownell, K.D. and Fairburn, C. (1998) *Eating Disorders and Obesity: A comprehensive handbook*, Guildford Press, Guildford

Fairburn, C.G. and Wilson, G.T. (1993) *Binge Eating: Nature, assessment and treatment*, Guildford Press, Guildford

Garner, D.M. and Garfinkel, P.E. (1997) *Handbook of Treatment for Eating Disorders*, Guildford Press, Guildford

Kaplan, A.S. and Garfinkel, P.E. (eds.) (1994) *Medical Issues and The Eating Disorders: The interface*, Brunner/Mazel, New York

Lask, B. and Bryant-Waugh, R. (1993) *Childhood Onset Anorexia Nervosa and Related Eating Disorders*, Lawrence Erlbaum, Hove

Vanderlinden, J. and Vanderlinden, W. (1997) *Trauma, Dissociation and Impulse Dyscontrol in Eating Disorders*, Brunner/Mazel, New York

6 A SOCIAL SERVICES PERSPECTIVE ON COLLABORATION IN MENTAL HEALTH CARE

Paul Craddock

Most enduring health problems have a social dimension and this is particularly true in severe and enduring mental illnesses. The often complex needs of people with such conditions can only be met in a co-ordinated fashion if health and social care providers work closely together. Fragmentation of services has too often resulted in poor care, inappropriate care and, in far too many instances, no care at all being provided for those most in need. This chapter describes collaborative mental health care from the perspective of a social services manager involved in delivering services within an inner-city locality. Care for people with mental health problems is largely driven by the government's agenda for the health service and delivered by NHS staff. There are, however, circumstances in which local authorities have a considerable direct or contractual input, providing services such as social work, home care, supported accommodation and day care. This chapter offers a social services perspective on how partnership-working with the health service and voluntary sector can meet the diverse needs of clients with severe and enduring mental illness, by extending workers' roles and encouraging and supporting staff to work in a multidisciplinary fashion. (Editors' note)

INTRODUCTION

Within North Birmingham, community mental health services are delivered by locality teams whose catchment is based upon GP registration. In the Small Heath area of Birmingham, entire GP patient lists are served by that locality's mental health team. People in Small Heath who are registered with GPs outside the locality are served by other teams. The adoption of this alignment of services, a change from the previous system of geographical patches, resulted in an increase in the population served from an actual population of 90 000 to a GP population of 112 000. Despite this increase of almost a quarter, service delivery was facilitated because of the clearer definition of who was being served.

Within this inner-city locality, which covers three electoral wards immediately to the north-east of the city centre, there is a highly mobile population. Some local schools report a 70% turnover in their reception classes in the first term, as families move from one form of local authority accommodation to another. Despite the best efforts of health care planners to make all services available to people within the locality, some do not receive the best from services because of having to relocate. GP attachment means that staff are not spending time transferring users to other teams if they move short distances, as, providing people retain their GP, mental health services also remain unchanged.

Reducing the rate of transfers between teams also preserves continuity of care and reduces the chance of people losing contact with the service.

Within the Community Mental Health Trust (CMHT), there are a number of smaller functional teams with similar structures, offering medical, nursing and social work services, which serve slightly different groups of users. When people are first referred by primary care, they will be in contact with either the Primary Care Liaison Team (PCLT) or the home treatment team. These operate as follows:

- The PCLTs serve all GP practices and are the first point of contact for the majority of new referrals.
- Home treatment teams respond to any urgent same-day assessments, where there is a possibility that a person might require admission to an in-patient facility. However, the primary objective is to care for the person at home. Frequently, users have problems with their accommodation and if the team cannot deal with these, they request and receive appropriate help from elsewhere. This is the one functional team that does not have any social worker deployed within it, although a social worker post is currently being advertised. The team comprises nurses and support workers.

Clients who continue to have care needs are directed either to the rehabilitation and recovery team or to the assertive outreach team. Clients who are served by both these teams generally have serious and enduring mental health problems, typically schizophrenia, but there are distinct differences in the types of client seen by the teams. The rehabilitation and recovery team cares for people who have a high level of need but a low level of social functioning. Typically, clients are reasonably compliant and the focus is upon enhancing their quality of life. The assertive outreach team also cares for people with low levels of social functioning and high levels of need, but who initially do not engage and have only periodic contact with services.

For both teams, the main focus is upon quality-of-life issues for people with severe mental illness. Between them, the teams have three social workers and one social work assistant. If clients are transferred to another team, the new team will meet all their care needs. In practice, the PCLT provides services for some users who should be served by other teams. However, it is not always possible to match users' needs with the types of services provided, and there are always far more demands on the assertive outreach team than on the home treatment service. Every primary care liaison worker has a mixture of clients, including some who should have progressed to other services, but have not.

We have learned over time that, no matter how much we try to develop services, there will always be some people whose needs will not be met. In addition, some clients with serious and enduring mental health problems persist in not engaging with services.

The PCLTs were designed specifically to operate at the interface between primary and secondary care; they have a 'gate-keeping role' in referring clients to secondary psychiatric services. The initial intention in establishing these teams was that they should respond swiftly to people's needs and, as far as possible, limit the intervention period to 12 months. At the end of this period, the person should either be discharged back to the GP or, if they have continuing needs, taken on by one of the other functional mental health teams (rehabilitation and recovery or assertive outreach).

CONTACT, LIAISON AND EXPECTATIONS OF COLLABORATION

Each of the PCLTs has at least one weekly meeting, to deal with incoming, ongoing and discharge work. This is supplemented by briefer duty handovers to update staff on a daily basis. This pattern of contact is replicated, though with fewer throughputs, in the assertive outreach and continuing care teams. The home treatment team has more formal contact and daily handovers, because of the nature of their work. At the management level, the senior manager meets with all the team managers at least twice a month to consider current and forthcoming work, but most business is carried on informally. All CMHT staff, whether NHS or local authority, are based at the same centre, so in addition to formal contact there is ample opportunity for less formal liaison. This arrangement is essential if staff are to be supported, and to feel supported, when working in the flexible and multidisciplinary manner that is expected by team managers.

Each team, whether rehabilitation or assertive outreach, has allocated social workers and community mental health nurses (CMHNs), but an independent management system. Social workers deployed within the mental health teams have a social services line manager, and the city council is their employer, while NHS staff have a health services manager. In practice, the manager of the NHS Mental Health Trust, who is responsible for the overall workings of the team, often determines day-to-day management. All CMHT social services and health services staff are based together, including managers. All the teams, apart from home treatment, have integrated nursing and social workers, and there are considerable overlaps in job descriptions. Notions of what is 'a social worker's job' and 'a nurse's job' have been deliberately downplayed, because users, staff and the organisation have gained no added value by maintaining discrete roles. Before integration, the needs of the individual were seen as partially medical, partially nursing and partially social; the revised system enables almost all needs to be addressed by one care co-ordinator, regardless of his or her professional background.

The care co-ordinator (key worker) takes total responsibility for a user, for his or her quality of life and for meeting all needs as far as possible. If one of the team of social workers is the care co-ordinator, that person is expected to understand symptomatology and treatment, and to have an adequate knowledge of medication. If the co-ordinator is a nurse, that person will check the benefits to which a user is entitled and ensure the user is receiving them. The result of this system is that referrals from nurses to social workers do not exist. The nurse (as care co-ordinator) simply says to the social worker, 'I don't know how to do this. How do you do it?' and the social worker can give advice. This method of working reduces the number of home visits, and the situation of service providers of different disciplines carrying out very similar assessments. It is more effective in terms of users' (and carers') time, practitioners' time and also helps reduce confusion for users, who may wonder why they are being asked the same questions several times over. (Some users interpret such repetition as a stalling tactic, to keep them waiting in the hope that they will eventually go away, or as evidence of indifference on the part of service providers.)

Social workers who are also care co-ordinators are expected to be responsible for all aspects of care, including symptom management, monitoring the side-effects of medication, keeping abreast of medication changes, and timing of outpatients' appointments. These responsibilities once belonged to the nurse and, in assuming them, social workers have an obligation to find out about them from their colleagues of all disciplines. Some formal training may be provided, but health-care personnel are expected to learn on the job. Learning is almost exclusively practice- and team-based, and staff learn more from their colleagues than from their managers. Managers have purposefully aimed to increase the permeability of professional boundaries, with the associated enhancement of skills and the ability of employees of each agency to assess and manage the services of the others. All social services and NHS managers have signed up to this way of working and see it as non-negotiable. This climate of reciprocity is essential for the effective delivery of services.

Newly appointed staff are aware of the ways in which the teams work before they take up their post, but some are surprised by the high level of integration and the blurring of professional boundaries, which they may not have experienced before. Initially, some may feel 'that's not my job and I have not been trained to do it', but both NHS and social services managers in the locality are firmly committed to encouraging more integrated working.

DEFINING MENTAL HEALTH NEEDS

Because no one has ever defined what a mental health need is, it is a feature of most of the inner-city teams that resources have never been allocated solely on the basis of need. It is difficult to know who should be defining mental health needs. Typically, we have a substantial referral rate from GPs. Quite often, people who are referred do have some mental health need, but that is not necessarily the reason for their referral, and neither is it what distinguishes them from others who have not been referred. Often it is other needs, such as housing problems, that cause the crisis and precipitate a referral.

In other settings, all GP referrals result in an outpatient appointment. However, the structure in North Birmingham has been designed to avoid this. Referrals continue to have access to medical personnel, but also have access to much more. In some instances, medical input may be unnecessary. One of the other team members will carry out a screening assessment, while the responsibility for the person's medical care remains with the GP. A high proportion of people referred have their care delivered in this way. This requires trust on the part of the medical staff within the mental health team, but they benefit hugely in terms of increased capacity as a result of not having to see everyone who has been referred by the GP. Psychiatrists have more time to spend with clients who really need their services.

One positive outcome of this is that psychiatrists are helped to redefine or re-state their role at a time of radical change in services. In the early days, difficulties arose when a GP expressed a wish for someone to see a psychiatrist and the person received a response from a social worker. A referral from primary care to secondary services was essentially a doctor-to-doctor referral. This has now changed as a result of persistence and a great deal of communication. We now have a service where respect for each other's skills is encouraged, and where time and effort are expended getting to know the skills of other members of the team.

NEW PATTERNS OF SERVICE PROVISION

Creation

The model for the current pattern of service provision was developed as a result of staff offering a duty service to users and carers at a voluntary day centre. The centre was under-resourced and medical cover was intermittent. Staff who operated the duty system came from a variety of disciplines and were therefore unable to respond to problems or queries that were outside their usual scope of professional practice. Staff realised that if they could access the expertise of their colleagues from other disciplines, they could extend their own knowledge base, enhance their roles and, consequently, respond promptly to users' needs. Changes were initiated by staff who insisted, 'We can't do this unless we do it this way', and were committed to responding to meeting the diverse needs of clients more efficiently. It soon became widely recognised that, when staff extended their roles, they were able to provide a better service and this set the standard for the rest of the locality work.

The major characteristic of this way of working is the merged health and social work agendas. Nowhere in the locality could social workers say to NHS staff, 'That's not our problem'; neither can the Trust staff say to social workers, 'That's your problem'. All staff now feel that any problem clients have is a problem for all of them. The model is one with which staff feel comfortable. Many of the original team still work in the locality, providing a degree of stability that is important for the support of more junior and new staff.

Adoption

It was the staff who had identified the need to extend their roles. They had also ideas about the changes that needed to be made and, because they 'owned' the ideas and had the confidence to make the changes, they proceeded with their implementation. Under these circumstances, more flexible roles were readily adopted. Change was facilitated because of a lack of clear management directives about how things should be done. The absence of a rigid and inflexible management structure allowed change to happen rapidly. CPA and care management were then in their infancy, and staff could see the results of their endeavours fairly quickly. This meant that their enthusiasm was maintained and burn-out was avoided. The organisational climate has since changed and has become far more prescriptive. Change on a similar scale would not now be achieved as easily because of the contract requirements that have been established between GPs and secondary services in the area of care management.

The modernisation of mental health care encompasses the integration of services, and also requires each participating organisation – health services, local authority and the voluntary sector – to review its own system of management and quality-assure its management practices. This means that change is taking place not just *within* organisations but also *between* them. Each organisation will be assessed by the Commission for Health Improvement on the extent to which it is participating with other organisations and sharing agendas.

With this in mind, Birmingham's mental health social workers were released from care management in order to become more involved and more skilled in CPA work. Indeed, after the experience of trying to implement care management within mental health – with little success – it was decided that pursuing further collaboration with health-care personnel to meet the expectations of users would be time well invested. There was ample evidence that maintaining both systems – care management and CPA – did not result in effective services. Clients were significantly disadvantaged when moving between systems because of the use of different approaches. To make a success of the implementation of CPA, the local authority agreed that mental health social workers should abandon care management and instead join with health services.

Why did this integration of services prove fairly easy to achieve? Perhaps the most significant factors were the presence of highly motivated individuals in both services, prepared to share methods of working, knowing their own roles, but not territorial about their skills, a management structure that allowed for innovation, and a culture that encouraged risk-taking and rewarded success. Health- and social-care professionals were committed to judging their success by how well they were able to respond to the needs of clients and their carers. The teams now feel that they are meeting the agenda of both the local authority and the Trust.

One of the difficulties faced by the team is the fact that social workers who have worked in a care management system have expectations of their role, which are not the same as those required by the current system. We are adamant that the care programme approach should mean that each care co-ordinator, regardless of professional background, can access the services of both agencies. Nurses within the team can request home care without going via a social worker, and social workers can arrange outpatient appointments. Flexibility of approach, combined with support for all members of the team, is the key to effective and progressive working. Even so, new members occasionally encounter resentment from other service providers, who complain that they 'haven't used the right form for that service' or 'haven't filled out the sections correctly'. Each new provider who comes on to the patch has to learn how to accommodate the care-planning processes, and ensure that referrals are managed with as little inconvenience to the user as possible.

Everything starts from the basis that, by operating the service in this way, we can deliver good-quality care. Users and other agencies appear to like what we provide.

ASSESSMENT

Performance indicators are increasingly important in public services, but at the moment there is an absence of robust systems for measuring performance in terms of meeting the needs of users and carers. If the number of people returned to the care of their GPs feeling satisfied with the care they have received is an indicator, the PCLT would appear to be quite good at doing what it is supposed to do. However, a more systematic approach to performance assessment is needed and is currently being developed. Indicators may include the following:

- time from referral to contact;
- appropriateness of referrals;
- quality of initial assessments (comprehensive, reliable and valid);
- effectiveness of interventions; and
- information about the quality of a user's contact with the service, and outcomes.

LIAISON AND COLLABORATION WITH OTHER BODIES

With PCGs and PCTs

At present, there is no formal interaction between social work and Primary Care Groups. This is primarily a consequence of recent changes in the way primary care is organised in the city, and the merger of smaller PCGs as a precursor to the formation of Primary Care Trusts. While primary health services have been engaged in this process, each of the mental health managers has maintained informal contacts. Now that the PCGs are bedding down, formal contacts and joint working must be established. PCTs are responsible for writing the mental health specifications to which mental health services will work, so it is vital that mental health services are involved in the assessment of service needs and planning. Joint work with PCG/Ts is essential to assist primary health services in formulating their specifications.

In the near future, health authorities as currently constituted will be replaced by strategic health authorities, with the commissioning of particular services devolved to the Primary Care Trusts. PCTs will determine what proportion of their resources to devote to mental health and will set out their specifications within the standards of the National Service Framework for Mental Health (Department of Health, 1999). Protocols for depression, starting with initial identification in primary care, post-natal depression, eating disorders, anxiety disorders and schizophrenia will also have to be jointly developed.

The newly formed Heart of Birmingham PCG covers nine electoral wards and the Small Heath locality provides services to one-third of the population covered by this enlarged PCG. The new PCG covers some of the most deprived populations in Birmingham. At the moment, these people are provided with secondary mental health services by three locality teams from two NHS Trusts, one of which offers its services on a resource centre basis. The PCG has already stated that it wants to deal with just one organisation for the delivery of mental health services, so it is likely that there will be mergers between localities and Trusts. Social services staff have to be part of this development if they are to continue to show improvement in service delivery.

The local authority allocates less than a quarter of the resources that the NHS allocates to mental health care. Nevertheless, as a result of the long-standing integration of social services and Trust mental health services, health service managers do not make commitments that social services would be unable to meet. Social services and the health service teams are aware of each other's agenda, and exchange information about developments on the horizon. We are therefore fairly confident in informing our own managers of the implications of various proposals. All personnel are aware that, despite the many changes that have already been achieved, many more are yet to come.

Between social services and health services

Within mental health services, collaboration between health and social services ebbs and flows. At present, social services, under the control of local authorities, have made considerable compromises in order to accommodate the NHS agenda. There have been other occasions when the opposite has been true. Whether the NHS agenda will continue to dominate is unsure, but there is a tendency within social services to view the merger of agendas as a step towards merging the organisations and already it appears that only one organisation is putting items on the agenda. Local authorities have not provided much of a lead in terms of what they are expecting mental health services to look like, allowing the driving force to be the NHS.

It is probably safe to predict that mental health services will eventually be within one organisation. Closer working with health services has implications for accessing other local authority services; it is, for example, becoming increasingly difficult to access child and family services. There are occasions when mental health social services staff must re-connect with the rest of social services. Should some mental health services be established in primary care, it might be the case that many social workers will find themselves isolated from their peers and distanced from their core values and beliefs.

With the voluntary sector

A high proportion of the day care and supported accommodation utilised by mental health services is provided by voluntary organisations. One person is responsible for setting up and monitoring the contracts with local groups and this person carries the lead for both the local authority and the NHS Trust. Robust service specifications and operational policies are in place and voluntary organisations have to demonstrate how they are going to work to these specifications. The local authority has a budget attached to the specifications, so contracted organisations are clear about what they are expected to do. In situations where care co-ordinators want to access service provision from voluntary organisations, they approach the approved providers first, because of the guarantees to deliver to an approved service specification.

With users

The issue of incorporating users and their views into service delivery and planning is an area that needs to be developed. A budget exists for the production of a local resource directory, to be compiled and updated by service-user groups. In addition, a sizeable sum is spent on ensuring that people are aware of services. However, there is a need for more structured user input into service planning and evaluation. Mental health services have considerable obligations in this area and sound ways must be found of tapping users' and carers' views of what an equitable service looks like, determining the hallmarks of good service provision, and measuring and evaluating services. Users must be involved in organising and operating audits. In health care there has been no tradition of user involvement, but social services has been associated with a different ethos, which must be rediscovered.

The contribution of users should be subjected to rigorous critique, because users are not a homogeneous group, nor will their reactions be constant over time. Effort is required to ensure that service planners understand what will be satisfactory to both the majority and the minority; inevitably, people will be heard, but not all will be responded to. Services have to be kept constantly under review and users are one of the best groups to undertake this task, although only a few may wish to be involved.

COLLABORATIVE RECORD-KEEPING

Joint record-keeping is one of the hallmarks of inter-agency collaboration, as each organisation demonstrates that it is willing to share ownership of records. This is only possible where team members are based together geographically. Currently, there is an expectation that both the NHS and social services department will maintain their own records. While this may suit the individual organisations, it does not work in practice for either service users or staff. It is pointless to have information in the nursing files that social workers are unable to access, or add to.

In practice within this locality, social services workers maintain the bare minimum of individual documentation (care plans, summaries and reviews) in a separate file to fulfil the administrative and statutory side of the social work department's requirements, and use the whole mental health team's records as the 'working record' for each user. The 'working record' is therefore integrated with the health record. Although this recording system is not supported by any formal inter-agency agreement, it was driven by the need to have a multidisciplinary chronological record. Some unresolved issues remain, relating to the ownership and retention of notes, and what happens if, in the event of a legal inquiry, records are required to provide an account of how decisions were made and what transpired with users.

LIMITATIONS AND POSSIBLE IMPROVEMENTS

The social care agenda is insufficiently developed at the moment, and social services could be helped by more guidance from the Department of Health on what it is expecting the NHS to deliver in relation to what local government currently delivers. Better measures of what constitute a good service are urgently required. Social workers within mental health are strongly influenced by the NHS agenda, but need to start agitating for the social care agenda to be incorporated into the NHS agenda; otherwise, the corpus of skills that has been built up over decades may be lost.

There are few disadvantages to our way of working and many advantages. So good is our team working now that it is highly unlikely that any member of staff who is underperforming could do so for very long. The team has to define what it is we do, because no one tells us how to operate. It requires courage to offer services in innovative ways, and team members have to take time to think about what they do, rather than merely doing what they are told to do. All the locality managers gain support from their shared conviction that this is the right way to offer services to this group of users; over the years, experience has shown the conviction to be correct.

Although many mental health managers have travelled an alarming distance beyond their original job description, they tend to be comfortable with it, because they feel that they are doing what they should be doing. Because team members have ownership of what they do and how they do it, as a consequence they take seriously the responsibility for what is done and there have been no incidents to date of express dissatisfaction. My job now bears little resemblance to the one to which I was appointed some years ago, but the creativity and innovation in which I have been involved have been stimulating and energising.

The system that we have developed has not come about as a result of directions from our own agency, but as a result of local agreements. Now, it appears that what we have done is becoming a model for elsewhere. We are grateful that we have found ourselves in tune with government thinking, or we would be having to unravel all that we have established, and return to separate agencies. In our reflective moments, we are able to acknowledge that we have taken some wrong turnings along the way, but we remain confident that we are getting to where we want to be.

This chapter describes the evolution of innovative services, set up specifically to meet the needs of a client group that had previously been poorly catered for. Ensuring that the principal team members share the same work location is shown to be an important first step. Once this was arranged, sharing practices and working collaboratively appear to have followed naturally. The importance of formal and informal contact between members of the team is stressed. (This is a major theme throughout this book; personnel who know each other work better together and are able to call on each other's services.) It is interesting to note that the teams seek to keep clients in the care of their GP for as long as possible. Primary care is acknowledged as the preferred place for care and treatment and referrals to secondary services are kept to a minimum. Members of the teams have learned how to support GPs in maintaining clients in primary care. Perhaps the most powerful message from this chapter is that, in establishing client-centred services, there should be as little organisational interference as possible. Local managers should have the authority to shape services that fulfil the aspirations of both clients and staff. The author takes pride in what has been achieved and reminds readers that having informed, involved and enthusiastic colleagues is an essential prerequisite to discovering and implementing what actually works on the ground. (Editors' summary)

REFERENCES

Department of Health (1999) *National Service Framework for Mental Health*, The Stationery Office, London

7 COLLABORATIVE CARE FOR PEOPLE WITH SEVERE AND ENDURING MENTAL ILLNESS

Helen Lester, Jim Cody and Neil Deuchar

This chapter examines the long-overlooked needs of people who suffer from severe and enduring mental illness (SEMI). It is entirely appropriate, given their historical neglect, that these clients have received much attention over the last two decades. Getting services right for them will inevitably improve services for everyone with mental health difficulties. The authors recognise that SEMI clients often have general health problems as well as multiple social disadvantages, and demonstrate what can be achieved for them through collaboration and teamworking. There is a strong sense of the commitment of the authors to developing good practice, and the pride and satisfaction they have experienced from their achievements. As the authors remark, vision and commitment are far more valuable than mere financial resources. There is nothing like success to sustain an initiative and the model of good practice described here represents a resounding success story, and should certainly be emulated elsewhere. (Editors' note)

INTRODUCTION

Twenty-five per cent of the adult population of the UK experience some kind of mental health problem in any one year; about half will present with the problem to the primary care team. Of these, the vast majority (around 98%) will have a common mental health problem (CMHP), and the remainder will be suffering from a severe mental illness (SMI); an even smaller number within this group will be suffering from a severe and enduring mental illness (SEMI) such as schizophrenia or bipolar affective disorder. SEMI is therefore an uncommon occurrence in primary care but, because of its chronicity, its prevalence in the community is disproportionately high – 0.5% to 1% depending on the location and methodology of the surveys (Goldberg and Huxley, 1980; Goldberg, 1991).

The average GP, with a list size of 2,000 people, can expect to see around 250 new cases per year of mental health problems, of whom five will have SMI and perhaps one will have SEMI. At any one time, however, there will be around 10 to 20 people registered with the GP who suffer SEMI.

The collaboration described here is between an inner-city group practice and a community mental health team (CMHT), both of which are committed to innovative and interactive models of mental health-care delivery across the primary/secondary care interface. The Colston Health Centre is a partnered practice in central Birmingham with a list size of 7400. The time covered by GPs (some full-time, some part-time) at the centre equates to that of four full-time GPs. The Ladywood Primary Care Liaison (PCL) CMHT is a functionalised team working alongside home treatment, assertive outreach and rehabilitation teams within the Ladywood locality of Northern Birmingham Mental Health Trust. Functionalised mental health teams are those that diversify into assertive outreach, rehabilitation, intensive home treatment and home liaison. This is in contrast to more traditional CMHTs, which carry out all these activities. The PCL team has an active caseload of approximately 950 clients, of whom around 400 were recently audited as suffering from SEMI. The team is well staffed, with community psychiatric nurses (CPNs) and social workers, and there are two nurse therapists and two occupational therapists as well. The Ladywood locality itself is one of the more deprived inner-city areas of Great Britain, with a Jarman index of 50.

This chapter briefly discusses current issues relating to the delivery of health care to people with SEMI in the primary care setting, then describes in more detail the anatomy of the process of collaboration between us and, finally, our plans for the future. For a formulation of our current interpretation of CMHP, SMI and SEMI, *see* Appendix I, page 265.

CASE STUDY MM

This client with complex problems, including SEMI, was helped by one manifestation of the process of collaboration between us – the development in the practice of a maintenance and monitoring clinic for clients with SEMI registered with the health centre.

MM is a 57-year-old divorced lady who lives with her eldest daughter in a semi-detached house in the north of the city of Birmingham. She was born in Jamaica but moved to England with her parents when she was eight years old. She worked in a shop after leaving school with few formal qualifications, and married when she was 22. Her two children were born when she was 23 and 25 years old. She had her first episode of psychotic illness when she was 27 years old and was admitted to a local psychiatric hospital for eight weeks. This was the first of three admissions, all of which occurred during the first five years of her illness. Her pharmacological treatment initially comprised chlorpromazine and a trial of lithium but her mental state continued to be unpredictable, the situation being exacerbated by her dislike of taking medication because of the side-effects. Her marriage broke down when the children were still young and she was divorced at 30. She never remarried.

MM has received a depot injection every two to four weeks and procyclidine tablets for potential side-effects for the past 15 years. Her mental state has been more stable for the past 10 years with no admissions or requirements for episodes of intensive home treatment. However, she continued to dislike having the depot injection and typically required considerable outreach by her community psychiatric nurse (CPN) when she missed appointments at the psychiatric hospital-based depot clinic.

MM developed non insulin-dependent diabetes eight years ago at the age of 49. She still has some difficulty in accepting the diagnosis and her adherence to tablets and diet has been erratic. Blood glucose and HbA1c results show that her diabetes control is less than optimal although monitoring is complicated by her dislike of having blood tests. MM is looked after by the practice-led diabetic team and attends yearly retinopathy screening checks.

The establishment of a maintenance and monitoring clinic at the Colston Health Centre in 1998 led to a number of positive changes in the care offered to MM and her family. The practice is closer to MM's house than the hospital-based depot clinic. Although MM still doesn't like having the injection, her attendance has improved since the start of the practice-based clinic, which may be a function of proximity and familiarity and perhaps of the less stigmatising setting of the practice. The decreased travelling time also means that her daughter now occasionally brings her to the depot clinic and her family feels more informed and involved in her care. Where possible, psychiatric, diabetic and general medical appointments are made on the same morning, enabling the daughter to see a number of health-care professionals about her mother's overall health in one visit. The receptionists, now more readily able to recognise MM as a depot clinic attendee with complex needs, can give her extra help in accessing other practice-based services if this is required.

The development of the depot clinic has also led to further collaboration between the CPNs and the primary care team, which has proved fruitful for MM's care. Her dislike of blood tests, for example, which had created some difficulty in monitoring her glucose control in the past, has been helped by the CPN occasionally taking the blood tests. MM seems more accepting of this. The practice nurses and GPs are also now more aware of MM's mental health and can monitor this during diabetes appointments. Concerns can then be discussed where appropriate with the family, with the CPNs in person on a weekly basis, at monthly consultation-liaison meetings with the consultant psychiatrist, or by writing in the medical notes. This collaboration between clinical teams has resulted in better communication and mutual education between the practice and community mental health teams. MM's primary care has also become more holistic, with mental health and physical health no longer seen as separate issues, or the compartmentalised responsibilities of different teams.

PRIMARY OR SECONDARY CARE?

The National Service Framework for Mental Health (Department of Health, 1999) articulates unambiguously that the majority of people suffering from CMHPs should have their needs assessed by a primary health-care team that can offer effective treatments and refer to specialist services if appropriate. Anyone suffering from SMI and SEMI, on the other hand, would invariably be appropriately referred to secondary mental health services, where they would come to be managed under the auspices of the Care Programme Approach. A consultant psychiatrist would become the responsible medical officer for the person's mental health care at the point of acceptance into specialist services.

This division of health service provision in the UK into primary and secondary care is probably efficient but poses the problem of where particular patients are best managed. While the NSF seeks to clarify this (and in this respect it is an extremely helpful document), a problem remains: once psychiatric patients are accepted into secondary care services, their primary health care needs often become overlooked. Alternatively, a reductionist model is adopted, whereby the responsibility for managing the various components of the person's difficulties become mutually abrogated between primary and secondary medical staff.

It seems to us to be a more reasonable proposition for primary and secondary carers to contribute in a collaborative fashion to the holistic and more seamless management of patients suffering SEMI.

There is no doubt that GPs have seen an increasing number of people with SEMI following the introduction of community care for the mentally ill (Kendrick *et al.*, 1991), and that a significant number of people with SEMI are only seen in primary care. Indeed, people with SEMI may exhibit a higher than average consultation rate in general practice (Kendrick *et al.*, 1994) and, furthermore, some 30% of such people may be receiving their overall medical care solely from GPs (Kendrick *et al.*, 2000). Despite this, there is a paucity of information relating to the best way to provide primary health care for people with SEMI (Burns and Kendrick, 1997) and fragmented opinion as to what kind of role GPs could have (Kendrick *et al.*, 1991). This is alarming and requires urgent attention as, in our view, primary care possesses a number of strengths that should be key to providing good quality of care for people with SEMI. The primary care team, for example, may have known the person before they became ill; they may be more alert to changes in behaviour that may precede a relapse; they may know the family; and they may be able to offer longer-term continuity of care. In addition, treatment in primary care may be more accessible and less stigmatising than that available in a community mental health resource centre.

ISSUES OF PHYSICAL ILLNESS

The other potential strength of a primary care-led approach to SEMI is the possibility of better physical health care for people with SEMI. Such patients are entitled to the full range of both mental and physical health care available to non-sufferers of SEMI, but they are also more likely than non-sufferers to suffer overt or undetected non-psychiatric disorders. It has been reported, for example, that 41% of a sample of patients receiving treatment for long-term mental illness at a psychiatric day care facility suffered medical problems requiring intervention; 44% of them appeared to have had their needs unmet, according to pathological screening (Brugha *et al.*, 1989). Furthermore, over half of a sample of people with long-term mental illness in a community support programme had previously undiagnosed medical problems; one-third of them had problems that, once detected, precipitated a refreshed episode of specialist medical intervention (Farmer, 1988). A high prevalence of complex neurological and other medical problems was reported in a cohort of long-stay psychiatric patients, deinstitutionalised into the community from three large psychiatric hospitals in Birmingham (Deuchar *et al.*, 1995).

Unrecognised and under-treated physical illness may help us to understand why there is both increased morbidity and mortality in people with long-term mental illness (Allebeck, 1989; Brown, 1997). Standardised mortality ratios for people with schizophrenia, for instance, are more than double the population norms. This has been found to be largely due to doubled cardiovascular and respiratory disorder mortality rates. Other relevant associations include higher rates of smoking, hypertension, side-effects of neuroleptic medication such as weight gain, and self-neglect or poor living conditions outside hospital confines (Brugha *et al.*, 1989).

Patients with SEMI fail to receive the level of physical health screening and education enjoyed by other patient groups within primary care. For example, GPs rarely intervene in or discuss cardiovascular and respiratory risk factors in this patient population (Kendrick, 1996). In addition, patients with SEMI may be reticent about discussing their general health because of the lack of self-confidence or the apathy that can characterise chronic mental illness (Wing, 1989). Part of the problem may also lie in the fact that, in contrast to the situation for patients with a chronic physical illness such as asthma, where practices are likely to keep patient disease registers, follow treatment protocols, and offer structured specialist clinic care, few practices keep registers of patients with SEMI, have specific policies or offer structured assessments to address their needs (Kendrick *et al.*, 1991).

ISSUES IN GENERAL PRACTICE

The role of the GP

The majority of GPs appear to regard their role in the care of people with SEMI as being limited to physical illness and prescribing, with only a fifth regarding themselves as involved in the monitoring and treatment of mental illness (Kendrick *et al.*, 1991; Bindman *et al.*, 1997). More worrying still, 10% of GPs seem not to want to accept responsibility even for the physical health care needs of the long-term mentally ill, with 22% declining to undertake medical screening procedures in this patient population (Kendrick *et al.*, 1991). This may be because GPs lack confidence in managing mental health issues (Kendrick *et al.*, 1995); this, in turn, may be a reflection of the fact that only 25% of GPs overall have held a postgraduate psychiatric post (Kendrick *et al.*, 1991).

It is not all bad news, however. GPs seem generally aware of the importance of improving their skills in the care of people with mental health problems, and some have identified management of psychiatric emergencies as a training priority (Kerwick *et al.*, 1997). Moreover, a recent study of GPs' views of the care of schizophrenia in general practice found that, overall, they wanted to make things better, and that they generally supported enhanced liaison with secondary mental health services (Nazareth *et al.*, 1995).

The relatively recent publication by the Primary Care Schizophrenia Consensus Group has also been encouraging. Its study of the management of schizophrenia in primary care takes as a model the structured care offered to people with a chronic physical illness (Burns and Kendrick, 1997). A first step in operationalising such a model of structured care might be the establishment of a register of practice patients identified as suffering from SEMI – the feasibility of this in a computerised and relatively well-organised practice has been demonstrated (Nazareth *et al.*, 1993). With such a register in place, it should be possible to check when the patient was last seen in secondary care, their current status (for example, are they on the supervision register? What is their CPA status?), to flag the primary care records appropriately and identify when a physical review last took place. Six-monthly structured assessments for those on the register would most probably enhance primary care involvement and positively affect the overall process of care.

If time constraints preclude undertaking such assessments in the course of routine practice, a separate clinic session model has been shown not only to be feasible, but also to have a measurable effect on clinical outcome (Nazareth *et al.*, 1996). Furthermore, it is known that paying GPs an item-of-service payment of £85 per annum for monitoring people with SEMI was successful in ensuring GPs undertook the assessments (Burns and Cohen, 1998). The most reliable method of expediting a chronic physical disease model of primary care management of people with SEMI has been found to be through a nurse-led specialist clinic (Burns *et al.*, 1998).

Assessments and client-held records

In our opinion, the content of regular assessments might logically comprise the checking of social and environmental factors such as events since last review, accommodation, the situation regarding carers and supporters, contact with social services, activities of daily living, employment and benefits; an assessment of the person's current mental state; an overview of their physical health, comprising health promotion and prevention, nutritional status, hearing, vision, dental and chiropody needs and contraception; and a review of medication with due attention to side-effects, polypharmacy and the patient's concordance with the pharmaco-logical strategy (adapted from the Sainsbury Centre review, 1998).

The views of mental health services users would tend to support such a strategy (Rogers and Pilgrim, 1993). Recent work in Birmingham found that one group of users – none of whom had had a specific review by their GP in the previous 12 months – were all in favour of a practice register of people with mental health problems, and all felt that guidelines for care were a good idea (Bailey, 1997).

There has been some optimism in respect of the development of client-held mental health records. These may be of particular value for patients taking lithium or those who have to interact with a large number of health and social services, and may represent a potential source of better communication between primary and secondary services, while investing in the client some badly needed ownership. A recent evaluation of such a scheme found that 80% of patients found the record useful and that 74% of contacts were recorded by professionals in the record (Laugherne and Stafford, 1996).

A randomised controlled trial of the use of a patient-held medical record for people with SEMI in Birmingham is about to be reported. The early signs are that the record has enhanced communication across the primary/secondary interface and has therefore encouraged the involvement of primary carers in the shared care of people with SEMI.

The role of the practice nurse

It may become appropriate to expand the role of practice nurses. In one large study, 61% of nurses were found to be administering depot injections and 44% were giving advice about antidepression medication (Gray and Plummer, 1997). In another study, 62% of practice nurses reported that up to 20% of their workload concerned mental health problems in consultations. A majority (80%) harboured concerns about their ability to address mental health problems effectively. However, 61% were keen to expand this role, if appropriate support and training were available (Crosland and Kai, 1998). This willingness, allied to the rapid expansion of practice nurses in primary care, may create practical opportunities for the expansion of the range of structured services available for people with SEMI in primary care.

THE COLSTON HEALTH CENTRE

There may be some justification, therefore, for suggesting not only that primary care becomes more involved with managing SEMI, but also that primary and secondary care teams should work together more effectively in this endeavour. We have attempted to respond to this perceived need by developing a multifaceted model of interaction across the primary/secondary interface at the Colston Health Centre.

The first step was for the general practitioner (HL) and the psychiatrist (ND) to get together on a regular basis to take things forward. This was undertaken in June 1998 within a consultation-liaison model (Creed and Marks, 1989; Gask *et al.*, 1997). Soon after his appointment as consultant psychiatrist in primary care liaison in the Ladywood locality of Birmingham, ND began visiting the practice on a monthly basis in order to meet and get to know the partners. He was able to offer support and advice about managing patients with mental health problems in primary care; consider potential referrals for specialist mental heath care; learn about the issues facing the GPs; and educate the GPs about the Trust, the kinds of services it offers, and how to access them. This soon led to excellent relations between the health centre and the consultant psychiatrist, with various new channels of communication being opened up (including use of a mobile phone for quick consultations or advice; written communications in the first person; e-mail dialogues; liaison with regard to undergraduate training in matters of mental health; and mutual invitations to teach each other's disciplines about mental health practice at a postgraduate level).

Two mental health professionals thereafter became attached to the practice as in the model described by Bailey and colleagues (1994). One was a CPN, whose initial role was to sift ('triage') patients presenting to the practice with CMHPs into the following groups:

- those whose problems did not require medicalisation (the CPN would then arrange for an appropriate community response, for example, giving advice to contact RELATE or CRUSE);
- those whose problems were appropriately medicalised in a primary care setting (the CPN would then work with the GPs in treating them); and

- those for whom specialist mental health input was thought to be potentially relevant (and bring them to ND's attention at one of two multidisciplinary clinical meetings held every week at the CMHT offices in Ladywood).

The other mental health worker was (and still is) a nurse therapist. This therapist began to practise a number of integrated therapies with clients with both CMHPs and emotionally unstable personality disorders at the practice, liaising closely with the partners at mutually convenient times. (Integrated therapies are those that use, or integrate, techniques from various different types of therapy; for example, cognitive analytical therapy espouses principles of both CBT and expressive psychodynamic therapy.)

After a while, the CPN and the practice nursing staff began to get to know one another and discussions between us all began to focus on the needs of registered clients who suffered with SEMI. We discussed the issues outlined above and decided to make a start with patients registered with the practice who were in receipt of depot medication, because they were relatively easy to identify and work with. A pilot scheme was initiated in November 1998, involving a total of 20 patients who had hitherto received their injections either at home or at a pre-existing monitoring and maintenance clinic located at All Saints Hospital (now closed), about 5 miles from the practice. The patients were advised that they would now be receiving their injections at the Colston Health Centre. The potential advantages (less stigma and an opportunity to benefit from greater holism in terms of the overall care) were explained to them.

For some figures relating to our experience of this service, *see* Table 7.1. After some initial teething problems and adjustments, there has virtually been a 100% attendance record since May 1999. This compares to a total attendance rate of around 70% at the depot clinic for other patients with SEMI at the CMHT offices in Ladywood.

Table 7.1 Maintenance and monitoring clinic, Colston Health Centre (start date 16.11.98)

Month	Attended	Failed to attend	Visited	Discharged	Admission/re-admission	Died
Nov 1998	16	3	3	0	0	0
Dec 1998	22	3	3	0	0	0
Jan 1999	19	4	4	0	0	0
Feb 1999	22	0	0	0	0	0
Mar 1999	25	1	1	0	0	0
Apr 1999	20	2	2	0	0	0
May 1999	21	0	0	0	0	0
Jun 1999	27	1	1	0	0	0
Jul 1999	22	0	0	0	0	0
Aug 1999	28	0	0	0	0	0
Sep 1999	18	1	1	0	0	0
Oct 1999	20	0	0	0	0	0
Nov 1999	25	0	0	0	0	0
Dec 1999	20	0	0	0	0	0
TOTAL	306	12	12	0	0	0

The depot injections are administered by the attached CPN and opportunities have arisen to discuss the patients with both the partners of the practice and with the primary care nursing staff. The nursing staff have, in turn, become more interested in and informed about not only the patients themselves but also wider issues pertaining to SEMI. We have eschewed the model of the shifted outpatient clinic (Strathdee and Williams, 1984), because we do not believe it encourages integration of management. In our view, shifted outpatient clinics merely perpetuate the compartmentalisation that bedevils traditional outpatient models in secondary care. In addition, not only do we suspect that health-care professionals conducting such clinics feel isolated from their specialist bases and less than integrated in the primary care setting, but we also feel that the vital ingredient of face-to-face interaction between primary and secondary staff is not encouraged by such a model.

BENEFITS OF THE COLLABORATION

Through the collaboration we believe we have achieved a better and more enjoyable working framework for both primary care and mental health staff. The new positivity has rubbed off on the clients, who are able to benefit from a more coherent and cohesive approach to their problems from their doctors and nurses, and have begun to perceive the health care services they receive as internally consistent and reliable. We believe that these benefits have extended not only to those patients we collectively manage with SEMI, but also to a number of other types of patients who present to primary care with a range of non-psychotic disorders. At one time, such patients would have had these problems managed in a disjointed style by a psychiatrist, communicating only in the form of long and predominantly irrelevant letters to the referring GP, who could not find the time to read them properly.

The outcome from our collaboration, in terms of benefits for both clients and for us, has far outweighed the time and effort invested. No massive additional resources have been necessary – the infrastructure has always been there and it was just a case of making some minor lifestyle adjustments at work. In essence, the change that was required was one of attitude and approach; the vital ingredient was reciprocity; and the driving force was a perception that things were not right and a sense of enthusiasm to correct the situation. The CPN finds the health centre a pleasant place to see clients but also benefits from retaining a sense of belonging to the specialist mental health team. The psychiatrist benefits from an easy-going relationship with a primary care team that has, through rational debate, acquired realistic expectations of what he can and can't provide. And the GPs have benefited from a much more meaningful and sensitive response from the specialist mental health team.

THE FUTURE

We now want to take things further. We plan to establish a computerised register of all patients registered with the practice who suffer from SEMI, and not just those receiving depot medication. As our use of atypical antipsychotics and the deployment of psychosocial strategies aimed at reintegrating patients with SEMI back into community life increases, our usage of injections will dwindle. We want to enable easier monitoring of patients with bipolar affective disorder by installing a desktop lithium assay in the practice, effectively negating the need for anyone suffering from this disorder to go anywhere near a hospital or mental health centre.

We want to build on our initial success in the use of client-held medical records, particularly for those who interact with a number of different agencies and/or who have complex mixes of both mental and physical disorder. We want to establish a protocol for the structured management of people with SEMI with proper contemporaneous multidisciplinary input (perhaps in the form of six-monthly CPA reviews under the control of an automatic recall system, which ensures that all relevant health and social services professionals are invited along with the patient).

We want to develop a model of shared responsibility between GP and psychiatrist (perhaps even abandoning the hackneyed term 'RMO', which, in our view, has little relevance away from an in-patient environment). We want to examine the evidence base and develop a shared vision for rational prescribing for all mental disorders; and agree about who prescribes what and push to have our decisions endorsed by the Trust and the Primary Care Group (PCG).

We are interested in seeing how such a pilot would work in other practices in the PCG. Duplicating the effort in other similarly sized group practices will be relatively simple, given the need for flexibility and appropriating the approach to suit the attitudes, temperaments and knowledge base of the primary care team involved. There are, however, a number of single-handed practices in the PCG and these represent a particular challenge, in terms of the logistics (particularly the time management of secondary care staff having to cover a number of different practices, each with relatively modest list sizes), and the high proportion of non-English speakers registered with these GPs.

ND is currently in the process of negotiating with these GPs on the subject of forming 'consortia' of four or five members who can collectively be 'serviced' by the mental health team (and particularly members of the team who speak several languages) in a very similar manner to that described for the group practice. In these cases, clients with SEMI registered with members of the consortia would attend a designated practice for the purposes of their care and reviews, perhaps with a 'lead GP' identified as either taking on the physical health needs of the clients or communicating to their own GP what needs to be done. Another possibility would be for patients on such a shared register to re-register with the lead GP, either for everything or perhaps just for their mental health care. (The problem with the latter strategy is that it invokes a built-in schism of just the kind that we are trying to eradicate.)

We are aware that, while at face value all these interventions have a great deal of potential, it will be vital to monitor our activities and measure the effects rigorously. We are therefore developing protocols for auditing and researching the changes; some of the research instruments used in previous surveys of the physical and emotional fate of those discharged from hospitals into the community will be helpful (after all, we are in essence attempting to dismantle the institution of outpatients along very similar lines). However, we will need to focus on ways of measuring levels of social and occupational integration in particular, as the process of 'normalisation' seems central to this effort.

A REINTEGRATIVE APPROACH

We are aware of the government's assertion that community care has 'failed'. Frankly, we disagree. We think that deinstitutionalisation has been a force for the good and that the majority of patients who suffer SEMI are incalculably better off outside a hospital environment. We feel that the majority of people who suffer from SEMI are, just as they have always been, more vulnerable to discrimination, persecution and marginalisation than they are dangerous. Proper and diligent risk assessment should continue to inform decision-making; this type of highly reintegrative approach should not only meet the needs of our patients but also defer appropriately to the interests of the public.

The implications of a reintegrative approach in terms of the general public's exposure to the mentally ill should be reframed, from an ostensibly negative viewpoint ('I don't want a schizophrenic sitting next to me') to a refreshed initiative espousing public education. Appropriate reassurance will reduce stigma, and primary prevention will be possible via mental health promotion, which should be everyone's business. The potential contribution of people with mental health problems and their carers to these strategies is enormous. Meaningful collaboration between 'them' and 'us' can only serve to facilitate the necessary culture change. However, if we, as their doctors and nurses, cannot find common ground and work together, what hope is there for change elsewhere?

The 'nuts and bolts' of providing more 'innovative' services for people with SEMI are already there. We need to break down the barriers of ignorance and fear, which appear to demotivate so many potential health-care providers. The process will need to espouse both undergraduate and postgraduate education, plenty of support and encouragement, and the broadcasting of simple but consistent messages about logical approaches to the problem.

The authors have shown how, with no extra resources, but with a great deal of vision, goodwill and regular face-to-face contact, services for people with SEMI can be transformed. Ample evidence is provided that services for such clients are best delivered in the primary care setting, where they can be arranged around the needs of the client, rather than in the cumbersome and complex structure of secondary care, where their primary health care needs are often neglected. It emphasises the potential that good relationships can unleash and the way they can lead to better education, better collaboration, better working relationships and, ultimately, better utilisation of the resources that reside in both primary and secondary care. The authors observe that the physical health care needs of clients are better addressed by primary care personnel and this can only result in better care for people whose physical health is known to be poor.

*Better collaboration between services can lead to a recognition of the impor-
tance of primary care receptionists and the vital part they can play in meeting the
needs of people with mental health problems and in health promotion. Where a
culture of collaboration is fostered, personnel appear to converse, consult and
seek help better than they do in environments where strict roles are adhered to
and disciplines operate separately. When GPs see the benefits of collaboration,
nurses begin to work more closely together, and the expertise of a community
psychiatrist enriches the service. The degree of collaboration reported above is
rendered much easier through the use of mobile phones; doubtless, future developments in technology will assist it even further. The strong message of this
chapter is that, where there is good collaboration, mutual respect for each other
and a recognition that the clients' welfare is the main objective, job satisfaction
increases and staff feel at ease with themselves and with each other. Perhaps the
most significant aspect of this chapter is the fact that the team members have
several areas that they wish to develop in the future. Realising that services can
be improved, and knowing that it is 'allowed', is one of the best ways of being a
stakeholder in those services. (Editors' summary)*

REFERENCES

Allebeck, P. (1989) Schizophrenia: a life-shortening disease, *Schizophrenia Bulletin*, **15**, 81–89

Bailey, D. (1997) What is the way forwards for a user-led approach to the delivery of mental health services in primary care? *Journal of Mental Health*, **6**, 101–105

Bailey, J., Black, M. and Wilkin, D. (1994) Specialist outreach clinics in general practice, *British Medical Journal*, **308**, 1083–1086

Bindman, J., Johnson, S., Wright S. *et al.* (1997) Integration between primary and secondary services in the care of the severely mentally ill: patients' and general practitioners' views, *British Journal of Psychiatry*, **171**, 169–174

Brown, S. (1997) Excess mortality of schizophrenia, *British Journal of Psychiatry*, **171**, 502–508

Brugha, T.S., Wing, J.K. and Smith, B. (1989) Physical health of the long-term mentally ill in the community – is there unmet need? *British Journal of Psychiatry*, **155**, 777–781

Burns, T. and Cohen, A. (1998) Item-of-service payments for GP care of severely mentally ill persons, *British Journal of General Practice*, **48**, 1415–1416

Burns, T. and Kendrick, T. (1997) The primary care of patients with schizophrenia: a search of good practice, *British Journal of General Practice*, **47**, 515–520

Burns, T., Millar, E., Garland, C., Kendrick, T., Chisholm, B. and Ross, F. (1998) Randomised controlled trial of teaching practice nurses to carry out structured assessment of patients receiving depot antipsychotic injections, *British Journal of General Practice*, **48**, 1845–1848

Creed, F. and Marks, B. (1989) Liaison psychiatry in general practice: a comparison of the liaison attachment scheme and shifted outpatient clinic models, *Journal of the Royal College of General Practitioners*, **39**, 514–517

Crosland, A. and Kai, J. (1998) 'They think they can talk to nurses': practice nurses' views of their roles in caring for mental health problems, *British Journal of General Practice*, **48**, 1383–1386

Department of Health (1999) *National Service Framework for Mental Health*, Department of Health, London

Deuchar, N., Cumella, S., Chung, M.C., Mohan, R. *et al.* (1995) Physical morbidity in a long-stay psychiatric population scheduled for relocation: the extent of the problem and its impact on successful placement, *European Journal of Psychiatry*, 9, 179–187

Farmer, S. (1988) Medical problems of chronic patients in a community support program, *Hospital and Community Psychiatry*, 38, 745–749

Gask, L., Sibbald, B. and Creed, F. (1997) Evaluating models of working at the interface between mental health services and primary care, *British Journal of Psychiatry*, 170, 6–11

Goldberg, D. (1991) Filters to care. In Jenkins, R. and Griffiths, S. (eds.) *Indicators for Mental Health in the Population*, HMSO, London

Goldberg, D. and Huxley, P. (1980) *Mental Illness in the Community: The pathway to psychiatric care*, Tavistock, London

Gray, R. and Plummer, S. (1997) *A national survey of practice nurse involvement in mental health interventions*, Institute of Psychiatry, London

Kendrick, A. (1996) Cardiovascular and respiratory risk factors and symptoms among general practice patients with a long-term mental illness, *British Journal of Psychiatry*, 169, 733–739

Kendrick, T., Sibbald, B., Burns, T. *et al.* (1991) Role of general practitioners in care of long-term mentally ill patients, *British Medical Journal*, 302, 508–510

Kendrick, T., Burns, T., Freeling, P. and Sibbald, B. (1994) Provision of care to general practice patients with disabling long-term mental illness: a survey of 16 practices, *British Journal of General Practice*, 44, 301–305

Kendrick, T., Burns, T. and Freeling, P. (1995) A randomised controlled trial of teaching general practitioners to carry out structured assessments of their long-term mentally ill patients, *British Medical Journal*, 311, 93–98

Kendrick, T., Burns, T., Garland, C., Greenwood, N. and Smith, P. (2000) Are specialist mental health services being targeted on the most needy patients? The effects of setting up special services in general practice, *British Journal of General Practice*, 50, 121–126

Kerwick, S., Jones, R., Mann, A. and Goldberg, D. (1997) Mental health training priorities in general practice, *British Journal of General Practice*, 47, 225-227

Laugherne, R. and Stafford, A. (1996) Access to records and client-held records for people with mental illness: a literature review, *Psychiatric Bulletin*, 20, 338–341

Nazareth, I., King, M., Haines, A., Rangel, L. and Myers, S. (1993) Accuracy of diagnosis of psychosis on general practice computer system, *British Medical Journal*, 307, 32–34

Nazareth, I., King, M. and Davies, S. (1995) Care of schizophrenia in general practice; the general practitioners and the patient, *British Journal of General Practice*, 45, 343–347

Nazareth, I., King, M. and Tai, S. (1996) Monitoring psychosis in general practice: a controlled trial, *British Journal of Psychiatry*, 169, 475–82

Rogers, A. and Pilgrim, D. (1993) *Experiencing Psychiatry: Users' views of services*, Macmillan Press, London

Sainsbury Centre for Mental Health (1998) *Keys to Engagement: review of care for people with severe mental illness who are hard to engage with services*, The Sainsbury Centre, London

Strathdee, G. and Williams, P. (1984) A survey of psychiatrists in primary care: the silent growth of a new service, *Journal of the Royal College of General Practitioners*, 34, 615–618

Wing, J.K. (1989) The concept of negative symptoms, *British Journal of Psychiatry*, 144, 10–14

8 TOWARDS ESTABLISHING MORE EFFECTIVE COLLABORATION IN THE CARE OF PEOPLE WITH PERSONALITY DISORDERS

Mary Tyson and James Briscoe

The concept of personality disorder has received an increasing amount of attention in recent years. However, controversy continues about the usefulness, the reliability and the validity of personality disorder diagnosis. People may stand on different sides of the debate, but it has to be recognised that clients who show patterns of thought, emotion and behaviour more or less consistent with personality disorder diagnostic criteria continue to present frequently to a range of statutory and voluntary services, often in crisis and apparently without benefiting substantially from any forms of intervention. They may suffer considerable emotional distress; they may cause distress to others; additionally, they cost a great deal of public money, because many of them are likely to become 'revolving-door' service users. Improving health workers' awareness of contemporary theoretical models and empirical studies, which trace the pathways to disruption in personality development, together with sustained efforts to collaborate across disciplines, may improve the care and management of people in this group. However, a number of impediments to collaboration need to be acknowledged and addressed. (Editors' note)

INTRODUCTION

Prior to about 1990, it was rare to see mention of the term 'personality disorder' in any British journal covering mental health issues; within the last decade, however, there has been a flurry of activity in the area, with a number of publications on the topic, conferences devoted to personality disorder and a growing demand for relevant training. Clearly, health professionals are recognising within their client group individuals who appear to fit the personality disorder rubric. These clients have long-standing difficulties, which pervade a number of areas of their life (such as occupational and social). While many of them do not appear to suffer from what is conventionally regarded as 'mental illness', they are likely to have episodic, recurrent anxiety and/or depression, or possibly transient psychotic-type experiences. It is not uncommon for them to present repeatedly with unexplained physical symptoms. Conventional treatments do not seem to work well. This can be a frustrating state of affairs for clients and health workers alike.

Unsurprisingly, some health professionals are eager to seize on the personality disorder label as a means of managing the frustration and the sense of impotence that working with these clients often engenders. Faced with a confusing problem, they feel better about it if they can 'get a handle' on it. However, detailed exploration of the personality construct reveals that it is fraught with difficulty in a whole host of ways:

- the diagnostic criteria laid out in psychiatric diagnostic manuals (World Health Organisation, 1992; American Psychiatric Association, 1994) leave room for considerable subjectivity of judgement on the part of any clinician looking to apply a personality disorder label;
- there is a diagnostic criteria overlap;
- the criteria are based on clinical consensus; they are not theory-derived or founded on a body of empirical research;
- getting two or more clinicians to agree on diagnosis, relying solely on their clinical judgement, is notoriously difficult;
- attempting to improve diagnostic reliability by using questionnaires or structured interviews brings in additional problems (such as over-diagnosis).

In addition to these problems with lack of adequately tight conceptualisation and statistical validity, practical objections to diagnosing personality disorder have been raised:

- applying a personality disorder diagnosis constitutes pejorative labelling;
- it is pointless to diagnose personality disorder because the diagnosis does not point the way towards treatments that can be used;
- the diagnosis is unhelpful because it does not convey anything about the cause or causes of the alleged disorder;
- a perusal of individual medical records often indicates that a label of personality disorder may be given, without the clinician checking to see whether the person's presentation meets the specified diagnostic criteria; in other words, the diagnosis may be applied in a less than systematic way.

For all these reasons, some argue in favour of jettisoning diagnosis of personality disorder altogether. Others would claim that the constellations of features described in the diagnostic criteria are indeed found in routine clinical practice. The latter group believe that, while the days of the personality disorder construct may be numbered, there is merit in retaining it for now, as it serves a purpose as a valuable organising principle, enabling thought about clients that might otherwise be neglected (Higgitt and Fonagy, 1992).

The jury is still out on the matter. In any case, it is clear that theoretical debates are not the sole or the main issue to which attention should be turned. The individuals currently grouped under the personality disorder umbrella need to be understood and cared for respectfully. To this end, using all the tools available, including diagnostic procedures (as long as they are followed carefully) may be the most circumspect approach at this point.

A diagnosis is like a snapshot – a *cross-sectional* approach to encapsulating an individual's difficulties. This is to be contrasted with a *longitudinal formulation* – an individual explanatory model, based on a lifespan approach, and incorporating all causal factors (drawing on existing clinical knowledge and empirical evidence) that appear to apply. In each individual case, such a formulation needs to be constructed, either alongside, or instead of a diagnosis. Arriving at a comprehensive formulation takes time and will often involve a pooling of the information available to a range of health professionals who have had (and perhaps are still having) contact with the client. When a formulation has been arrived at, collaborative working will often be essential to the successful implementation of the care plan. All those involved need to have an accurate, up-to-date picture of the current state of knowledge about personality disorder, to inform their thinking about the client, and their responses to that person.

Throughout the processes of assessment, formulation, construction of a care plan, and putting the care plan into action, there are numerous pitfalls. This chapter highlights some of these and offers suggestions about how they might be tackled. A number of general considerations might be borne in mind by health professionals seeking to relate productively to clients with personality disorder. The focus we adopt is based on ideas from attachment theory (Bowlby, 1980), cognitive therapy (Beck and Freeman, 1990) and cognitive analytic therapy (Ryle, 1997). Our argument throughout is that the following tenets lie at the core of care and management of this group of people:

- understanding the beliefs about self and others held by people with personality disorders, initially developed in significant early relationships and perpetuated through processes of selective attention and reinforcement;
- tracing the interpersonal behavioural patterns related to these beliefs; and
- paying close attention to our responses as professionals.

For an understanding of the technical aspects of current approaches to assessment and treatment of personality disorder, refer to works by Millon and Davis (2000) and to the clinical practice guideline published by the Department of Health (2001).

CHARACTERISTICS OF CLIENTS WITH PERSONALITY DISORDERS: CASE STUDIES

Largely because of the publicity surrounding recent high-profile murder cases in Britain (Fred and Rosemary West, Thomas Hamilton, Michael Stone), the image that most people have of an individual with personality disorder is of a 'psychopath' – a term that roughly corresponds to the category of 'antisocial personality disorder'. However, the personality disorder concept is much wider than this, as the following case studies illustrate.

CASE STUDY JOHN

John's difficulties came to the attention of health services when his brother contacted his GP requesting a domiciliary psychiatric visit. It was reported that John, aged 34 at the time, was becoming even more socially withdrawn than usual, increasingly unwilling to engage in any interaction with his mother and his brother, with whom he lived. He had recently been suspended from his job as a college computer technician, for allegedly assaulting a male colleague.

When John spoke to the psychiatrist who conducted the domiciliary visit, he insisted that he had struck the male colleague for a 'good reason' – the colleague was 'showing off'. John went on to tell the psychiatrist that he was attracted to his colleague's girlfriend and was jealous of him. He had secretly followed the woman home from work a couple of times. He had also followed other women in the past. As the consultation unfolded, John tried to explain what he called his 'main preoccupation'. This was a rather unusual system of thought revolving around football. Depending on which party was in government at any given time, John altered his allegiance to particular teams worldwide. The precise manner in which his preferences varied was elaborately documented on numerous scraps of paper, which he kept filed in a locked briefcase.

Unable to make sense of John's presentation, the psychiatrist requested further assessment by the community mental health team. After the psychiatrist's visit, John made a formal complaint, apparently furious because the psychiatrist had not been able to understand his 'preoccupation'.

Further assessment indicated that John had always been suspicious and mistrustful of others; he was a loner, with fantasies about taking revenge on all those he perceived as having been unjust to him. He revealed that he had a plan to flood the Internet with pornographic material. John instigated, or threatened to instigate, formal complaints against everyone in the mental health service with whom he came into contact . Eventually, he was prescribed low-dose neuroleptic medication and seen fortnightly for supportive therapy and monitoring of his mental state.

Commentary on John's case study

Prior to experiencing a stressor that exceeded his resources, and tipped him over from coping mode to not coping, John had had no contact with statutory services; his difficulties had been contained within the family and the community. While being seen as 'a bit of an oddball', no one expressed serious concerns about his wellbeing or about his potential risk to the wellbeing of others. In common with a number of people who are subsequently diagnosed with personality disorder (in this case, paranoid personality disorder with schizotypal features), John had a turbulent personal history. He had repeatedly been dismissed from jobs on account of his interpersonal difficulties and had never been able to sustain a close relationship. Further on in his contact with mental health services, it emerged that, in childhood, he had been in a family where the children were left to their own devices, with little adult supervision or support. He was physically beaten on a regular basis and had frequently witnessed domestic violence.

CASE STUDY   BRENDA

Brenda, aged 39, consulted her GP some months after the tragic death of her 21-year-old daughter in a house fire. The police had concluded that the death was due to suicide. Brenda was troubled by flashbacks, suicidal urges and uncontrollable anger.

This anger was leading her to avoid any dealings with people, so that she found it difficult to go into supermarkets or be in crowds of people. She was sent for bereavement counselling, but dropped out after a couple of sessions. The counsellor reported great difficulty in getting Brenda to engage; she repeatedly made and then cancelled appointments.

Some time later, Brenda went back to the GP, complaining of depression. Cognitive-behavioural therapy with a psychologist was suggested but, once again, Brenda dropped out prematurely. She subsequently returned to the GP about a year later, and was sent to a community mental health team for re-assessment. On this occasion, the assessing clinician, noting Brenda's apparent 'approach-avoidance' pattern of engaging with helping agents – she initiated contact, broke it off and then resumed help-seeking behaviour once more – decided that persistence was needed. Predictably, Brenda was equivocal about attending her appointments. By adopting an 'assertive outreach' approach (mainly through telephone contacts), consistently seeking to validate her current difficulties and instil a sense of hope that talking about her difficulties may help, the team encouraged Brenda to attend for several sessions where her life history was explored.

In these sessions, it emerged that Brenda's father had subjected her to childhood sexual abuse. She had developed a drug and alcohol habit as a young teenager. In her mid-teens, she became involved with a man by whom she had two daughters, both of whom claimed, at the ages of 10 and 11, that their father had sexually abused them. Social services had become involved, but Brenda persuaded her daughters to drop all charges. Brenda ended her relationship with her partner a couple of years later.

In the assessment sessions, Brenda started to talk about feeling guilty and responsible for her daughter's death. She made a connection between her own abuse and that of her daughters, voicing the view that perhaps she had stifled her daughters' revelations because they threatened to bring back her own abuse experiences and she was frightened of being overwhelmed by traumatic memories. Following this assessment, Brenda expressed a wish to undergo therapy to reflect on her own abuse and to understand the life choices that she had made in the wake of it.

Commentary on Brenda's case study

Brenda's case illustrates what can happen when health workers do not put information into a lifespan context. Taking a snapshot of her recent experience at the point at which she first presented to her GP, where 'problem onset' was defined as the point at which she suffered the loss of her daughter, led to a diagnosis of 'abnormal grieving reaction'; the suggested remedy was 'bereavement counselling'. The point at which she dropped out of the counselling was when the counsellor tried to persuade her that many people feel responsible when a loved one dies, but this is not real and she was not responsible for her daughter's death. This conflicted with Brenda's belief that she *did* bear genuine responsibility for her daughter's life going 'off course'. At this point, a breach occurred in the tenuous therapeutic bond that she had developed with the counsellor.

Similarly, when she presented with depression and the solution was seen as cognitive-behavioural therapy, Brenda felt that what she was trying to communicate, somewhat obliquely, was not being understood. Her frustration about this led her to drop out. In diagnostic terms, Brenda showed some features of borderline personality disorder, although at the time of her latest presentation, she did not meet enough diagnostic criteria for this diagnosis to be applied.

Brenda's case illustrates the use of dissociation in the face of trauma. Dissociation involves cutting out traumatic experiences from conscious awareness, in order to avoid being confronted by unmanageable emotions. Initially, it is a productive strategy for survival, but used habitually in the longer term it can often rebound on the individual. Following her abusive experiences, Brenda tried to 'blank out' what had happened to her by recourse to drugs and alcohol, both of which can be viewed as dissociative mechanisms. Through these means, she was able to prevent her consciousness from being flooded by painful memories. When in this blanked-out state, though, she inadvertently became involved with another abuser, and a further cycle of abuse began.

CASE STUDY   COLIN

Colin was a frequent visitor to his GP. From the age of 10, his medical history included investigations for chronic bronchitis, ulcers, irritable bowel syndrome, unexplained fits and a chronic back problem. He described himself as having been 'very close' to his mother and, shortly after her death, he took an overdose. The precipitating circumstances, according to Colin, were that his siblings were leaving him with all the responsibility for dealing with the funeral arrangements and his mother's estate, and that his partner, Will, was being very unsupportive of his predicament.

The GP referred him to a local mental health team, where he was seen by a CPN. The CPN tried to support Colin through the aftermath of his mother's death, but felt drained by the demands Colin made on her. Attempts to encourage Colin to verbalise his needs to his partner did not progress. At this point, the CPN asked another member of her team to see him, to offer an independent opinion about how he might be helped at this stage. The team decided that a psychological assessment might be helpful in informing the way forward.

The psychologist who saw Colin administered a number of personality profiling and interpersonal functioning questionnaires. In addition, in-depth interviews, exploring Colin's entire life history, were conducted. The following picture emerged: Colin was one of 18 children in his family of origin. His earliest memories were of his father, an army sergeant, cruelly teasing him. When he was five, his father died, leaving the family homeless, because they lived in accommodation provided by the military. Colin had not been told of the death. He only knew that he, his mother, and his 17 siblings had hurriedly moved from one part of the country to another; he vaguely recalled that social workers had wanted to split the family up, believing his mother to be incapable of looking after the children on her own. From the age of seven, he was expected by his mother to take time off school to look after the younger children in the family. His mother told Colin (and any educational welfare officers who enquired) that the reason he was away from school was because he was 'poorly, with chest problems'. His mother went on, over the years, to show problems with alcohol abuse. The cause of her death had been cirrhosis of the liver.

While his brothers and sisters had established independent adult lives beyond their family of origin, Colin had remained geographically and emotionally close to his mother, with contact at least once daily. She had made major decisions in his life, including those relating to a business that he set up, which subsequently went bankrupt. Although at interview he referred a number of times to episodes when both his mother and his current partner had done things to let him down, he expressed no anger about this, stating that he loved them and so would do 'whatever they wished', because 'they are my life blood – I need them to be there for me'.

Commentary on Colin's case study

Diagnostically, Colin met the criteria for dependent personality disorder. He showed a pattern of marked submissiveness in relation to others, clinging emotionally to them and being extremely fearful of being alone. He was unable to make life decisions without relying on others to take the lead.

Common ground

What do John, Brenda and Colin have in common? First, they all came into contact with health services following a crisis. They had achieved some kind of precarious equilibrium in their life, until a particular event revealed that they had neither the internal nor the social resources to cope beyond a certain point. Second, in all cases there was a risk of harm to themselves (notably Brenda and Colin) or to others (John) on account of their inability to modulate their internal emotional states.

Third, they all presented in a manner such that health professionals found it hard to 'get to the bottom of' their core difficulties. It is as if they presented in code and the task of the professionals was to use their skills to decode the meaning. Fourth, all of them had difficulties that appeared to be traceable in some way to early-life adversity.

Finally, all of them had difficulties in interpersonal relationships, although these emerged in different patterns in the different cases. John's main difficulty was in being unable to make usual social approaches to others, coupled with a tendency to be highly socially avoidant in times of distress. Brenda showed a marked, sometimes rapid oscillation between approach and avoidance behaviour in relation to others. In Colin's case, there was in a sense 'too much' approach behaviour, to the point where he was unable to function day to day without having someone else constantly at his side.

The implications of these patterns for health workers are considerable, because they are likely to be re-enacted in contacts with professionals, as they are with others in the individual's personal life. An understanding of the patterns, and a reasonably good grasp of their origins, may avoid repeats of interpersonal sequences that are doomed to end in disaster. The professionals' main aim is not to become part of the problem instead of part of the solution. Careful trawling of medical records, together with close observation of an individual's behaviour at interview (or in contacts pre-interview) may give clues to a client's particular 'interpersonal blueprint'. This information should then be used to devise appropriate, individually tailored strategies, to increase the probability of engaging people like John, Brenda and Colin.

UNDERSTANDING CAUSAL FACTORS IN THE DEVELOPMENT OF PERSONALITY DISORDERS

There has been a considerable amount of theorising about causes of personality disorder, together with some empirical studies that highlight common background factors in the lives of individuals affected by it. However, the theorists are still a long way from identifying with any certainty the pathways to personality disorders. These conditions are complex and variable and it is increasingly apparent that any further understanding will depend on taking into account multiple, interacting causes, and weaving them into integrated explanatory models.

This section outlines the findings from a number of empirical studies. It is useful to see where theoretical speculations converge, in order to arrive at a view of the current position of the evidence relating to causes of personality disorders.

'Mad' or 'bad'?

Opinions – lay and professional – are divided as to whether those who show signs of personality disorder are 'mad' or 'bad', and whether they are 'in control' or 'out of control'. Certainly, the average person in the street would be inclined to see John's 'preoccupation' as verging on the 'mad'. Some would regard Brenda's ambivalent behaviour – for example, sometimes turning up for appointments and sometimes not – as 'wilful manipulation'. This sort of judgement is neither helpful nor scientifically warranted. The 'mad/bad' and 'in control/out of control' divides are oversimplifications. The question is not whether people like John are (potentially) 'damaging' or 'damaged'; he is clearly both. Likewise, the hypothesis that Brenda is deliberately setting out to be difficult cannot be conclusively proven, either way.

Many clinical errors seem to occur because individual clinicians align themselves too closely with certain aspects of the individual with personality disorder, while screening out awareness of others. This can give rise to situations where clinicians in the same team split into positions. One person (aligned with the 'damaged' aspects) may attempt heroic rescue or therapy work, trying to save the client from the distress caused by their past, and often going to great lengths – well beyond the boundaries that they would normally apply – in order to achieve this. In the mean time, others in the team may stress the 'damaging' features of the client's attitudes and behaviours. It will probably be impossible for the team to agree a common management strategy.

As an alternative to this state of affairs, all team members should adopt, and work to maintain, a position of *equidistance between the polarities* of 'damaging/damaged' and 'controlling/controlled', in which the whole person, with all their disparate facets, is borne in mind. Ryle's (1997) approach to working with people with borderline personality disorder is founded on a stance similar to this.

Biological or environmental factors?

Another kind of split comes to light within the causal research literature. Some have proposed biologically based models of personality disorder, while others have emphasised the role of early abuse, neglect and trauma.

Biologically based models have been proposed because of findings indicating that incidence of certain kinds of personality disorder are higher in those with relatives with that disorder. On the basis of these findings, it has been suggested that there may be a genetic basis to schizoid, schizotypal and antisocial personality disorders (McGuffin and Thapar, 1992). Other biologically based research has implicated birth trauma and early head injury as putative causes, although method-ologically sound research, in which adequate control cases are compared with the experimental (diagnosed as personality-disordered) cases, is hard to come by. In a review of biological factors in the development of personality disorders, Paris (1996) states that studies to date point to the conclusion that certain personality *traits* may be under biological influence, but not *disorders*. He goes on to say that

> *...biological factors are insufficient by themselves to cause disorders. The explanation would be that even in the presence of biological risks, personality disorders will not develop unless individuals are also exposed to psychosocial risk factors. (pp. 38–39)*

Studies of neurochemical abnormalities in individuals with personality disorder led Siever and Davis (1991) to suggest a theory of personality disorder, in which these abnormalities were viewed as primary causes. However, later work has shown that abuse and trauma in childhood can alter brain functioning, thus raising the possi-bility that neurochemical abnormalities may be secondary to abuse, rather than primary causal factors in personality disorder development (Glaser, 2000; Perry, 1995).

A prominent strand of research has been the focus on the role of childhood neglect and abuse, particularly in the background of women with a diagnosis of borderline personality disorder (thought to be the most common of the personality disorders and hence the subject of the most study so far). Studies suggest that 60–80% of women with this diagnosis report abuse in childhood, most often sexual abuse. However, the data is problematic for a number of reasons. First, it is based on retrospective self-report, with all the potential for distortion and bias that can creep in with such a study design; considering the rates of reported abuse with this in mind, one may be inclined to query whether they are inflated. However, there may also be reasons to regard these rates as underestimates. We know that dissociation is common following abuse and trauma (van der Kolk *et al.*, 1996), so that the information about abuse may not be available to the individual's conscious awareness and hence may not be reported to researchers or clinicians. Also, if abuse has occurred and the individual has subsequently become extremely wary of others, they may be unlikely to disclose deep, personal information to anyone who asks them about their childhood experiences, professionals included.

Theoretic models

Turning from research to theory, there are a number of models from which to draw in an attempt to trace the development of personality disorder. Cognitive conceptualisations have tended of late to emphasise the maladaptive schemas (belief systems linked with propensities to action), which individuals with personality disorders learn as they are growing up (Davidson, 2000). These individuals show a preponderance of deeply entrenched negative self (and other) schemas, such as 'I am fundamentally unlovable'; 'Others will always let me down'. Armed with these beliefs, they are likely to be on the alert for information that confirms their schemas, and to ignore information that contradicts them; in other words, they show *selective attention* in relation to their own thought processes and to incoming information from the interpersonal environment. Their beliefs are likely to guide their actions in such a way that they inadvertently create the very scenario they dread. For example, someone who holds the belief that they are unlovable may push the limits in a relationship until they exhaust the patience of the other person involved; when the other withdraws, defeated in their attempts to relate, this is read as 'proof' of unlovability. Repeated over time, the belief becomes reinforced and harder to modify.

The general trend that appears to be emerging in this area, though, is away from models that focus largely on one domain of functioning (thinking, feeling, relating, neurophysiological activity). There is an attempt to synthesise what is known or hypothesised about some or all of these areas, so as to begin building more comprehensive explanatory models. Three recent attempts at integrated models are described briefly below.

1 Linehan's (1993) 'biosocial' model of the development of borderline personality disorder holds that temperamental biological vulnerability combines with what she believes is an 'invalidating environment' for the child; the end product is an inability to learn emotional self-regulation. An invalidating environment is one in which all failures are seen as due to the inadequacy of the child's problem-solving capacity; no allowance is made to take account of their developmental emotional immaturity and limited cognitive problem-solving capacity. Noting the frequency with which sexual abuse is reported by these individuals, Linehan views this sort of abuse as an extreme form of invalidation.

2 Ryle's (1997) account of the development of borderline personality disorder gives prominence to parental failure, actual abuse and the subsequent development of dissociation. This is said to lead to the development of a number of 'multiple self-states', in which identity is fragmented; the individual cannot link up their experiences into a coherent whole, because of their proneness to dissociate in times of stress. The rapid switching between self-states is thought to be the basis for the sometimes sudden and apparently contradictory changes in

behaviour (for example, from intense love and idealisation to equally intense hate and denigration) shown by the individual.

3 In a complex theory relevant to the development of dependent personality disorder and the tendency towards somatisation, Taylor (1987) suggests that, in infancy, in a 'good-enough' relationship, the primary care-giver, by being empathically attuned to the infant's emotional needs, intervenes to regulate the level of arousal and that this is the basis for later learning of emotional self-regulation. Drawing on a theory of how emotion-processing develops throughout childhood (proposed by Lane and Schwartz, 1987), Taylor argues that, where the care-giver is not empathically 'tuned in', the cognitive-affective developmental progress of the infant may be inhibited. The infant may remain in a position where emotion-processing capacity sticks at an early stage – that of 'somatic representation', where affect is experienced as bodily sensation, rather than being able to be symbolically (verbally) encoded. Unable to learn to voice emotions, the child (and, later, the adult) in this position is apt to focus on their physical being and to experience distress in physiological terms. Unable to mobilise cognitive resources for dealing with difficult emotion (that is, to label the emotion and to select an effective strategy to deal with it), they go on relying on external resources – people, or maybe drugs – in an attempt to provide the regulation that they cannot provide for themselves.

Tentative conclusions

These three theories, although different in many respects, all stress the importance of early experiences of significant others as creating a fundamental platform for learning emotional self-management. From our consideration of the literature, and from our own and our colleagues' clinical experience, we have reached some tentative conclusions about the factors influencing the development of personality disorder. We do not regard these as amounting to a causal theory, mindful as we are of our own potential for selective, biased interpretation of the literature. These conclusions merely serve to guide our clinical approach to this client group, in the hope that we can deliver a more needs-led service. They are as follows:

1 Ideas of 'biological vulnerability' or of 'predisposition' remain speculative, although advances in neurophysiological research techniques may shed light on this issue in the future. Some (for example, Linehan, 1993) suggest that we have to invoke biological vulnerability to explain why certain individuals go on to develop features of personality disorder following abuse, while others do not. However, it is possible that the answer to this question lies elsewhere; for example, it may be that access to protective factors, such as having a good relationship with one supportive adult, prevents the development of personality disorder following abuse. One concern we have is that if clinicians and researchers rush to embark on a 'hunt for the biological basis of personality disorder', this may lead them to overlook the extent of the problems that early abuse alone may cause.

2 In both research and clinical evidence, abuse, neglect and trauma early in life seem to emerge consistently as important precursors of personality disorder.

Attachment disruption, brought about by the absence of a primary care-giver (literally or emotionally) is usually found in clinical practice to accompany active forms of chronic childhood abuse.

3 New ideas emerging indicate that the capacity for emotional self-regulation, the development of social cognitive function, and the learning of relationship skills are all dependent on the quality of early attachment bonds. The infant brain grows rapidly and many neural connections are established in the course of the first five years. This may be a crucial period for learning and it could be that, if there is a serious environmental failure at this stage, it will lead to deficits that may be harder to overcome later in life. This is not to say that that they can never be overcome; the plasticity of the human brain, as we keep discovering, is impressive.

4 It is becoming increasingly obvious that the way forward involves integration beyond that attempted in explanatory attempts so far, and that 'biopsychosocial' models need to be generated to account for the varied manifestations of personality disorder.

GENERAL PRINCIPLES FOR WORKING WITH CLIENTS WITH PERSONALITY DISORDER

We have found it helpful to seek to adhere to a number of inter-related principles in our work with this client group. First, it is our belief that the work has to be underpinned by *respect*. Respect for fellow workers, even though they may hold different opinions from our own (mainly because their training base is different), can be difficult in paranoia-inducing 'cut-back' climates. Our inclination may be to band together with our own discipline and see other disciplines as rivals, threatening our professional self-esteem and even our livelihood. If our efforts with clients with personality disorders are to stand any chance of success, we have to find ways of rising above such divisive influences, and of developing and maintaining productive working relationships with other professionals.

Respect for clients and their needs can also be difficult to sustain, in the face of non-engagement, verbal (and maybe also physical) aggression, lack of progress, and so on. However, bearing in mind the likelihood of them having been the victims of abuse can aid our attempts to preserve an empathic and respectful stance.

All professionals involved with individuals with personality disorder need to cultivate the habit of being *reflective rather than reactive*. Often, these clients evoke strong emotions, sometimes on account of their behaviour and sometimes also on account of our own interpersonal history. These emotions can interfere with sound clinical planning.

Containment has to be offered to the client. Especially if they have a history of being abused, these clients will be hypervigilant about change, since abuse often leads to a heightened scanning of the environment in order to detect changes that may signal danger. Their need for consistency and for clear explanations about what we intend to do in relation to them may be greater than average.

We firmly believe that staff undertaking this work need *support*, in the form of adequate supervision, training and opportunities for sharing the care of clients with personality disorder.

Finally, we need to radically alter our concept of 'referral on', so that we stop the feeling of being involved in a game of pass-the-parcel. Collective, genuinely shared responsibility can lighten the weight of responsibility that comes with personality disorder clients, particularly those at risk of self-harm and/or harm to others.

THE 'TEAM HOLDING' APPROACH

We devised the 'team holding' approach as a framework for the care of people with personality disorder. We have tried it out with one or two clients, but no attempt has yet been made to evaluate it systematically; it is very much 'work in progress', at a preliminary stage of development. The approach arose out of multidisciplinary discussions about clients who were high service users. We felt we were not making any progress with these clients, despite months and sometimes years of input from an array of professionals.

The framework is summarised in Table 8.1. It involves a number of steps, with aims, and the considerations that may have to be borne in mind at each stage. The overarching aim is to find a means of introducing greater collectivism and stability into work with clients with personality disorder. Within the framework, the concept of 'team' does not necessarily refer to a specific, already established team, such as a community mental health team, but to the grouping of all professionals currently involved with the client.

Table 8.1 The 'team holding' approach to personality disorder

Step		Aims	Considerations
Step 1	**Team contract:** agree to collaborate	Reduce risk of individual burn-out in client management	Inter-disciplinary rivalry; medico-legal clarity
Step 2	**Assessment:** symptoms, mental state, type of PD, physical health, risk, neurological, patterns of service use	Collect comprehensive, individually relevant information to aid clinical planning	Co-ordination; time; training
Step 3	**Formulation:** diagnostic/ cross-sectional, plus lifespan/longitudinal	Aid selection of treatment; predict likely future behaviour	Achieving consensus
Step 4	**Consensual care plan**	Promote clarity re individual roles; set boundaries	Management backing
Step 5	**Contingency planning**	Anticipate crisis, have strategies in place	Involvement of client, carers, other agencies
Step 6	**Monitoring**	Assess outcome; reformulate if required, change Steps 4 and 5	Clearly clarify who is responsible for this; choice of measures for assessing outcome

The six steps

Step 1 involves all those actively involved with the client contracting to collaborate, basing their clinical responses to the client on the principles outlined earlier. Information about current thinking regarding the development and maintenance of personality disorder features is provided and an attempt is made to abide by an 'evidence-informed' approach. Collectivism is emphasised, while clarity about medico-legal responsibility is maintained. All members of the team are offered access to consultation and supervision.

Step 2 will vary according to particular client needs (for example, for neuropsychological assessment) and may involve a variety of clinicians.

At Step 3, an attempt is made to draw the information gathered into a formulation: a statement of the client's core difficulties, together with hypotheses about their origins and their implications for the wellbeing of the client and others in the present and the future. We have found it useful to use cognitive analytic therapy techniques (Ryle, 1997) at this stage, including constructing a diagrammatic representation of the formulation. It is essential that the formulation is 'owned' by everyone in the team, so that uniformity of approach, based on a shared understanding, is maximised.

Step 4 is primarily about making decisions about appropriate care and management and delineation of roles of team members. It can be helpful to consult with managers in finalising this, particularly in the case of clients who are at risk of self-harm or of harming others.

Contingency planning (Step 5) is conducted with reference to the client's past patterns of behaviour when in crisis. It affords the team the opportunity, having spotted patterns in this behaviour, to put in place crisis management strategies before any further crisis arises. Again, the purpose is to maximise consistency of response. It may also provide a chance to 'coach' the client about new behaviours to deal with crises, if they are involved in this process.

The final, monitoring step (Step 6) requires a designated individual to take responsibility for tracking the progress of the care plan. This is done by coordinating and disseminating information from all workers involved, calling meetings to keep the care plan under review and ensuring that the indices of progress are clearly spelled out and are relevant to the client's needs; for example, one individual marker of progress may be 'reduced frequency of visits to A&E'; another may be 'relies less on medication', compared with the time before the care plan was implemented.

Impediments to implementing the 'team holding' approach

The 'seamlessness' of care implied by the 'team holding' approach is, of course, an ideal that we are far from delivering. As we see it, the main obstacles to achieving such integrated services are the following:

- *Resources (time and money)* – the 'team holding' approach is labour-intensive, demanding a considerable amount of time, especially in the early stages. However, in theory, it should mean that, once the care plan is up and running, less service time will be required. In the long term, time input and costs should reduce. This remains to be tested; it could be put to the test by comparing the costs (in time and money) to services incurred in, say, the year prior to implementing the 'team holding' approach, compared with the costs in the year afterwards. In our limited experience to date, we have found that, where planning ahead for crises was undertaken, management of such crises proved smoother and shorter.

- *Training* – until such time as all professionals are brought 'up to speed' with emerging knowledge about the development and the manifestations of personality disorder, coupled with heightened awareness of the common impacts on professionals that this group of people have, there will continue to be splits within groups of health professionals about how best to approach these sufferers. If health professionals are to grasp the complexities of personality disorder, training needs to be multi-model, rather than rooted in one paradigm (such as medical, cognitive or psychodynamic). Joint training at core professional level has the potential to do much to foster later collaboration: social psychological research on inter-group prejudices would tend to suggest that exposure to members of what might be regarded as 'out-groups' diminishes negative attributions.

- *Professional support* – the importance of clinical supervision for all of those working with individuals with personality disorder cannot be underestimated. Joint care plans can easily flounder where one member of a team 'acts out' their responses, rather than having space and time to reflect on them. This again has time and cost implications.

CONCLUSION

Understanding (in both the intellectual and emotional sense of the word) of personality disorder is not widespread among health professionals. This seems to derive primarily from training deficits and resource limitations, as well as a degree of understandable scepticism engendered by the amount of conceptual disarray surrounding the personality disorder construct. It may well be that the construct will be radically modified or discarded in the light of future thinking and research. However, as we enter an era in which treatments of personality disorder are beginning to be described as 'promising' (Roth and Fonagy, 1996; Department of Health, 2001), there is justified hope that at least some of the symptoms and/or difficulties of people with personality disorder can be addressed.

Given the multiple domains of problems experienced by this group, an inter-disciplinary approach would be expected to enhance the chances of treatment success. Such an approach also models integration for clients whose inner world and life experiences are often marked by chaos and fragmentation. Our 'team holding' approach is in the early stages of development and remains, for the moment, largely untested, but it is a valid attempt to offer more 'joined-up care', premised on what we hope are needs-led principles and practices.

This chapter has much to contribute to an understanding of the current theoretical assumptions that are used to explain personality disorder. Clearly, clients who are deemed to have this condition encounter many difficulties. The case studies sensitively present the degree to which clients suffer and the fact that this may continue throughout their life. The extent of sexual abuse of children seems to be considerable and the fact that it can give rise to multiple problems later in life should warrant more concern than it currently receives. Though it is not mentioned in this chapter, it is vitally important that such people are properly assessed when they first approach health services and that effective help is identified. For this to happen, primary care practitioners, who by their nature are generalists, need to have a working knowledge of the complex nature of inter-actions with this client group. This chapter provides a valuable introduction.

This group has multiple needs, and suffers not only at the hands of a hostile media but often also because of the attitude of professionals by whom they expect to be helped. Because several factors are thought to be both causative and explanatory in this condition, good teamwork is necessary for effective interven-tions. Initial assessments, as the authors point out, should be conducted by more than one professional; interventions should be multidisciplinary; and there should be several aims to the interventions (seeking to assist in emotional control, seeking to assist in developing cognitive awareness and assisting the person in achieving social competence). The importance of respect for clients and for other disciplines is emphasised, especially as it is suspected that many factors are involved in the causation of personality disorder. Rivalries between theoretical positions and professional groups can cause untold harm to the management of this client group. As with other complex conditions, it is important to recognise that no one discipline has all the solutions and honest collaboration is always beneficial to the client.

This chapter provides a good overview of the theoretical models that purport to explain this condition and the recent research in this area, and proposes a helpful model of how a team could set about approaching these clients. (Editors' summary)

REFERENCES

American Psychiatric Association (1994) *Diagnostic and statistical manual of mental disorders*, 4th edition, American Psychiatric Press, Washington, DC

Beck, A.T. and Freeman, A. (1990) *Cognitive therapy of personality disorders*, Guilford, New York

Bowlby, J. (1980) *Attachment and Loss, Vol. 3, Loss: Sadness and depression*, Hogarth Press, London

Davidson, K.M. (2000) *Cognitive Therapy for Personality Disorders*, Butterworth-Heinemann, Oxford

Department of Health (2001) *Treatment choice in psychological therapies and counselling: Evidence-based clinical practice guideline*, Department of Health, London

Glaser, D. (2000) Child abuse and neglect and the brain: a review, *Journal of Child Psychology and Psychiatry*, **41**(I), 97–116

Higgitt, A. and Fonagy, P. (1992) Psychotherapy in narcissistic and borderline personality disorder, *British Journal of Psychiatry*, **161**, 23–43

van der Kolk, B.A., McFarlane, A.C. and Weiseath L. (eds.) (1996) *Traumatic Stress: The effects of overwhelming experience on mind, body and society*, Guilford, New York

Lane, R.D. and Schwartz, G.E. (1987) Levels of emotional awareness: a cognitive developmental theory and its application to psychopathology, *American Journal of Psychiatry*, **144**, 133–143

Linehan, M.M. (1993) *Cognitive-Behavioural Treatment of Borderline Personality Disorder*, Guilford, New York

McGuffin, P. and Thapar, A. (1992) The genetics of personality disorder, *British Journal of Psychiatry*, **160**, 12–23

Millon, T. and Davis, R. (2000) *Personality Disorders in Everyday Life*, Wiley, New York

Paris, J. (1996) *Social Factors in the Personality Disorders*, Cambridge University Press, Cambridge

Perry, B.D. (1995) Childhood trauma, the neurobiology of adaptation and use-dependent development of the brain, *Infant Mental Health Journal*, **16**, 271–291

Roth, A. and Fonagy, P. (1996) *What Works for Whom? A Critical Review of Psychotherapy Research*, Guilford, New York

Ryle, A. (1997) *Cognitive Analytic Therapy in Borderline Personality Disorder: The model and the method*, Wiley, London

Siever, L.J. and Davis, L. (1991) A psychobiological perspective on the personality disorders, *American Journal of Psychiatry*, **148**, 1647–1658

Taylor, G.J. (1987) *Psychosomatic Medicine and Contemporary Psychoanalysis*, International Universities Press, Madison, NJ

World Health Organisation [WHO] (1992) *International classification of diseases*, 10th edition, WHO, Geneva

9 PREVENTION, DETECTION AND TREATMENT OF PERINATAL MENTAL ILLNESS

Gillian Wainscott

For the majority of newly delivered mothers the arrival of a new baby is a time of great joy, but a minority may experience a range of emotional, psychological or psychiatric conditions, which, if not treated promptly, can have far-reaching consequences for whole families, in particular children. These include bonding disorders, post-natal psychosis, post-natal depression, severe anxiety, adjustment reactions and post-traumatic stress disorders. Routine use of the Edinburgh Post-Natal Depression Rating Scale (EPDRS) has broken through the reluctance of mothers to admit their real feelings, which may be less than overwhelming joy, wellbeing and confidence. Use of the EPDRS has also heightened awareness of professionals working in primary care to the possibility of problems in this area. There remains a danger though that all post-natal mental illness may be assumed to be depression, with early signs of other conditions being missed. This chapter introduces the range of perinatal mental illness and describes how care in the primary and secondary sectors can be delivered. Health visitors and general practitioners have a key role but need more support and information. Additional areas to which more attention should be paid include the mental health of mothers who have a child with a serious or prolonged illness in the first year of life, and the ante-natal identification of mothers who may be at risk of developing post-natal mental illness. (Editors' note)

INTRODUCTION

It is quite apparent that over the last decade there has been an increasing awareness that the post-partum period – the first year after the birth of an infant – is a time of increased risk of mental health problems for the mother. Much of this enlightenment has been due to the efforts of dedicated professionals working in the area in specialist mother and baby units, including, among many others, Professors Ian Brockington in Birmingham, John Cox in Stoke, and the late Channi Kumar in London.

The potential seriousness of mental health problems, with respect to the mother, has been highlighted particularly with the publication of *Why mothers die: Report on confidential enquiries into maternal deaths in the United Kingdom 1994–96* (Department of Health, 1998). Detailed investigation into the causes of maternal deaths during this three-year period revealed that psychiatric illness leading to suicide was a significant factor in at least 10% of maternal deaths. Suicide was the second most common cause of death in mothers during the first year after the birth of a baby but the most recent report (Department of Health, 2001) indicates that it is now the main cause of death.

During the 1990s, the impact of maternal illness on the development of the infant and its effect on the remainder of the family became increasingly recognised. There is much published work from the 1990s, which describes in detail the detrimental long-term effects on later social attachments and cognitive development of the child (particularly boys) that remain, even after resolution of the illness. In May 1998, in an edition of the *British Medical Journal* dealing solely with the health of children, the first editorial reported on the effects of maternal depression on the subsequent development of the child (Hoghughi, 1998). The authors also drew attention to the fact that primary care workers were best placed to identify vulnerable women. This is because the ante-natal and post-partum periods are times when the mother has access to care from a variety of different professionals from a multitude of disciplines, but the emphasis of care lies in the primary sector.

Towards the end of the decade, we saw the emergence of a determination to address the problem from the perspective of both the mothers and their infants. *The National Service Framework for Mental Health* (Department of Health, 1999) focuses on the incidence of mental illness post-natally, emphasising the potential seriousness of depression, reiterating the suicide risk as evaluated in the confidential enquiry into maternal deaths (Department of Health, 2001), and advocates the introduction of measures to reduce its incidence and minimise its adverse consequences. The Royal College of Psychiatrists' detailed report on perinatal maternal mental health services (Royal College of Psychiatrists, 2000), provides an excellent synopsis of the wide spectrum of perinatal mental health issues, predicting the needs of mothers within health authorities of differing sizes and setting out the case for the provision of specialist perinatal psychiatry services.

EPIDEMIOLOGY

Typically, textbooks teach that there are three major categories of post-partum psychiatric morbidity: the 'baby blues', puerperal psychosis and post-natal depression. There is currently an emphasis on post-natal depression and, while it is clear that mood disorders constitute the major component of psychiatric morbidity, it is all too easy to label all cases of mental distress occurring post partum as 'post-natal depression'.

The 'baby blues' is a transient state of emotional lability, with onset during the first week after delivery. It rarely lasts more than seven or 10 days and occurs so frequently (in 60–70% of all mothers delivered) that it is considered to be part of normal experience. Tearfulness is often a marked feature of the baby blues, but the hallmarks of a depressive illness – profound, sustained and pervasive mood changes, and a lack of enjoyment in all aspects of life – are lacking. The condition resolves spontaneously. There is a suggestion that mothers who suffer more intensely from the baby blues are more at risk of developing a depressive illness. If the symptoms are unduly prolonged and become more deeply entrenched, suspicions should be raised that a more serious illness is developing.

Puerperal psychosis is a relatively rare condition (occurring in two per 1000 deliveries), but it can cause considerable distress. It is characterised also by emotional lability, ranging from depression to elation, and frequent tearfulness is also a feature. The mother may be perplexed and confused, and show signs of other more obviously psychiatric symptoms, including the expression of delusional beliefs and perceptual disturbances in the form of hallucinatory experiences (such as hearing voices or seeing things that others do not).

While the distinction between puerperal psychosis and 'post-natal depression' should be easy to make, the latter term has become so common that confusions do occur. Disappointingly, one consultant community paediatrician recently referred in a court report to a woman who had suffered a severe psychotic illness after the birth of her baby as having had 'post-natal depression'. In this situation, the clinical picture was clear; the mother had showed features of hypomania with hyper-activity, pressure of speech, disinhibited behaviour, and the expression of grandiose and paranoid delusional beliefs. In another case, eventually referred to Birmingham Mother and Baby Service, a health visitor quite rightly recognised that a mother was unwell. She labelled the illness as 'post-natal depression', and recommended counselling as the right approach. In fact, she had failed to appre-ciate that the woman was acutely psychotic; a week later, the mother walked into her local police station at midnight, barefoot, and in night clothes, saying that she believed that her baby had turned into a snake.

Post-partum mood disorders comprise the majority of the psychiatric morbidity, and most authorities would quote an incidence of 'post-natal depression' occurring in 10–15% of all mothers delivered. However, the emphasis on this condition – and on the classical triad of baby blues, puerperal psychosis and post-natal depression – fails to take into account the many other forms of mental distress or illness that may occur post partum. Newly delivered mothers are at risk of devel-oping many different forms of mental disorder after childbirth. Other perinatal mental health problems may include the following:

- new episodes of mental illness or recurrence of pre-existing psychiatric illness;
- varying degrees of anxiety, sometimes of such intense severity that 'puerperal panic' would be a better descriptive term;
- post-traumatic stress disorders following particularly difficult deliveries, which may lead to secondary tokophobia (a pathological fear of the process of giving birth, first described by Dr K. Hofberg);
- obsessive-compulsive states; and
- increased stress or adversity in the response of vulnerable women to motherhood.

Clearly, blanket use of the term 'post-natal depression' can hide the true nature of the problem and hinder the effective delivery of care.

Bonding disorders have also been recognised as a distinct problem area. Typically, these include a lack of interest in the baby, a failure to feel the expected maternal love, and a progress through hostility and rejection, to the extent that the mother comes to fear or even hate any contact with her baby. In extreme cases, the mother will run away, in an attempt to avoid such contact, or will try to harm the infant. At the other end of the spectrum there may be an unhealthy over-dependence on the baby, with hyper-vigilance and fear of sudden infant death syndrome (cot death). Bonding disorders may be co-morbid with other illness, including 'post-natal depression', but may exist as a primary condition. Unless it is part of a depressive illness, its presence may be missed. It is often a condition that mothers are reluctant to volunteer, for obvious reasons. A screening instrument is currently being developed in Birmingham to allow easier disclosure by the mother and to heighten the awareness of professionals to this possibility.

THE MYTH OF POST-NATAL DEPRESSION

There is no doubt that the use of the term 'post-natal depression' has done much to raise consciousness that emotional distress can occur after giving birth, and that this distress is not the 'fault' of the mother concerned. In this context, the use of the label has proved helpful. However, its use also fails to acknowledge that the depressive illness may have its origins earlier, or start during pregnancy itself. It can lead to rather muddled thinking – one article in a well-known women's magazine was entitled 'I suffered from post-natal depression before my baby was born'. In the past, there was a somewhat fanciful view that a woman is protected from mood disorders during pregnancy, but there is now a greater acceptance that depression may occur during pregnancy. The screening instrument that has been developed to detect depression post-natally (*see* page 136) has its use ante-natally as well. Published work has confirmed its validity in this respect and suggestions have been made that 'Edinburgh Perinatal Depression Rating Scale' is a better name for it.

There is no real difference clinically between a depressive illness occurring post partum and one occurring at any other time. Women are sometimes unsure whether they are suffering from post-natal depression or whether their symptoms reflect a relapse of a recurrent depression. There is little mileage in attempting such a differentiation; it is the impact of the illness on the mother-infant relationship that must always be considered.

The following case study, based very closely on the story of a mother referred to the Mother and Baby Services (although names have been changed) illustrates many of the above points. Studying clinical cases gives a better understanding of the issues involved, and points to ways in which management and treatment can be improved. In this case, collaborative care between the primary health care team and the specialist service did work in some areas, but there were other areas where it could have been improved. Clearly, there are a number of lessons to be learned.

CASE STUDY   DW

D is a 25-year-old married woman. At the time of referral, she was the mother of two children, Katie aged two months and Martin aged 16 months. Her husband worked in Birmingham's jewellery quarter.

Referral

The referral letter from D's GP was detailed and perceptive. She said D had been increasingly depressed since the birth of her second child and validated this diagnosis by describing symptoms of lowness of mood and tearfulness. These symptoms were accompanied by a fear of going out, which in turn was associated with a feeling of morbid dread that something terrible would happen to her children.

The GP also mentioned D's past history of anxiety and an 'eating disorder', which was treated by her local psychiatric team. She said that after the birth of her first child she suffered from the 'baby blues' for a few days but 'nothing more severe than that'.

Assessment

The first assessment took place at the mother's home, when the consultant psychiatrist undertook a domiciliary visit. A diagnosis of a moderate depressive disorder based on clinical features was made and other risk factors were identified. D admitted to the pregnancy being unplanned and described her own ambivalent feelings about this. She said she became reconciled slowly to the idea of having a second child as the pregnancy progressed. She became hypertensive towards the end of the pregnancy and was admitted to hospital because of this one week before her due date of delivery. This coincided with the start of her depressed mood and in retrospect she felt that this imposed separation from her 15-month-old son was probably the reason. Labour was induced and her daughter was born weighing nearly 6 lb. D said she loved her immediately and had no trouble establishing breast-feeding.

In spite of her good feelings towards her daughter, D's mood deteriorated gradually after the birth. She felt her depressive symptoms were putting a strain on her relationship with her husband and her feelings towards him. She believed that he was unsupportive and not putting her first.

Treatment

It was confirmed that D was suffering from a moderate depressive illness of sufficient severity to justify treatment with antidepressants. It was also thought that she would benefit from attendance at the specialist mother and baby day service, where her vulnerability factors could be clarified both through individual therapy and in a group setting. It could also help her look at her continued feelings of rejection by her husband, which were perpetuating her depressed mood.

Much information emerged regarding her early life experiences, which illuminated the reasons behind her low self-esteem. She also disclosed more about her more recent life, including the guilt she felt following a termination of pregnancy she underwent one year before she became pregnant with her first child.

Further information came from observation. During her first assessment, D had commented that she felt that the imposed separation from her son, when she had been admitted to the maternity hospital during the later stages of her second pregnancy, was a probable factor in the onset of her depression. When she attended the day service, together with both her children, it was very obvious that she was reluctant to allow Martin out of her sight, holding his hand constantly. He became very distressed if she was absent from his sight even for a second when she attended to her own personal needs. She had no such difficulty separating from her younger daughter and her daughter in turn exhibited no separation anxiety.

When this was discussed with D she became very tearful and hesitantly told her therapist that, after Martin was born, he had to be admitted to neonatal intensive care. D became convinced that he had died and that this was a punishment to her because she had previously had a termination. When her baby was returned to her, she refused to believe that he was her son, although she did not voice her worries to any members of staff. From then on, she lived in constant fear that the 'real' mother would appear to reclaim her child. She felt no such anxieties after the birth of Katie, whom she accepted without any difficulty as her own daughter. She found it difficult to understand why her mood had deteriorated so significantly.

Treatment with antidepressants continued, and psychological therapy intensified. Psychological therapy was directed towards the following:

- helping D to come to terms with her early life experiences and to understand the effect this had on her self-esteem, her fear of rejection and feelings of lack of support, together with her continued feelings of guilt since her earlier termination;
- working on D's feelings towards her son. This proved very difficult, as she held the belief with delusional intensity and any attempts at separation, even for the shortest of periods, were met with antagonism and resistance; it was readily apparent that this was having a detrimental effect on her son's development;
- working with her husband, to help him understand the difficulties that his wife was encountering. He appeared to be a reasonably helpful and understanding man and certainly not the ogre D had first described. He benefited from counselling, which helped him understand D's feelings and enabled him to help her feel more supported.

Slowly, D's depression lifted and gradually she learnt to tolerate separation from her son for short periods. It was much more difficult to help her with her deeply entrenched feelings of low self-esteem. In the medium term, the outcome was good; D felt brighter in mood and generally better about herself, and was able to talk more to her husband. He shared in the child care more and D was able to embark on activities for herself, including evening classes. Martin was enrolled in a local nursery, which he began to enjoy. Much of his early clinginess resolved and D was discharged back to the care of her GP.

LESSONS FOR COLLABORATION

D's case illustrates how there can be much more to what at first sight appears to be a relatively straightforward case of 'post-natal depression'. D was fortunate to have a GP who recognised her distress when she presented at the surgery and made an accurate diagnosis. The GP felt that her whole situation was probably more complex than it appeared on the surface, and referred her for specialist management.

Nevertheless, if collaboration had been better at an earlier stage, the outcome in D's case could have been better. During her first pregnancy, D was experiencing guilt about her previous termination. This was intense in her case, particularly because termination was regarded as sinful by the strict religious sect in which she had been brought up, and against which she had rebelled. She was probably depressed as a consequence and this had not been recognised. Because of the intense guilt she felt, she was reluctant to discuss her feelings with a professional.

The illness of a new-born baby is a very powerful factor in the causation of post-partum depression. D did not display any classical features of depression at the time, but she was acutely anxious and too embarrassed to communicate her fears spontaneously to staff. Indeed, her worry that the baby would be taken was sufficient to have prevented her from talking about her belief that he was not her son. After his birth, D was said to have suffered from the 'baby blues'. This was well recognised and appropriate, but her more deeply entrenched anxiety was not, neither were the clinginess and over-dependency on her child. Rejection and hostility on the part of a mother towards her baby quite rightly raise alarm and concern in health-care professionals, who apply the label of bonding disorder. The problems of over-protectiveness and dysfunctional dependency are less well appreciated, but can have an equally devastating effect on child development.

Retrospection is a very powerful and irritating clinical tool. Had there been better collaboration, her mental health problems might have been identified much earlier. Guilt following a termination of pregnancy is very common and stays with a woman for many years. There is much published data to suggest that if a further pregnancy is started within a year of a termination (or less than a year following miscarriage or stillbirth), there will be an increase in various mental health problems, including anxiety and depression. This can occur both during the pregnancy and after delivery, and even if the second pregnancy is a much-wanted one. Better collaboration with obstetric staff (doctors and midwives) and better communication regarding previous obstetric history might have enabled D's vulnerability to be identified earlier. D's reaction to Martin's illness as a baby was extreme, requiring better therapeutic services. Other warning signs were evident in D's complete dependency on Martin and a better awareness among health visitors relating to dysfunctions of mother-infant bonding might have brought these difficulties to light earlier.

PREVENTION OF POST-NATAL MENTAL ILLNESS

'Prevention' is an all-encompassing term, which has been further defined and categorised by a number of workers in different fields:

- 'Primary prevention' is now accepted as a means of preventing the incidence of mental disorder by counterbalancing adverse factors before they can create a disorder.

- 'Secondary prevention' refers to early diagnosis and intervention, thus limiting the adverse consequences of the disorder and reducing the prevalence of the condition (*see* page 136, on detection).

Primary prevention

An enormous amount of research has been undertaken to identify factors associated with the development of depression after childbirth. Many of these factors are applicable to vulnerability to depressive illness in general, including a family history of depression, a personal history of depression, a previous post-partum episode, and personality factors. The latter include low self-esteem, which may have its origins in early-life experiences; these may in turn be traced to a lack of satisfying nurturing during the mother's own childhood, death of her mother at an early age, or actual neglect or abuse, including childhood sexual abuse.

Other personality factors can comprise an obsessional, perfectionist personality, which is not sufficiently flexible to allow for the disruption in routine that invariably accompanies the arrival of a baby.

Psychosocial factors are of considerable importance and can be identified by primary care workers ante-natally. As with all forms of depressive illness, these include housing or financial problems, relationship crises, and other adverse life events. Of particular importance perhaps in the aetiology of post-natal depression is bereavement, especially the death of the mother's own mother, if this is temporally related to the birth of a child.

Added to a general list of vulnerability factors are those that are specifically 'baby-related'. Numerous publications indicate adverse events such as previous obstetric catastrophes – stillbirth, miscarriage or termination – painful or harrowing experiences of previous labours and deliveries, ambivalence about the most recent pregnancy, lack of commitment to the infant, teenage pregnancy, and obstetric problems associated with the current pregnancy, especially worries about the health of the unborn child and realistic worries about the health of the baby after its birth.

Much of this information is readily available to primary care workers and can be communicated from specialist services by a series of didactic lectures, but sharing of information in this way can hardly be regarded as collaborative. The information does need to be shared, but a lecture identifying vulnerability factors is often met with the response that most expectant mothers would match this pattern, and some mothers are faced with ostensibly insurmountable problems in this respect.

Identification of these vulnerability factors does not in itself equate to prevention, but more detailed knowledge of background risk can lead to an effective preventive intervention. The negative aspect is that heightening awareness in primary care workers in this manner can lead to more anxiety, and an increase in the number of referrals to a specialist service. This is not the objective of the didactic lectures. Referral should not be discouraged, but it is not always the best answer. Women often feel that a referral to psychiatric services is stigmatising.

They do not attend outpatient appointments because they are frightened of 'the mad house', and even refuse domiciliary visits for fear of the neighbours seeing a psychiatrist at the door.

The attitude towards collaboration between specialist services and primary care needs to be much more proactive. One way that better liaison can be achieved is by the specialist moving physically into the primary care setting. Individual cases can be discussed between all workers involved, and care plans devised in a spirit of working together in the best interests of mother and child. This is a move away from the tradition of referring only the most difficult patients, whose needs are felt to be beyond the scope of primary care. The specialist can set up clinics actually within the primary care setting, usually the GP surgery, to make an initial assessment, and work on the care plan together with the primary care team. Various options can be discussed more constructively, ranging from in-patient admission, home treatment from the specialist service, attendance at the day hospital or more practical support from social services or from the various voluntary agencies.

Secondary prevention and detection screening

The Edinburgh Post-Natal Depression Rating Scale (EPDRS) (Cox et al., 1987; see Appendix II) has broken through the reluctance of mothers to admit their real feelings. Its routine use has also heightened the awareness of all professionals involved of the possibility of problems.

Traditionally, women are supposed to 'blossom' during pregnancy, as they prepare themselves for their ultimate purpose. Childbirth is a time of fulfilment for women; the travails of labour are forgotten, to be replaced by the joy of a child being born. Partner, family and friends are ecstatic as they look forward to the new addition to the family.

In the face of these traditional images, it is not easy for a woman to admit to others – or to herself – that pregnancy and childbirth have not lived up to her expectations. The pregnancy itself may not have been wanted or planned; the mother may be troubled by sickness during the pregnancy; the partner may not be overjoyed to add further responsibilities; and the current trend is for new families to be further away from their own nuclear family than before. There may be additional financial pressures and the question of child care to be considered. Labour and delivery may be particularly traumatic and fail to go according to plan. Deviations from pre-determined birth plans are frequently poorly tolerated by mothers, even in an emergency, as they fear losing control. In the euphoria that is supposed to follow childbirth, the mother may be reluctant to disclose that she feels unwell, that motherhood does not live up to her expectations, or that she remains tormented by nightmares during which she re-lives the horrors of her delivery. In the universal delight of seeing a cute baby, professionals also have an understandable tendency to assume that everything is well.

The self-rating EPDRS, devised and validated by Professor Cox (Cox et al., 1987), has contributed much to a change in the assumptions. Its use is now almost universal and on a routine basis, making it apparent to the mother that the professionals do *not* expect everything to be well. Mothers clearly find it easier to admit to an anonymous piece of paper that, while being aware that they 'should' feel on top of the world, they actually feel dreadful, low in mood, constantly tearful. Actions that should bring them pleasure are undertaken robotically, and the bundle of joy in the corner assumes monster-like proportions, with its constant demands to be fed and washed, and sleep interruptions. The expected maternal bond may not have developed; a lack of bonding can range from indifference to hostility and rejection, or an intense desire to run away. It is easy to understand why mothers may be reluctant to discuss such feelings. They assume that they will be judged as lazy, inadequate or bad (or even mad). They worry that, if they seek help, the ultimate sanction may follow – the removal of their child by social services.

Use of the EPDRS is not without problems. The scale is a screening instrument. It does not diagnose depression but should raise awareness that there are mental health problems. A high score on the scale frequently does point to a depressive illness but it is the patient who should be treated, not the score, and the matter is one of clinical judgement. High scores can raise anxiety levels in professionals who administer rating scales, and this anxiety can lead to a refusal to take part in this sort of detection. But the problem may still exist and early detection does give a better chance of more effective therapeutic intervention. It is clear that professionals involved at the sharp end need to be offered adequate support, perhaps through planned de-briefing sessions. They need to be more readily available, at least for consultation, rather than wait for emergencies to arise.

TREATMENT OF POST-NATAL MENTAL ILLNESS

It is generally accepted that 80% of all women suffering from post-natal depression are adequately treated in the primary care setting and that a 'counselling' approach is the preferred treatment option. While there is published evidence to suggest that this might be the case, it is important not to attempt to apply it to *all* mothers. The danger of this approach is the possible implication that the distress is not serious and does not merit a more specialist intervention.

The preliminary therapeutic intervention – the first time a mother discloses that all is not well in the way she feels about herself, or towards her baby, to a detached, non-judgemental, outside professional – is crucial. It can determine consequent therapeutic success. The feeling of being understood, and not judged to be mad, bad or plain lazy, gives enormous relief and this allows for further ventilation of feelings. It has been suggested that a series of 'listening sessions' with a trained health visitor at this stage can consolidate the improvement in wellbeing. There is clear merit in this concept. The health visitor is the one who is closest to the mother in need and the whole family, and will probably be the professional to suggest that other services might be helpful to resolve more entrenched difficulties. Sessions with the health visitor must also be used to firm up diagnosis and to identify the exact nature of the difficulties that may be present. It cannot be emphasised too strongly that the health visitor should be adequately supported in this role, by other colleagues from the primary care setting and by specialist services.

At what stage should a mother be referred for further help? There is no definitive answer to this question. Obvious indications could include the presence of psychotic features, severe bonding difficulties and persistent suicidal ideation with intent. Complicating symptoms will probably also lead to referral to specialist services. These might include those of post-traumatic stress disorder, or more deeply entrenched personality issues, such as those that might be subsequent to re-awakened memories of trauma from the mother's own childhood, including childhood sexual abuse.

A more contentious issue is when to treat a depressive illness with antidepressants. The use of antidepressants in the treatment of post-natal depression is sometimes regarded as a controversial issue. It has been reported that the majority of mothers are best treated in primary care and respond to a counselling approach. This form of intervention is probably also best favoured by mothers. It is also said, with some justification, that there are few good controlled trials of the use of antidepressants in this situation. Breast feeding is also cited as a contra-indication to the prescription of antidepressants. While this is undoubtedly best practice for the majority (perhaps up to 80%) of mothers suffering from the more common mixed anxiety/depressive state, it highlights the importance of judging carefully the nature and the severity of the illness. It is unlikely that a depressive illness of more than moderate severity will respond to psychological therapies quickly without the prescription of an antidepressant and this holds true for a depressive illness occurring post-partum as well as at any other time. It cannot be emphasised enough that untreated or inadequately treated depression holds considerably more risk to the mother and has a more detrimental impact on the wellbeing and development of the infant than any speculative risk from the antidepressant itself.

THE TAKE-HOME MESSAGES

The time around pregnancy and the first year post partum is a vulnerable time in the life of any woman, when many risk factors accumulate to increase the potential for many different types of mental distress, to the detriment of mother, baby and the family. Mental health problems that occur around the time of pregnancy and after delivery may have potentially serious consequences to both mother and child.

The term 'post-natal depression' is useful in that its use has highlighted the possibility of illness occurring at that time, and it has provided a diagnostic term that is not stigmatising and is easily understood. It is less helpful when it is used as an all-encompassing term, excluding the possibility of other psychiatric disorders. Its use also restricts the understanding that many 'post-natal' mood disorders may start during pregnancy, or earlier.

Many vulnerability factors for post-natal mental illness have been identified, and mothers at risk of developing problems can be recognised. Early detection of mental health problems may be facilitated with the use of validated screening instruments during pregnancy and after delivery. Collaborative practice means offering support to primary health-care workers who use these instruments, to defuse the anxieties that arise as increased morbidity is detected.

Collaborative practice means moving away from traditional referral practice – the specialist service and consultant reacting to emergency or difficult situations – and working proactively with primary care workers within primary care settings to formulate comprehensive care plans for mothers. These care plans should take into account all aspects of a mother's distress, including treatment of any depressive illness. This includes intervention at earlier stages than may traditionally have been envisaged, and this includes a more vigorous liaison with obstetric services.

*The author has raised a number of points that have relevance not only to care of mother and child, but to health care generally. The issue of the 'labelling' of conditions is contentious and can lead to delay in providing care and, in some instances, a failure to assist people in need. Maximum benefit from collaboration between secondary and primary care requires that professionals own a common language and shared meanings, to prevent misunderstandings between different professional groups and between members of the same profession. Having a baby may give rise to problems that can be anticipated, but it may also cause some that are unexpected, and hence unprepared for. Collaboration must exist between people or agencies that can provide relevant and immediate help. Collaboration for the sake of collaboration without a clear understanding of the client's needs is pointless, because inappropriate collaboration undermines the client's confidence in the health worker, and her self-esteem if she feels she has been offloaded on to someone else because the original carer was ill chosen. Appropriate collaboration enables a fuller picture of the client to emerge. People from different backgrounds see different aspects of the client and enable a clearer focus on how to achieve the best outcomes. The author reminds us that, while there is a place for measurement scales in the care of the post-natal mother, it is the professional's ability to foster equality in the relationship with the client that is by far the most important aspect of care. If the client feels that she is an equal partner in her care, she can bring her understanding to bear on the often complex problems facing her and help identify what she needs from her carers. (**Editors' summary**)*

REFERENCES

Cox, J.L., Holden, J.M., Sagovsky, R. (1987) Detection of postnatal depression: development of the 10-item Edinburgh Postnatal Depression Scale, *British Journal of Psychiatry*, **150**, 782–786

Department of Health (1998) *Why Mothers Die: Report on confidential enquiries into maternal deaths in the United Kingdom 1994–96*, HSC 1998/211, HMSO, London

Department of Health (1999) *National Service Framework for Mental Health*, Department of Health, London

Department of Health (2001) *Why Mothers Die: Report on confidential enquiries into maternal death in the United Kingdom 1997–99*, Department of Health, London

Hoghughi, M. (1998) The importance of parenting in child health, *British Medical Journal*, **316**, 1545

Royal College of Psychiatrists (2000) *Perinatal Maternal Mental Health Services*, Council Report CR88, Royal College of Psychiatrists, London

10 CHILD MENTAL HEALTH PROBLEMS IN PRIMARY CARE

Jon Arcelus, Fiona Gale and Panos Vostanis

*In this chapter, Arcelus, Gale and Vostanis provide an introduction to the range, incidence and aetiology of child mental health problems, and discuss the recently established role of the primary mental health worker (PMHW). Historically, child and adolescent mental health services have been a hidden part of the NHS. A major review was commissioned in the mid-1990s, and concluded that lack of liaison and joint working was hindering effective service provision for children and their families. Arcelus and colleagues highlight the multi-factorial nature of mental health problems in children, and argue that a multi-agency approach is required. PMHWs can come from a variety of mental health disciplines; in-depth knowledge of agencies involved in children's wellbeing and mental health, and the ability to promote and support joint working are as important as the worker's professional background. (**Editors' note**)*

INTRODUCTION

There are approximately 15 million children and young people under 20 years old in the UK, representing 25% of the population (Mental Health Foundation, 1999). An increasing number of them are developing complex and enduring mental health problems. Mental health problems in children are a major concern for families, schools, social services, child and adolescent psychiatrists, and society in general, as they can predict a wide range of poor prognoses in adult life. These might include poor job history and consequent financial dependency, poor interpersonal relationships, high rates of marital break-up, and parenting of children with an elevated risk of developing behavioural problems.

Different cultures have varying views about what is seen as 'mentally healthy' behaviour in young people. In general, children who are mentally healthy will have the ability to develop psychologically, emotionally, intellectually and spiritually; will initiate, develop and sustain mutually satisfying personal relationships; will use and enjoy solitude; will become aware of others and empathise with them; will play and learn; will develop sense of right and wrong; and will face problems and setbacks and learn from them, in ways appropriate for that child's age.

Mental health problems in childhood and adolescence can be described as a disturbance of function in one area of relationships, mood, behaviour, or the development of difficulties of sufficient severity to require professional intervention. The term 'disorder' describes a number of more persistent and severe mental health problems, and generally implies the presence of a clinically recognisable set of symptoms or behaviours, usually in the presence of several risk factors (Mental Health Foundation, 1999).

MENTAL HEALTH PROBLEMS IN CHILDREN AND ADOLESCENTS

According to a survey carried out in 1999 by the Office for National Statistics (ONS), around 10% of children aged 5–15 years in England, Scotland and Wales present with some form of mental health problem (Office for National Statistics, 1999). It is well established that behavioural problems are one of the most common forms of psychopathology in children and adolescents, and constitute a significant proportion of clinic-referred children. Although early studies suggested more behavioural problems in socially deprived areas, not all studies have found major geographical differences (Offord *et al.*, 1991). However, gender differences are consistent, with a ratio of about 3:1, male to female (Office for National Statistics, 1999).

Children with behavioural problems present with a pattern of negativistic, hostile and defiant behaviour. Negativistic feelings are often expressed by adolescents, especially before they come to treatment, because they are frightened of the implications for themselves and their families. The young adolescent's lack of objectivity coupled with an upsurge of multiple impulses, as well as the tendency to confuse fantasy with reality, make the discussion of feelings threatening. In older children, the behavioural problems can escalate to a point at which they present with severe aggression towards people, property or animals. When behaviour is so extreme and dangerous, including delinquency in adolescence, the term 'conduct disorder' is used.

Attention deficit hyperactivity disorder (ADHD)

Children with ADHD present with symptoms of inattention, impulsivity and hyperactivity, which have persisted for at least six months, to a degree that is maladaptive and inconsistent with their developmental level. Such children often fail to pay attention to details, and make careless errors in schoolwork; have difficulty in sustaining attention in tasks or play activities; and are easily distracted by external stimuli. The prevalence of the disorder has been estimated at 2–9% in children of primary school age (Sidane *et al.*, 1998), and at 5.8% in adolescents (Rhode *et al.*, 1999). Some doctors and professionals, particularly in Europe, refer to people with these symptoms as having hyperkinetic disorder. However, there are some differences between the two terms.

Emotional problems

The manifestation of emotional symptoms will vary in relation to the child's development. Young children present with non-specific symptoms such as physical complaints, irritability and withdrawal. Older children and adolescents often present with symptoms that are similar to those of adults; they will usually suffer from depressed mood, loss of interest and enjoyment, reduced energy and fatigue. Other common symptoms are reduced concentration and attention, low self-esteem, ideas of guilt and unworthiness, bleak and pessimistic views of the future, disturbed sleep, diminished appetite, and ideas or acts of self-harm or attempted suicide. The ONS study found that around 4% of 5- to 15-year-olds presented with emotional problems, predominantly anxiety and depression (Office for National Statistics, 1999).

AETIOLOGY

There is a range of theories on the development of mental health problems. In most conditions, a multi-factorial aetiology – an interaction of biological and environmental factors – is considered. Research has identified several risk factors, in other words, those circumstances that increase the probability of a child developing a mental health problem. These factors can be divided into two main groups: factors intrinsic to the child, and environmental factors; *see* Table 10.1.

Table 10.1   Risk factors for the development of mental health problems in children and adolescents

In the child	In the family	In the environment
Genetic influences	Inconsistent discipline	Socio-economic disadvantage
Low IQ	Poor parental relationship	Homelessness
Developmental delays	Abuse	Poor support network
Difficult temperament	Parental psychiatric illness	
Chronic illness	Parental criminality	

MHF (1999)

Most of the risk factors are inter-related. This makes the understanding of why a child develops mental health problems very difficult and the treatment of those disorders extremely complicated. Risk factors are *cumulative*: if a child is only exposed to one risk factor, the likelihood of ever developing a mental health problem has been defined as being 1–2%; with three risk factors, it is thought that the likelihood increases to 8%; with four or more risk factors, it increases to 20% (Mental Health Foundation, 1999). There are also certain factors that *protect* children against the development of mental health problems. Those factors may also be child-related, within the family, or within the broader environment; *see* Table 10.2.

Table 10.2   Protective factors against developing mental health problems in children and adolescents

In the child	In the family	In the environment
Being female	Good parent–child relationship	Wide support network
Intelligence	Good parental relationship	Good housing
Secure attachment	Parental warmth and affection	High standard of living
Good communication skills	Consistent discipline	Positive attitude
Easy temperament	Support for education	Leisure opportunities
Good coping mechanisms		Supportive peer relationships

Kaplan et al., (1994); Mental Health Foundation (1999)

Services for children and adolescents with mental health problems

Development of child and adolescent mental health services

In the UK, child and adolescent mental health services (CAMHS) have developed in a very different way from adult mental health services. It has taken a long time for society to acknowledge that children also have mental health needs and problems. In 1995, the Health Advisory Service (HAS) published a national review of CAMHS. The report highlighted a concerning picture, in which the needs of children and their families were largely unmet, primary care professionals were unsupported in dealing with mental health problems in children, and statutory agencies did not give priority to providing such services (NHS Health Advisory Service, 1995). The central message from the report was that there was a pressing need for agencies to work more closely together, both in providing a more co-ordinated service and in jointly commissioning such services.

The report also provided a four-tier strategic framework for examining the provision of services, which has received widespread support among CAMHS and forms the basis of many joint commissioning strategies (*see* Table 10.3).

Table 10.3 Child and adolescent mental health services – the four-tier framework

Tier 1	Professionals with whom children and adolescents with mental health problems first come into contact	GPs, health visitors, residential social workers, juvenile justice workers, school nurses, teachers
Tier 2	Specialist child and adolescent mental health professionals working individually to provide assessment and intervention to families	Individually working: clinical child psychologists, educational psychologists, paediatricians, community child psychiatric nurses, child psychiatrists
Tier 3	Mental health professionals in specialist multidisciplinary teams established to assess and treat problems	Multidisciplinary team: social workers, clinical psychologists, community psychiatric nurses, art, music and drama therapists, child psychotherapists, occupational therapists, child psychiatrists
Tier 4	Highly specialised services	Day units, highly specialised outpatient teams, in-patient units

HAS (1995)

Development of primary mental health service

In 1997, the House of Commons Health Committee published its report (House of Commons, 1997) on child and adolescent mental health services. Its findings, summarised here, paint the backdrop to developing local frameworks for collaborative work.

The report reiterates the findings of previous studies, describing current provision of CAMHS as 'inadequate in quality and geographical spread', and CAMHS as having suffered historical neglect as a priority within the NHS. It observes weaknesses in both the commissioning and provision of CAMHS. The absence of specific goals in the existing *Health of the Nation* targets is highlighted.

The report recommends that the Department of Health adopt new *Health of the Nation* indicators and targets specifically relating to child and adolescent mental health. There is also an observed lack of close co-operation between agencies and professionals and a reiteration of the importance of the development of children's services plans in improving this situation. It recommends that CAMHS professionals should be actively involved in the production of services plans, together with other professionals from a variety of agencies.

The report reinforces the HAS four-tier model of CAMHS as a 'rational blueprint for service provision'. It recommends that the DoH should make the model obligatory for health authorities as a way of highlighting areas for improvement, particularly in cross-boundary working.

The document pronounces on a number of specific issues related to the development of services in primary care, all of which reiterate the original recommendations of the HAS report, including:

- support for the concept of primary child and adolescent mental health workers, as a cost-effective way of improving prevention and early diagnosis of mental health problems; it recommends that purchasers develop such a role locally, combining it with a process of collaboration with and support to primary care professionals;
- support for voluntary-sector schemes such as HomeStart and Newpin (community parent support initiatives) in respect of prevention of mental health problems in children.

PRIMARY MENTAL HEALTH WORKERS

Who are they?

Following the recommendations of the NHS Health Advisory Service, a number of CAMHS have established primary mental health worker (PMHW) posts. Their objective is to enhance service provision at Tier 1 through collaborative work. This is achieved by a combination of support, consultation, training, liaison and joint work with Tier 1 professionals (health visitors, general practitioners, school nurses, social workers and the voluntary sector). The aim is to close the gap between Tier 1 and more specialised child and adolescent mental health services.

A recent national survey showed that 25% of NHS Trusts that provided CAMHS were developing this role and 40% were considering such posts (Lacey, 1998). The developments fall into a number of quarters – within an existing professional's role, as a full-time post, as a small-scale community initiative, or as a CAMH service within primary care. In Warwickshire CAMHS, for example, the clinical nurse specialist provides designated time for telephone and face-to-face consultation, on a part-time basis (Lacey, 1998). In Portsmouth, a specialist mental health worker provides support and advice to general practices (Neira-Munoz and Ward, 1998). Full-time posts have been developed in the West Midlands. In Leicestershire and Rutland, a large team of PMHWs links in with small community-based multi-agency teams developed from a joint strategy with social services, education and the voluntary sector, with the aim of providing early intervention for children with emotional or behavioural difficulties, and for their families.

In some instances, child mental health services have been developed within primary care, which operate at Tier 1. These initiatives involve child mental health specialists, who operate within small areas and are based within the local infrastructure such as primary schools and general practices. The specialists within such services are linked primarily with that community, rather than with the Tier 2 CAMHS, and focus to a greater extent on providing early intervention to children and their families, as well as helping to strengthen existing resources at Tier 1.

Characteristics of the primary mental health worker

The HAS report advocates that the PMHW role should be undertaken by a senior professional from a mental health background (nursing, social work, psychology, occupational therapy or medicine). The importance of this is the need for the professional to have autonomy, accountability and the ability to utilise specialist knowledge to assist other professionals in making decisions or in working with children's mental health.

The core attributes of a PMHW are:

- specialist knowledge of child and adolescent mental health;
- experience of working in a community setting with children, adolescents and their families;
- a senior level within their profession, with the ability to take responsibility for decision-making;
- assessment skills;
- an ability to provide clinical supervision and consultation to other professionals on a variety of levels;
- excellent communication and networking skills; and
- a range of direct work/therapeutic skills.

ROLES OF THE PMHW

The fundamentals of the PMHW role encompass the provision of specialised consultation, training, supervision and support to primary care professionals, with the principal aim of strengthening child mental health services within primary care. One important facet of the role is the undertaking of liaison and joint working with cases that have complex issues and require a multi-agency approach in order to meet the needs of children and families.

The PMHW should develop and undertake initial assessments and brief focused treatment interventions, with children and families who do not respond to initial management in primary care. Direct work may also be appropriate where issues have become too complex for the primary care setting, but do not require the intervention of the specialist child and adolescent mental health team; for example, with children who exhibit behavioural or low-level emotional difficulties, such as night-time fears or social anxieties. The aim is not to replicate services that are already available. The important feature is that, once intervention is complete, the child can be managed successfully by primary care professionals, with ongoing support from the PMHW.

Essentially, the role provides a link between primary and specialist tiers and is proactive in the filtering of all referrals to specialist CAMHS, directing children towards the most appropriate service for their needs and advising referrers of the same. This enables a 'whole-service' approach, while at the same time providing vital education to primary care professionals and acting as a resource for what is available in the locality.

When developing working protocols for the PMHW relationship with primary care professionals, the principles must be based on the following targets:

- active promotion of the mental health of children and young people through positive preventative strategies and approaches, in partnership with primary care professionals;
- addressing mental health issues within local communities through encouragement, empowerment and education, in respect of children, families and primary care professionals;
- the provision of an appropriate, accessible service to children, young people and families when necessary;
- assessment of children and young people in order to formulate a needs-based, multi-factorial approach to care offered;
- working in a seamless inter-agency way, within the local community;
- advocation at all levels of the importance of prevention within child and adolescent mental health approaches;
- offering valuable consultation, education, support and supervision to those working directly with children and young people;
- enabling and aiding primary care professionals and parents/carers in the early recognition of mental health issues in children and young people;
- identification of the skills of primary care professionals in working with the mental health needs of children and young people;
- working jointly with agencies in meeting the mental health needs of children and young people in the community. Identification, where appropriate, of the need for intervention by the specialist CAMHS team and support and facilitation of the child's and family's access to this;
- facilitation of access to the agency or agencies best placed to meet the child's and family's identified needs.

Liaison

Within mental health services, the use of the word 'liaison' typically implies contact between psychiatric and non-psychiatric services, and is seen as collaboration between professionals. Skills and knowledge are incorporated into the interventions of the non-psychiatric team, and notions of networking and collaboration between agencies and professionals are also included (Roberts, 1997). These aspects are seen as integral to the PMHW role; in the past, an established lack of inter-agency collaboration has resulted in the isolation of primary care professionals.

When developing the role in a locality, the PMHW should prioritise networking and liaison, developing a more seamless approach to care. It is important to 'map' services available to children within a locality, taking time to visit and discuss service provision and ways of working together. This has been found to be a useful approach in understanding the role of the agencies, and how they might fit together. It is often useful to create a directory of services from the mapping process. This will aid all professionals to think strategically when they are deciding on the best programme of care for a child. Such liaison activities also provide primary care professionals with a co-ordinated link with CAMHS.

In whatever form, liaison aims to achieve the following:

- a reduction of duplication in service provision;
- aiding professionals in making informed decisions about a child's care;
- the education of the professionals in what is appropriate to refer to CAMHS;
- the development of a strategic approach to planning care for children and families.

A supportive inter-agency network can instil in front-line staff a confidence in their knowledge and clinical skills.

Until recently, the liaison role was little developed in the UK. It was originally introduced in the 1970s, when there was concern for the increasing number of suicide attempts and deliberate self-harm in the adult population (Catalan *et al.*, 1980). Initially, it was a crisis intervention initiative, predominantly based in accident and emergency departments (Department of Health, 1997). Nursing staff usually undertake such posts, with the aim of assessing the person at the time of crisis, undertaking short-term interventions, and referring to a more specialist service where necessary. This work can be applied to the early recognition of children's mental health difficulties within the primary care setting.

Within primary care, liaison with CAMHS regarding children's mental health needs can take place on a number of levels, including direct liaison between a PMHW and a referrer, to discuss the services that may be most appropriate to meet a child's needs. For example, a child referred to CAMHS, who is upset following the death of an aunt, would benefit most from intervention from an agency specialising in bereavement issues. Liaison with the referrer would reveal that the child did not present with mental health difficulties, as such, but required some help to get over his (understandable) grief. The referrer might have referred to CAMHS because of a lack of knowledge about other agencies available. Without effective liaison, the case might conceivably languish on a waiting list for some time.

Another important liaison approach relates to the organisation of and attendance at multi-agency meetings to plan for a child's care. Frequently, children who have presented with long-standing behavioural difficulties are found to have a number of agencies already involved with their care. Often, none of the agencies has communicated its concerns, or indeed its interventions, to any other. Work is replicated, or there may be gaps in what is being offered. For example, one boy of seven was referred to CAMHS by a concerned social worker after a short bout of fire-setting within the family home. After liaison with the social worker, it became apparent that the child had difficulties in school, which were spilling over to the home environment. He already had the involvement of the educational psychologist, and was receiving help from an educational welfare officer, because of limited attendance at school. His mother also had support from HomeStart, a charitable organisation that provides volunteers to support the parent in the home. After the organisation of a multi-agency meeting, care was planned in a more co-ordinated way. All concerned agreed that there was no need for the involvement of CAMHS, but that the agencies would benefit from continued support from the PMHW, regarding advice about children's mental health and interventions most appropriate to the child's needs.

Consultation and advice

The origins of consultation within this context lie within the nursing role and were developed during the 1930s (Roberts, 1997). The fundamentals of consultation have parallels with consultation/liaison psychiatry – a role historically undertaken by psychiatrists in a general medical setting. Access to such skills is considered to be essential in collaboration with primary care professionals and aids in the management of psychological problems and decision-making about treatment directions for children. Consultation is an important part of the PMHW role and a vital component of multi-agency work. The importance of collaboration has been emphasised in the government Green Paper on developing partnerships in mental health (Department of Health, 1997).

Consultation work can be carried out on a number of levels:

- the consultant may work indirectly on a problem with the consultee;
- the consultee is an autonomous practitioner who may accept or reject advice;
- the consultee is regarded as a competent professional within their own area of practice; and
- consultation may be considered to be educative or formal training may be undertaken.

Consultation is viewed as being on a continuum, ranging from telephone and face-to-face consultation, to regular consultation/supervision groups and training of practitioners, and is seen as the specialist facet of the consultation-liaison of the PMHW roles (Hobbs and Murray, 1999).

The PMHW can provide consultation to primary care professionals in the form of telephone and face-to-face consultation, where a discussion surrounding a case takes place. This is usually when a professional has concerns regarding a child's mental wellbeing, is unsure where to refer, or is uncertain about what services are available. Primary care professionals can benefit from regular supervision groups set up in the locality, undertaken with health visitors, school nurses and also within GP surgeries. Individual cases can be presented or general issues relating to mental health difficulties in children may be discussed. The PMHW acts mainly as a facilitator for discussion and also provides advice where necessary.

It can also be useful for the PMHW to work closely with professional community forums and voluntary agencies (such as parenting networks, HomeStart, special needs forums, volunteer groups, local voluntary action forums or domestic violence forums). The aim should be to provide education, support and information, and to inform discussion on children's mental health issues, thereby strengthening the confidence of these professionals to recognise and tackle mental health difficulties early.

Joint work with primary care professionals and direct work with children and families

Joint work between primary care professionals and PMHWs is important and can be undertaken in a number of ways. It may be in the form of a joint assessment with a practitioner already involved in a case, for the purpose of understanding the needs of the child or the family in relation to mental health. Alternatively, the PMHW can support practitioners in the work they are already undertaking, assisting them in developing choices for intervention, or educating them in the assessment process.

It is imperative that joint work is negotiated through the process of consultation and that it should be seen as educative. It will serve to enhance the existing skills of primary care professionals and improve their confidence in the work they do with children. The process should be a two-way learning activity, with both workers setting agreed aims and objectives for the piece of work, both in service and professional development. If the workers collaborate in this way, there will be greater understanding of roles and skills and a development of joint responsibility for children's mental health. Such collaboration should be an interactive process that enables professionals with different expertise to generate solutions to mutually defined problems.

Once the joint working process has ended, it is important that supportive or supervisory plans are put into place for the professional, who continues the work with the case, thereby enabling ongoing communication and management.

In some cases, which have been seen during joint work, it may be necessary for the PMHW to undertake assessment and direct work with the child and the family. This might happen when it is decided during the joint assessment that the child's difficulties are not responding to methods and interventions tried by the primary care worker, or through support from the PMHW, and where the primary care professional has concerns regarding the child's mental health needs, which cannot be supported through consultation. The cases selected for direct work have usually proved to be intervention-resistive at a primary care level, but are not considered appropriate for a more specialist intervention from CAMHS. The child must also be suitable for management by primary care professionals once the intervention is complete. This is an important principle in maintaining continuity with Tier 1 staff, as it is envisaged that many children and families will either require lengthier but a similar kind of intervention, or may suffer future relapse episodes (Visser *et al.*, 1999), and require further intervention without referral to specialist CAMHS.

In such cases, the PMHW offers direct work in the form of brief focused intervention of approximately six to eight treatment sessions, followed by a formal review with the child and the family. Direct work is tailored to meet the needs of the child and family, with such activities as parenting training, cognitive-behavioural therapy, solution-focused brief therapy, and anger management. Each child and family should be seen for an assessment session, to ensure screening for mental health problems that may require intervention from specialist CAMHS. The assessment should look at the child and the family from a holistic viewpoint, while undertaking a full assessment of the child's mental health needs. A management plan should be agreed with the child and family, incorporating the need to collaborate and communicate with other appropriate agencies. Intervention is then related to the identified needs and implemented in partnership with other agencies, where possible, and with permission from the family.

One of the strengths of PMHW interventions is that they can be locally based, for example, at community health centres. This will increase access to both professionals and families and put the PMHW in a prime position to network with all agencies available to that locality, while maintaining a co-ordinated link with CAMHS. An intervention in the community and family environment can also help to reduce the perception of stigma of mental illness.

PMHWs can advise on simple behavioural techniques for behavioural problems such as temper tantrums, other oppositional behaviour, sleep problems or bed-wetting, to both the professional and to families. While this is often the remit of the primary care professional, such problems can be found commonly to defy intervention. They can also offer intervention for families dealing with stress, which may include maternal depression and/or loss of confidence in the ability to parent, or advice on concerns regarding school.

Training

Training is an important aspect of the role of the PMHW. In an evaluative study undertaken with 116 primary care professionals, examining their perceptions of the PMHW role (Gale, 1999), 76% considered training by a PMHW as appropriate and necessary for their needs, in relation to working with mental health difficulties in children.

Training offered to primary care professionals should enable them to develop their understanding of children's mental health issues and should consolidate their existing knowledge through experiential learning. It should not seek to turn front-line staff into specialists, but enable them to recognise and manage child mental health problems at an early stage. Also, it should provide them with a broad knowledge base and a theoretical framework to make informed choices on the best care approach for each child.

CHALLENGES IN IMPLEMENTING THE PMHW ROLE

The importance of primary care interventions, such as those provided by PMHWs, will increase with the establishment of Primary Care Groups in the UK. However, there are many challenges in the successful implementation of the PMHW role.

First, that role is contrary to the previous working experience of many professionals. It can be be a difficult role to introduce, as professionals are historically used to seeing all referrals, or working with waiting lists. The post-holder needs to be versed in the process and function of consultation and support of other professionals, to have confidence in his or her own skills, and have the ability to instill confidence in others. It is important to have in-depth understanding of the child mental health strategy within which the post-holder is working, and to have the ability to 'sell it to others'. Regular supervision should also be provided for staff. There may be concerns regarding clinical supervision by a practitioner from a different professional background.

The PMHW should be thought of as a member of a multidisciplinary team and managed in the same way, with leadership from a professional who has a vision of the direction of the team and model of working, and of how it fits within the overall CAMHS strategy.

It is possible to be quickly overwhelmed by demand, so it is vital for the PMHW to build networks and working protocols with primary care professionals, and to have flexible ways of working. How close should the PMHW be to specialist CAMHS? There are many emerging models of primary mental health work throughout the UK, coupled with arguments for either being separate from or being part of the CAMH team. In some areas, PMHWs are managed by local authorities (education or social services) rather than a Trust. Regardless of the model developed, the support of CAMHS is paramount from the outset. Without this understanding, it is difficult to provide the interface between tiers, and the team can become a satellite service.

Primary care professionals sometimes see the PMHW role as one that blocks access to CAMHS. It should be emphasised to them that access to CAMHS will be more efficient for those children who need it, and that access should be seen as a continuum; it begins with the very first contact with the PMHW. One similar concern is that the team has been developed in order to protect CAMHS from insurmountable demand; the impression may be that families are deliberately being denied a service, or that the team is in competition with the CAMH team. Instead, there should be emphasis on the benefits for the specialist team of working with and educating primary care professionals. There should be reiteration of the promotion of early recognition of children's mental health problems, and of appropriate, considered referrals to CAMHS. Such a process will enable CAMHS to undertake work with those children who need the service, reducing the numbers of children who develop entrenched and severe mental health disorders.

The real challenge for debate within primary mental health work is that patients and tiers are not static. It is crucial to consider how to deal with the overlap between specialist CAMHS and primary care. Children may be prone to relapse episodes, or make a significant improvement that merits a referral from CAMHS to the primary care level. It is important to think how these anomalies may be challenged, in order to streamline the services.

TIERS 2 AND 3: THE CHANGING ROLE OF SPECIALIST SERVICES

Specialist CAMHS provide secondary and tertiary care. They should have an appropriate balance and mix of professional expertise. This should be reflected in the disciplines represented within the service and in the experience (grading) of the team members. A typical service should include representation from child and adolescent psychiatry, clinical child psychology and child mental health nursing. Some services may include other specialists such as child psychotherapists, occupational therapists, art therapists, and speech and language therapists. Social workers have been placed routinely at child and family guidance clinics, and there are still many CAMHS with specialist social work mental health input. Members of the specialist CAMH teams may act alone with a child or family, or as consultants to another agency or service.

TREATMENT MODALITIES APPLIED TO CHILDREN WITH MENTAL HEALTH PROBLEMS

Cognitive therapy

Cognitive therapy is based on the theory that, through practice, the young person will be able to identify and correct the cognitive distortion that makes him or her depressed or aggressive (Rutter *et al.*, 1994). Cognitive therapy was initially developed for treating depression; however, its remit has gradually expanded. It has been shown to be effective in reducing aggressive and antisocial behaviour at home, at school and in the community (Baer and Nietzel, 1991). It has also been shown to be feasible and effective in treating emotional problems both at specialist and at primary care level (Bernstein and Kinlan, 1997).

Behaviour therapy: parent training

Behaviour therapy has been used effectively for many groups of children, including those with severe learning disabilities (Cunningham *et al.*, 1995) or sleep problems (Scott and Richard, 1990). However, it has been found to be particularly useful in helping parents with children with behavioural problems (Webster-Stratton, 1991).

Parent training programmes were first described in the 1960s. They initially focused on teaching techniques to individual parents to ameliorate specific child behaviours. Parent training refers to procedures in which parents are trained to alter the child's behaviour (Patterson *et al.*, 1992). It is based on the assumption that parents often inadvertently reward the undesired behaviour:

> *Coercion refers to deviant behaviour on the part of one person (eg the child) that is rewarded by another person (eg the parent).*
>
> (Kazdin, 1997)

Sometimes, in attempting to stop the unwanted behaviour, parents inadvertently reinforce it and may increase the frequency with which it occurs. For example, a child who enjoys playing on the computer in his bedroom, rather than sitting quietly and talking with visitors, might behave in such a way that his parents are compelled to 'punish' him. They may choose to respond to the undesired behaviour by sending their child to his bedroom; they may find that the child continues to misbehave in the same way. The child will not see the 'time out' in his bedroom as a punishment but as a reward. The child will continue to misbehave in order to be sent to his room, to play on the computer.

It is always important to look into the consequences of a child's behaviour. In order to change the unwanted behaviour, therapists can work with parents using the 'ABC' analysis. This is based on the notion that the expression of most behaviour is influenced by Antecedent events (what happened before the Behaviour) and the Consequent response (what happened following the behaviour). Altering the antecedents or consequences of any unwanted behaviour may change the frequency of occurrence. The therapists will ask parents to record the events happening before the child's unwanted behaviour. Then the therapist and parents together need to look into any kind of pattern that may illustrate how the child exhibits the unwanted behaviour in certain circumstances. Altering the parental pattern of behaviour that maintains the child's behaviour can reduce the unwanted behaviour. This requires the development of different parenting styles, such as establishing clear and consistent rules for the child to follow, providing positive reinforcement for appropriate behaviour, and other techniques and strategies.

Family therapy and family work

Various schools of thought in family therapy have evolved over time and have influenced each other. Three schools are particularly well known: Structural (Minuchin, 1974), Strategic (Haley, 1963), and Systemic or Milan (Palazzoli *et al.*, 1977). Family therapists will usually regard the child's mental health problem as a shared family problem, rather than one that belongs only to the identified child. In family therapy, a problem is viewed as part of a repetitive sequence of interaction, which maintains and is maintained by the problem. Family therapists aim to identify and change the meaning and function of a presenting problem within the context of the family system (Burnham, 1994).

Individual work (psychodynamic therapy)

This treatment has been applied particularly to children and adolescents with emotional problems. The therapist works with the patient on the here-and-now relationship, in the light of past history and external relationships. This is an opportunity to allow the child to explore his or her thoughts, feelings, relationships and experiences in privacy, without the risk of upsetting parents or other adult carers. The therapist may use play, art, or drama (in the form of role-play), to facilitate young children, or those who have difficulty in putting feelings into words.

Pharmacological treatment

Different types of medication can be used to help children and adolescents with severe mental health problems. Medication should always be part of a comprehensive treatment plan arrived at after a thorough psychiatric assessment. The indications for drug use in children are often different from those relating to adults.

For children with moderate to severe ADHD, for example, medication (usually the stimulant methylphenidate) can improve physical restlessness and attention capacity. Although it does not directly target behaviour, improvement in these areas can facilitate the implementation of psychological and educational interventions (Overmeyer and Taylor, 1999). Medication can also be used for the treatment of severe emotional disorders, particularly depression (Martin *et al.*, 2000; Velosa and Riddle, 2000).

THE FUTURE

The future development of CAMHS lies in the development of comprehensive services that begin within primary care and have a co-ordinated link with the more specialist tiers. The Audit Commission's report *With Children in Mind* (2000) recommends the strengthening of links between Tier 1 and specialist CAMHS, by paying particular attention to the support available to professionals within Tier1. This can be achieved through development of strategic relationships with local health professionals, social services, education departments and voluntary agencies, to enable establishment of effective ways of meeting the needs of children. The report also indicates that 64% of health authorities have now undertaken a local 'mapping' process, which highlights the areas of particular need in relation to children's mental health, child protection issues and exclusions from schools. However, the quality of the multi-agency response to this varies greatly. Most of the relationships developed did not include GPs, who still continue to make a large number of referrals to specialist CAMHS.

The Mental Health Foundation report *Bright Futures* (1999) emphasises the importance of invoking a perspective from all agencies that has clarity and flexibility. Agencies should challenge poor and ineffective channels of communication and ways of working, and build upon support networks, skills and links. The ownership of children's mental health by all professionals is crucial and is the present challenge to all agencies. Professionals in Tier 1 possess many skills, but it is important to raise awareness of children's mental health and to provide support that seeks to build knowledge and confidence in tackling such issues. Such provision should be on the agenda of all CAMHS.

The prime objective is for all professionals who work with children to develop a basic understanding of mental health, enabling early identification of such difficulties and early intervention for those who require it. The mental health needs of children are wide-ranging and complex. They do not exist in isolation and can affect the child's daily quality of life in all areas. Research has shown that early intervention has a significant impact on the reduction in severity of children's problems (Target and Fognay, 1996). The Mental Health Foundation (1999) suggests that services for children should provide a continuum of help and support, indicating the development of multi-agency initiatives that provide greater access to a range of advice and interventions, encompassing all aspects of the child's life. This could be achieved through a programme of training, support and intervention to professionals and, in time, families.

The CAMHS agenda for development should embrace easier access for professionals and families to services that offer a range of information, resources and help. The Audit Commission (2000) recommends that specialist CAMHS should seek to demystify their entrance criteria, so that referring professionals can make more appropriate referrals, reducing waiting times and the need for waiting lists. Gaps in service provision between agencies should be identified and service specifications should be more transparent, so that new services can be planned strategically. It is important for agencies to catalogue the available resources and to become familiar with provision so that there is no duplication or wastage of provision.

The importance of reducing the stigma associated with mental ill health has been recognised by the government. This can only be achieved via a change in the attitudes of the public perception. However, it has to begin with the professionals, through the development of new and existing services, increased knowledge and understanding of children's mental health and a commitment from agencies to develop ways of working together. It is a challenge that is the responsibility of all professionals who come into contact with children and their families.

This chapter impresses on the reader the magnitude of the problems surrounding the delivery of child and adolescent mental health services. It discusses the new role of the primary mental health worker and how this might contribute to improving child and adolescent services. The authors feel that these workers will assist in the early identification of clients, by improving communication with and between other services. There is, however, an ever-present danger that far more will be expected of them than they can reasonably deliver. Support is vital if they are to make a significant difference to services. The most important message to emerge from this chapter is that all professionals working with children need a basic understanding of mental health, to ensure early intervention for those who require it. The mental health needs of children are wide-ranging and complex and do not exist in isolation from the other areas of the child's life. A growing body of knowledge reveals that early intervention significantly reduces the severity of a child's problems. Recognising and responding to the mental health needs of children should be seen as an important means of reducing the prevalence of mental health problems in adults. (Editors' summary)

REFERENCES

Audit Commission (2000) *With Children in Mind: Child and adolescent mental health services*, Audit Commission Publications, Oxford

Baer, R.A. and Nietzel, M.T. (1991) Cognitive and behavioural treatment of impulsivity in children: a meta-analytic review of the outcome literature, *Journal of Clinical Child Psychology*, **20**, 400–412

Bernstein, G. and Kinlan, J. (1997) Summary of the practice parameters for the assessment and treatment of children and adolescents with anxiety disorders, *Journal of the American Academy of Child and Adolescent Psychiatry*, 36, 1639–1641

Burnham, J.B. (1994) *Family Therapy*, Routledge, London

Catalan, J., Hewlett, J., Kenner, C. and McPherson, J. (1980) The role of the nurse in the management of deliberate self-poisoning in the general hospital, *International Journal of Nursing Studies*, 17, 275–282

Cunningham, C.E., Bremner, R. and Boyle, M. (1995) Large group community-based parenting programs for families of pre-schoolers at risk of disruptive behaviour disorders: utilisation, cost effectiveness and outcome, *Journal of Child Psychology and Psychiatry*, 36, 1141–1159

Department of Health (1997) *Developing Partnerships in Mental Health*, HMSO, London

Gale, F. (1999) When tiers are not enough: an evaluation of the perception and experiences amongst primary care professionals of the primary mental health worker role within CAMHS [unpublished MA thesis], University of Central England, Birmingham

Haley, J. (1963) *Strategies of Psychotherapy*, Grune Stratton, New York

Hobbs, R. and Murray, E.T. (1999) Specialist liaison nurses, *British Medical Journal.* 318, 683–684

House of Commons (1997) *Health Committee Report: Child and Adolescent Health Services*, HMSO, London

Kaplan, H.I., Sadock, B.J and Grebb, J.A. (1994) *Synopsis of Psychiatry*, 7th edition, Williams & Wilkins, Maryland, MA

Kazdin, A.E. (1997) Practitioner review: psychosocial treatments for conduct disorder in children, *Journal of Child Psychology and Psychiatry*, 38, 161–178

Lacey, I. (1998) The role of the primary mental health worker – national survey and local development [unpublished dissertation, Master in Health Science] University of Birmingham, Birmingham

Martin, A., Kaufman, J. and Charney, D. (2000) Pharmacotherapy of early-onset depression, update and new directions, *Child and Adolescent Psychiatric Clinics of North America*, 9, 135–157

Mental Health Foundation (MHF) (1999) *Bright Futures: Promoting children and young people's mental health*, Mental Health Foundation, London

Minuchin, S. (1974) *Families and Family Therapy*, Tavistock, London

Neira-Munoz, E. and Ward, D. (1998) Side by side, *Health Service Journal*, 13, 26–27

NHS Health Advisory Service (1995) *Child and Adolescent Mental Health Service: Together we stand: the commissioning, role and management of child and adolescent mental health services*, HMSO, London

Offord, D.R., Boyle, M.C. and Racine, Y.A. (1991) The epidemiology of antisocial behaviour in childhood and adolescence. In Perpler, D.J. and Rubin, K.H. (eds.) *The development and treatment of childhood aggression*, Lawrence Erlbaum, Hillsdale, NJ

Office for National Statistics (1999) *Mental Health of Children and Adolescents*, ONS, London

Overmeyer, S. and Taylor, E. (1999) Annotation: principles of treatment for hyperkinetic disorder: practice approaches for the UK, *Journal of Child Psychology and Psychiatry*, 40, 1147–1157

Palazzoli, M.S, Boscolo, L., Cecchin, G.F. and Prata, G. (1977) Family rituals and powerful tools in family therapy, *Family Process*, 16, 445–453

Patterson, G.R., Reid, J.B. and Dishion, T.J. (1992) *Antisocial Boys*, Eugene, OR: Castalia

Rhode, L.A., Biederman, J., Busnello, E.A., Zimmermann, H., Schitz, M., Martins, S. and Traumontina, S. (1999) ADHD in school sample of Brazilian adolescents: a study of prevalence in comorbid conditions and impairments, *Journal of American Academy of Child and Adolescent Psychiatry*, 38, 716–722

Roberts, D. (1997) Liaison mental health nursing: origins, definition and prospects, *Journal of Advanced Nursing*, 25,101–108

Rutter, M., Taylor, E. and Hersov, L. (1994) *Child and Adolescent Psychiatry: Modern approaches*, Blackwell Science, Oxford

Scott, G. and Richard, M.P.M. (1990) Night walking in infants: effect of providing advice and support for parents, *Journal of Child Psychology and Psychiatry*, 31, 551–567

Sidane, A., Bhatia, M.S., and Choudary, S. (1998) Prevalence and patterns of psychiatric morbidity in children, *Indian Journal of Medical Sciences*, 52, 556–558

Target, M. and Fognay, P. (1996) The psychological treatment of children and adolescent mental health problems. In Roth, A. and Fognay, P. (eds.) *What Works for Whom: Implications and limitations of the research literature*, Guilford Press, New York

Velosa, J.F. and Riddle, M.A. (2000) Pharmacologic treatment of anxiety disorders in children and adolescents, *Child and Adolescent Psychiatric Clinic of North America*, 9, 119–133

Visser, J.H., Van der Ende, J., Koot, H. and Verhulst, F. (1999) Continuity of psychopathology in youths referred to mental health services, *Journal of the American Academy of Child and Adolescent Psychiatry*, 38, 1560–1568

Webster-Stratton, C. (1991) Annotation: strategies for helping families with conduct disordered children, *Journal of Child Psychology and Psychiatry*, 32, 1047–1062

11 Working with People Who Use Illicit Drugs

John Macleod

*This chapter explains the scope of the challenge confronting GPs in relation to substance abuse. Readers may conclude that the figures seen in reports under-estimate the real extent of the problem. The author explains why attempting to define a 'typical' substance abuser is pointless; victims come from very varied backgrounds, succumb to substance abuse for different reasons, and have different pretexts for wanting help. If professionals are to be effective, they must abandon the stereotyping of abusers, and rid themselves of prejudice. Many GPs are currently unaided in their work with substance abusers. The author considers whether GPs should collaborate, how and with whom. Collaboration is time-consuming and patients may not wish other agencies to be involved in their care and treatment. Collaboration is difficult when there is no agreement on the nature of substance abuse, or whether it is a medical or a social problem. More research is needed in the field, as well as more resources and a far more realistic and less guarded discussion about how to approach the problem of substance abuse sensibly and humanely. (**Editors' note**)*

SETTING THE SCENE

Workers trying to help people whose problems are categorised under the heading of mental health often face two difficulties that are not always important issues for health workers as a whole. They may have to deal with problems that some might argue are not true illnesses in a strictly patho-physiological sense; and they almost invariably find themselves relying on a scientific evidence base that is, at best, incomplete. This general truth is particularly pertinent to those who work with people who use illicit drugs.

The use of psychoactive drugs is hardly new but the 'drug problem' only came to the fore, in the UK at least, in the latter part of the twentieth century. From being viewed as a minor personal issue – of delinquency, weakness, misfortune or choice – drug use, and particularly drug dependency, came to be seen as part of a funda-mental and threatening social malaise. The reasons behind this paradigm shift are, inevitably, complicated. Interested readers are directed to some of the many comprehensive accounts available (Royal College of Psychiatrists and Royal College of Physicians, 2000).

Before considering the 'nuts and bolts' of trying to help people with drug problems in the primary care setting, it is vital to acknowledge the huge social stigma that attaches to drug use. Many 'initiatives' in this area have not been motivated primarily by concern for the welfare of the drug user. Instead, they were part of a strategy designed to contain the social threat that drug users were perceived to pose. These considerations are important, because they continue to shape much of our work.

Around 50% of people between the ages of 16 and 25 have used an illegal drug (Ramsay *et al.*, 2001). A significant minority use drugs regularly – once a week, or more frequently. A small number experience the extremely debilitating problems traditionally seen among clients of 'drug services'. Increasingly, it is this latter group of 'problem drug users' that is presenting for help in primary care (there are several reasons for this; *see below*). Because of this, this chapter will concentrate on working with these adolescents and younger adults who are 'problem drug users'. While it is probably true that problematic, health-damaging use can be associated with any psychoactive substance, most users presenting in primary care have problems with the following:

- opiates (principally heroin, methadone, morphine, buprenorphine and dihydrocodeine);
- stimulants (the various forms of cocaine and the amphetamines); and
- benzodiazepines (temazepam, diazepam, and others).

The method by which a drug is used also influences the type of problems likely to be experienced. In general, injection drug use is associated with more serious problems. However, users who smoke, 'snort' and swallow drugs can also experience significant problems.

Drug problems can be divided (roughly) into problems associated with the drug itself (its pharmacological effects, problems associated with the way it is taken), and those that arise out of the fact that, since drug use is illegal, users are inevitably criminalised. There is an important point to make in relation to this criminalisation. All drug users are criminals because they purchase and consume an illegal substance. However, the relationship between drug use and crime is more complex than that. This complexity is often not acknowledged and statistics relating to the issue are often presented in a misleading way (Stimson *et al.*, 1998). In some subcultures, drug use may be more common than in society generally. For example, it appears that many criminals take drugs, and they also (by definition) commit crimes. It is naïve to believe (as many politicians and journalists often seem to) that this is a simple relationship of cause and effect. It is much more likely to be due in a large part to what epidemiologists call 'confounding'. Both taking drugs and committing crimes are associated with being a criminal but it does not follow that taking drugs causes criminals to commit most of their crimes; furthermore, the criminality of most drug users is confined to their drug use. Importantly, from the point of view of primary care treatment services, it also does not mean that treating a criminal's drug use will stop them committing crimes; it is more realistic to hope that it may reduce the amount of crime they commit.

Problem drug use does not just affect problem drug users. It affects the communities in which they live and, more significantly, it also affects the people close to them – their partners, siblings, parents, children and other family members. Help for these 'significant others' has often not been high on the treatment agenda.

In terms of proportional impact on population health, the most damaging psychoactive substances are of course tobacco and alcohol. Problems associated with use of these drugs will not be considered here.

COLLABORATION – ASPIRATIONS AND REALITIES

Since problem drug use is a multi-factorial social problem, helping problem drug users should ideally involve a range of professionals and agencies. Inter-agency and inter-professional co-ordination, liaison and 'shared care' are all important issues. Nowhere is the theme of collaboration more challenging than in the service response to drug problems. Part of this challenge lies in the diversity of the people whose work ostensibly is to help problem drug users, or to reduce the harm to individuals and communities associated with drug use.

The group of 'professionals' includes health workers from various disciplines, social workers and probation officers, the police, educationalists and also various advocacy groups. Each of these constituencies has its own traditions, experience and agenda – sometimes the overlap may be slight, representing a philosophical barrier to collaboration. There is also a serious practical barrier, based on a lack of resources. For example, in Edinburgh in the late 1980s and early 1990s, the perceived urgency of the local situation meant that community drug services were extremely well resourced; innovative, collaborative practice flourished. However, as concerns about the threat to the general population receded, funding was cut.

In the current reality for most practitioners, the greatest barrier to collaboration is the difficulty of finding someone willing and able to collaborate. Most 'specialist' agencies measure their waiting lists in months and have little to offer in terms of 'emergency' support. It is also true that most primary care 'drug services' would be more accurately described as 'prescribing services'; their main function is the delivery of decriminalised substitute drugs. The service-use patterns of most drug users appear to reflect this reality. Even when opportunities for involving others in collaborative care exist (and they generally do not), some clients may be reluctant to engage with workers other than those closely related to the provision of their prescription. This chapter reflects this reality. The consequent lack of description of 'collaborative practice in action' is not intended to suggest any philosophical disagreement with the *principle* of collaboration.

Tables 11.1 and 11.2 list some of the agencies that may collaborate in the care of any individual problem drug user. Co-ordination of their efforts is, in theory, the responsibility of social services and in practice this can usually be achieved through letters and telephone contact. Occasionally, 'case conferences' may be called, to allow more in-depth discussions. In the following accounts it may at times appear that the GP is 'doing everything'. Again this is simply a reflection of the practical reality that currently exists in much of the UK, rather than an anxiety that the involvement of too many collaborators might upset a special relationship between the drug user and their GP. Most GPs working with drug users are likely to be happy to enter into shared-care relationships where the opportunity to do so exists.

Table 11.1 Potential collaborative relationships in David's care

Professional agency	Role
Probation officer/social worker	Assessment and identification of needs Development, implementation and supervision of care plan Co-ordination and liaison with all professionals involved in care
Welfare rights officer	Welfare rights, benefits advice and advocacy
General practitioner	Assessment and identification of needs Referral and liaison with other professionals Substitute prescribing Ongoing general medical care
Practice nurse	Hepatitis B immunisation
Pharmacist	Dispensing of substitute prescription – supervision of consumption Daily contact point – in some circumstances may provide ad hoc psychological support
Housing officer	Housing needs
Specialist drug agency	Assessment, tolerance testing, ongoing shared care Extended support services Prescription advice
Needle exchange	Provision of clean injection equipment, advice on safer injection technique
Drug users peer-support agency	Peer support, perhaps advocacy in relation to contact with statutory services
Crisis centres	Crisis and respite care

Table 11.2 Potential collaborative relationships in Sandra's care

Professional agency	Role
Social worker	Assessment and identification of needs Development, implementation and supervision of care plan Co-ordination and liaison with all professionals involved in care Help and advice around issues related to child care
Welfare rights officer	Welfare rights, benefits advice and advocacy
General practitioner	Assessment and identification of needs Referral and liaison with other professionals Substitute prescribing Ongoing general medical care for patient and children
Practice nurse	Hepatitis B immunisation
Pharmacist	Dispensing of substitute prescription
Housing officer	Housing needs
Hospital Department of Infectious Diseases	Specialist monitoring and treatment advice around HIV infection, including in-patient care as appropriate Liaison with other hospital-based therapists, eg, occupational therapists
Community psychiatric services	Assessment, support, counselling and treatment advice
Sex-workers peer-support agency	Peer support, perhaps advocacy in relation to contact with statutory services
Hospice services	Crisis and respite care, bereavement counselling May run structured day-care programmes

A 'TYPICAL' PROBLEM DRUG USER?

It is vital to understand that there is no such thing as a typical problem drug user. Stereotypes do exist and in general these are unhelpful. Many problem drug users come from a background characterised by multiple social deprivation, horrendous experiences of sexual and physical abuse in early life, and criminality of various sorts. Many have enduring difficulties in the areas of making and sustaining close personal relationships, concomitant mental health problems and ongoing difficulties in managing most aspects of their life in general. *However*, others do not. Problem drug users can be male or female, of any age, from any social or ethnic group. Within this variety it is fair to say that – like most forms of ill health – problem drug use is strongly socially patterned and problem users are certainly over-represented among people who are socially disadvantaged.

This chapter will consider three hypothetical 'patients' but these are *not* typical problem drug users. They are composite fictional characters, created to illustrate some of the issues that are involved in work in this area. All of their problems have been experienced by people who have been seen in primary care.

CASE STUDY DAVID

David is 26. He has been 'diverted' into treatment from the criminal justice system. His lawyer has advised him that, in demonstrating a commitment to rehabilitation, he may avoid a custodial sentence from an imminent court appearance. He has been in prison on numerous occasions before, generally for crimes involving theft or violence. He has been using illegal drugs since his early teens – he takes anything he can get his hands on via a variety of routes. His childhood was characterised by violence at the hands of his alcoholic father, who left the family home when David was 10. David never got on with his mother's subsequent partner. He has no formal educational qualifications and most of his schooling was in 'list D' schools. He has had frequent contact with mental health services and has been labelled as having a 'psychopathic personality disorder'. His elder brother died from a heroin overdose, he also has a younger sister and a daughter with whom he has no contact. He lives with his mother. David currently mainly uses heroin, cocaine and temazepam (which he mainly injects), along with cannabis (which he smokes). He has lost two fingers as a consequence of intra-arterial injection. He was removed from his last GP's list because he assaulted one of the doctors.

CASE STUDY SANDRA

Sandra is 36 and is HIV positive. She found out she was infected when her second son was born. Both her sons (aged 18 and 14) are HIV negative, she has a younger daughter (aged 7) who is HIV positive. She is a lone parent; the children have different fathers who occasionally make contact but provide little support. Sandra is unsure how she acquired HIV infection – it may have been through her injection drug use or her involvement in prostitution. She no longer injects drugs. Her previous GP prescribed her 25 30-mg dihydrocodeine tablets daily and 50 mg of diazepam – she occasionally uses cannabis. She has had to change GPs due to re-housing. She regularly takes her daughter to hospital for check-ups but tends to neglect her own HIV infection. She takes antidepressants but despite this is frequently depressed. She was sexually abused by her father as a child and was thrown out of the family home when she disclosed this at the age of 16. Her family has 'disowned' her.

CASE STUDY FAWZIA

Fawzia is 17. Her parents are both doctors, Moslems, who came to the UK from Pakistan in the 1970s. Her elder brother is at medical school. There has been a family assumption that Fawzia will also go to university although her grades in her 'mock' A-levels were disappointing. Her family has always been a close and supportive one. Despite this, Fawzia has always lacked confidence and felt to some extent in her brother's shadow. Fawzia started occasionally using amphetamines and ecstasy when she began to go 'clubbing' at 15 – she felt they increased her confidence, helping her to enjoy herself more. After one night out she was offered heroin, and she started using it intermittently. For the past six months, she has been using it on a daily basis. She smokes it and has never injected. Her parents are unaware of her drug use. She has never been in trouble with the police.

CURRENT BEST PRACTICE

Clinical governance and the promotion of adherence to best practice guidelines are currently high on the primary care agenda. Despite this, the recent *National Service Framework for Mental Health* (Department of Health, 1999a) did not specifically refer to management of problem drug users. Best practice is, arguably, that which is supported by best evidence for effectiveness. Unfortunately, evidence of the effectiveness of most management strategies that might be used in this context is limited. Guidelines for best practice, based on expert consensus and the limited evidence available, were published by the Department of Health (1999b).

INITIAL ASSESSMENT

The three fictional (although not particularly unusual) case studies present to their GP in an emergency surgery on a Friday afternoon; the GP has no previous notes for guidance. Fawzia has been a patient of the practice since she was a small child but her notes simply indicate intermittent attendance for vaccinations and trivial illnesses. David and Sandra are new patients who have registered with the practice that day. David was 'allocated' by the health authority.

The aim of the initial assessment is to determine the nature of the problem and to establish what is likely to be an ongoing relationship. In practice, it is seldom as difficult as might be expected to establish a healthy relationship with problem drug users. Because of the general public opinion of drug users (particularly someone like Sandra – a single mother, a 'junkie' and an HIV-infected prostitute), users often expect to be held in unconditional negative regard. (Unfortunately, many professionals reinforce this expectation.) Consequently, a professional who treats a user with simple civility may find that a rapport can be established remarkably quickly. This is not always true, however; for example, David might present difficulties in this regard.

One issue often comes up at this stage – behavioural contracts. There are arguments for and against these, but it is clear that they encourage a certain degree of infantilism and are generally also hostages to fortune. In practice, a professional health worker has the same 'contract' with problem drug users as with any patient: 'Behave in a civil and reasonable way towards me and I will behave similarly towards you.'

At this point, readers are directed to three publications that cover many of the relevant issues: the Department of Health guidelines on clinical management of drug misuse and dependence (Department of Health, 1999b); *Management of Drug Users in the Community* (Robertson, 1998); and *Care of Drug Users in General Practice* (Beaumont, 1997).

Assessing David

David will present a challenge to the person initially assessing him – the GP (or other 'front-line' member of the primary care team) running the Friday-evening emergency surgery. David attends alone and it is two weeks before a court appearance, at which he will be invited to enter a plea on charges including those relating to assault of his previous GP. Fortunately, this doctor suffered no serious physical harm from the assault, which resulted from an argument over a prescription. He had a particular interest in working with problem drug users, and a caring and informed approach, but, understandably, he felt unable to work with David following the incident. Somewhat reluctantly, he decided to press charges. David is currently not on any prescribed drugs. He had a double appointment with another doctor in the practice yesterday but failed to keep this, for reasons that are not entirely clear.

There are several issues that should be addressed at this first meeting; the following are the most important general points:

- You are here to help David be healthier and you will do anything that is reasonable towards this.
- Within this, you will be honest and explicit about where you feel you can help and where you feel you can't.
- David has a right to be treated courteously and competently and to complain if he feels that his care does not reflect this.
- You expect your relationship to be based on mutual respect; go through any other 'ground rules'.
- Complex problems need complex solutions, and these take time – more than

one consultation will be necessary. You may prescribe for David, but it is unlikely to be on your first meeting.

The following specific points should be addressed at the first meeting:

- What sort of 'help' does David want? (Supported detoxification? A substitute prescription? Help with other health problems? Help with social problems? A 'sick line'? A letter? A referral? Something else?)
- What made him come to see you now?
- What is the history of his drug use? (Which drugs, how, how often, how much does he spend on them, where does he get the money?)
- What is his previous experience of drug services or of trying to address his 'drug problem'?
- Past health – ask specifically about problems related to drug use (for example, blood-borne viruses, Hepatitis B vaccination).
- What are his social circumstances?
- What is his forensic history?

David wants two things: free legal drugs and a chance to improve his sentencing prospects through demonstrating a commitment to rehabilitation. If he is using free legal drugs he has less incentive to use expensive illegal ones – with all the associated consequences. Imprisonment will contain David (at great public expense). All evidence suggests it will do little to rehabilitate him. In addition, unless he is contained indefinitely, when he returns to the community his problems and the problems he causes for other people are likely to be worse. There is a basis of 'harm reduction' for you to work within. But before he gets a prescription (as he probably eventually will), you need to assess him further. The points above form the basis of that assessment but you also need to know the following:

- What is his probable opiate tolerance (how much can you safely give him)?
- Are you sure he is not receiving a prescription elsewhere? (Get the details of his last doctor; you should also check with local prescribing services such as community 'drug' clinics.)
- Does urine toxicology confirm his story of recent drug use?

It would be best to make an appointment to see David again the following week. Exactly what happens next will depend on your local services (statutory or non-statutory). If they can see people as an emergency (within the next two weeks), arrange an appointment for full assessment and tell David to phone you on Monday to find out when and where. In reality, they are unlikely to be able to respond in this time, and care is therefore the responsibility of the primary care team. The next decision, if you are a doctor, is whether to prescribe. Use your judgement. The harm-reduction pros of a prescription are well rehearsed; the cons are that David may be lying to you. He may not really be addicted and then you will potentially be *creating* addiction; alternatively, he may sell his prescription. If you do decide to prescribe, use the right books to convert street drugs into methadone equivalents. If you are unsure, 40 mg of methadone mixture is a reasonable amount (more would run the risk of killing someone who is, in fact, opiate-naïve) to be dispensed daily. Diazepam is the substitute benzodiazepine of choice, initially at no more than 30 mg daily. Prescribing stimulants is probably best left to specialists – antidepressants may help in cocaine withdrawal.

If David says he wants to stop using, the accepted strategy is outlined on pages 169–70.

Assessing Sandra

Sandra has also presented in an emergency surgery. She missed an earlier booked appointment because her daughter developed a cough and high temperature and Sandra took her straight to the children's hospital. It turned out to be a simple viral respiratory infection. Sandra's 'presenting complaint' is that she needs a new prescription. You have no previous information about her. She tells you that her previous GP prescribed her 750 mg (30 mg x 25) of dihydrocodeine, 50 mg of diazepam (10 mg x 5) and 50 mg of sertraline daily – her prescription 'runs out' tomorrow. If you decline to prescribe, one of two things will happen. Either Sandra will have no drugs and within the next 24–48 hours will experience withdrawal symptoms. In the case of opiates these will be extremely unpleasant but not life-threatening; in the case of benzodiazepines these may include seizures associated with permanent brain injury, or (rarely) death. Sandra knows this, and is likely to try to buy expensive illegal drugs and will have to find the money somehow. Apart from her occasional purchase of cannabis and her occasional prostitution this will be her first contact with the criminal sub-culture since her previous GP put her on a substitute prescription.

In view of these considerations, arguably the healthiest approach in this situation is to give Sandra a prescription. It is normally straightforward enough to corroborate the details (doses, when last dispensed) by phoning the pharmacy she last picked up from (the number will be on the medicine bottle). Her previous surgery can also be contacted, although possibly not late on a Friday. If no information can be obtained that evening, she can be given a prescription for the weekend only. The doses she states are high but unlikely to be lethal; some practitioners may prefer to 'cover themselves' by not prescribing above the BNF maximum (240 mg of dihydrocodeine and 30 mg of diazepam). This is essentially a personal decision.

When asked about past serious illnesses, Sandra states that she 'has the virus', as does her daughter. She has no idea what her viral load or CD4 count is. She has been on various medicines in relation to her HIV infection in the past; the only names she can remember are AZT and Septrin, and they didn't agree with her. Her daughter is on various anti-virals, anti-infectives and 'build-up' drinks. Sandra has brought a list, as she needs a repeat prescription for the child (who has also just registered with the practice). She also has an appointment card indicating regular attendance at the local paediatric infectious disease clinic. When you ask Sandra about her own hospital attendance she is vague and indicates that she has been advised to return if she feels unwell. She states that, as long as she has her prescription and 'keeps busy', she is fine. She denies suicidal feelings, although she acknowledges that she often feels 'low'. She cut her wrists many years ago but dismisses this as 'stupid' and doesn't go into details. She feels the sertraline 'probably' helps. She tells you about her other children and states that she has no contact with their father or with any of her own family.

She tells you she has not injected drugs in many years but assumes this is how she acquired her infection. She also mentions 'working' in the past but seems embarrassed and does not elaborate. She denies drug use other than her prescription (she doesn't mention cannabis) and is not in contact with any services other than in relation to her daughter. She was going to apply for Disability Living Allowance on the advice of her previous doctor but never got this organised. Her daughter gets DLA at the 'middle' rate.

Examining Sandra you note that she seems thin (you weigh her) and that she has some thrush in her mouth. There is nothing else specific to find. You notice that while you are trying to talk to her about her own problems, once she realises you are going to give her a prescription, she seems more inclined to talk about her daughter. Your assessment this evening is inevitably superficial and incomplete. You make a double appointment for Sandra and her daughter in your next available surgery. By then you will hopefully have obtained information from her previous doctor. You can also contact your local health authority and ask them to prioritise the forwarding of her notes. You give her a prescription that will run out on the day of the appointment.

Assessing Fawzia

Fawzia arrives at 2pm stating that she needs to see a doctor today and that she is prepared to wait. It is now 4pm. She presents as a healthy-looking, fashionably dressed young woman. She appears nervous and uncomfortable. She also appears assertive, perhaps even inappropriately so. She states she is a 'heroin addict' and she 'wants help'. She also says that she has telephoned a drug 'helpline' and that their advice, in synopsis, was to see her GP, who will 'sort her out'. Somewhat tactlessly and aggressively you ask her what sort of help she has in mind; she bursts into tears.

Everybody who works with people who misuse illegal drugs must be aware of their own prejudices and the impact these may have on their practice. David and Sandra may provoke predictable negative judgements around ideas of socially responsible behaviour and morality; however, these may be tempered by (somewhat paternalistic) sympathy, based on their obvious social disadvantage. Fawzia, on the other hand, appears to come from a privileged, solidly middle-class background. This can lead to several possible unhelpful assumptions on the part of the professional. There is a temptation to see her as a 'silly girl', who is risking ruining her life through some adolescent foolishness. You may feel that she ought to 'pull herself together'. You may have children of around the same age. Fawzia's predicament may play to anxieties you already have about them. It may be more difficult to distance yourself socially from Fawzia. Alternatively, you may feel that Fawzia has had advantages that you yourself never had as a child. You may contrast your own strength with Fawzia's 'weakness'. All these attitudes are unhelpful.

Fawzia is a person with a 'drug problem' who is new to 'drug services'. She has described herself as a heroin addict. You need to determine whether this is the case, or whether she is someone who occasionally uses heroin and perceives they have a problem with it. She describes daily use and typical withdrawal symptoms (basically a severe flu-like illness) if she abstains for much more than 12 hours. She has never injected. She spends around £20–30 a day on heroin. She gets the heroin from a friend of her boyfriend. She finances her use mainly from her own money (she has a weekend job) or from money stolen from her parents. Recently she has also stolen some jewellery from her mother and a credit card from her father. Her boyfriend's friend took these in lieu of cash. Her parents are obviously suspicious but have not confronted Fawzia directly – she is terrified of the consequences if her thefts are discovered.

Fawzia's boyfriend is 24. He comes from a similar middle-class background, but purports to eschew the values of his own parents (who are doctors and friends of Fawzia's parents). He deals small amounts of cannabis and stimulants (but not heroin) to his friends. Fawzia occasionally sells on cannabis from him to her friends and makes a small profit. Fawzia's boyfriend has alluded to a time in the past when he injected drugs but has never gone into details. He now appears to tolerate, though disapprove of, heroin use; Fawzia has hidden her addiction from him and led him to believe her use is occasional and controlled. This has put her in a difficult position with her supplier who has suggested that he may disclose her use to her boyfriend. Recently she has started a sexual relationship with this person (also in his mid-20s), at his suggestion. She is on the Pill (her notes confirm this) and never uses condoms. Fawzia's parents are aware of her relationship with her boyfriend. They disapprove, and see the relationship as the main reason for Fawzia's deteriorating academic performance, but they feel she must make her own decisions. There is considerable tension in the home but the underlying issues are never openly articulated.

Physical examination of Fawzia is normal and she is happy to provide you with a urine specimen. She states that in terms of 'help' she has heard of people who are prescribed methadone in a gradually reducing regime. She states a wish to be drug-free as soon as possible and has assumed that, in order to achieve this, you will prescribe her methadone tonight. She says that she now feels relieved that she has taken the 'big step' of disclosing her drug problem.

There are issues around prescribing at first contact. In the circumstances she has described it is unlikely that you will prescribe her methadone tonight. She may feel angry and disappointed at what she perceives to be your unhelpful and suspicious attitude, no matter how carefully you explain the reasons for your decision.

One thing you can truthfully tell her is that withdrawal from methadone is likely to be harder than withdrawal from heroin. If she wants to be drug-free, arguably her best initial option is to stop using today. You can give her a prescription for 30mg diazepam a day (explaining that this will be short-term only), you may augment this with lofexidine depending on your experience in using this drug (regimes are described in the Department of Health 'orange book'). There are other sources of help towards which you can direct her– but probably not tonight.

There are other health issues that you want to pick up on in the future, in particular relating to sexual health. Again, following this initial management, a longer appointment will probably be needed in the near future. You give her a prescription to last till then and possibly also a short-term sickness certificate specifying a 'situational problem'.

PLANS OF TREATMENT

David

David's treatment plan has the same aim as any treatment plan for any problem drug user: the reduction of drug-related harm to David and to people on whom David's behaviour could potentially have an impact. This plan is likely to have several elements:

- prescription of opiates in a form incompatible with injection (usually oral methadone), in an amount that minimises the likelihood of additional use of illegal opiates and within a regime that minimises the likelihood of bingeing and diversion to the black market (usually daily dispensing, perhaps supervised by a pharmacist);
- possible prescription of diazepam, according to the above principles;
- confirmation of tolerance to the doses of drugs prescribed through supervised consumption;
- possible prescription of another opiate if oral methadone is 'unacceptable' (injectable methadone, buprenorphine, dihydrocodeine and diamorphine all have their advocates);
- ongoing general physical and social care.

Doses and prescribing regimes are likely to change with time. Doses may rise as tolerance develops, prescribing schedules may relax as trust develops.

If David was not using drugs at all, drug-related harm would not be an issue. One much-discussed model looks at the relationship substance users have to their substance use (Prochaska and DiClemente, 1986). The model has face validity, as it seems to accord with the steps that many go through when trying to change an addictive behaviour (stopping smoking, for example). Change is contemplated, then action is taken to make change, with varying degrees of success. Lessons are learned from any setbacks and eventually it may be possible to sustain the change, until there is a relapse. However, this 'transtheoretical' model does not seem to predict what people will do or not do, and so far it has been disappointing as a basis for effective interventions. In the terms of the model, David could be described as being at the 'pre-contemplative' stage in relation to changing his behaviour. In other words, abstinence from drugs is not currently a realistic aim of his treatment plan. If it were, opiate withdrawal would be managed in the same way as described for Fawzia, above.

Methadone has been described as 'the glue that sticks people to sources of help'. In many situations this is a somewhat idealistic view. Picking up a substitute prescription does entail regular contact with a health service, but in many cases this contact will not involve any additional care. David is likely to have many and complex additional needs in the area of his physical, psychological and social health (*see* Table 11.1 on page 161, for details of the different agencies that might be able to meet these). In addition, David lives with his mother. Research suggests that people close to problem substance (legal and illegal) users often experience significant psychological morbidity themselves. Brief behavioural interventions have recently been developed that seem to be effective in helping such people to cope better.

Sandra

In the context of her overall health, the treatment of Sandra's 'drug problem' is relatively straightforward. She is already on a substitute prescription and from that point of view appears to be relatively stable. This stability is evidenced by several apparent facts: she is not using additional drugs in a problematic way; her functioning as a person does not seem to be impaired by her drug use; she is not making frequent requests for changes to her prescription; and she does not appear either intoxicated or in withdrawal when she is seen at the surgery for her booked appointments. This stability could be threatened by changes to her prescription – for example, changing her from dihydrocodeine to methadone, as most guidelines would suggest. Perhaps in this case 'guidelines' should be taken simply as a guide rather than a directive.

This does not mean that all her health needs, or those of the family, have been met. Both Sandra and her children are likely to have complex needs outside of the immediate context of Sandra's 'drug problem'. These and the collaborative services that might be required to meet them are described in Table 11.2 (*see* page 161). In particular, aspects of the management of Sandra's HIV infection are likely to be most effectively approached through collaboration with other agencies. These agencies might have expertise related to infectious diseases and to the complex problems that someone with Sandra's particular life experiences may encounter.

Fawzia

In some aspects the plan of treatment for Fawzia is the most straightforward, since her current problems are almost exclusively confined to the area of her drug use. This fact, along with her youth, the relatively short duration of her non-injection dependency, the apparent lack of other serious physical health problems and her social background, mean that her prognosis is relatively good. There may be less need for collaboration, or certain forms of collaboration may be less appropriate. For example, some people might argue that introducing Fawzia to a 'typical' community-based drug agency (and agencies are probably more typical than the clients who use them) would be likely to socialise her into drug sub-culture in a new way. This is not because her social background might be different from that of many agency users (although in truth it probably would be), but because so far her contact with drug sub-culture appears to have been largely peripheral. The argument against referral would be the same in the case of any relatively naïve problem drug user; in many ways, it is similar to the argument against a custodial sentence for a relatively minor first criminal offence.

Similarly, the 'harm reduction' argument for a maintenance substitute prescription for Fawzia is perhaps less compelling. So far she has not experienced any major consequences of her criminal activity. However, her luck in this regard is unlikely to last indefinitely. Although initial treatment strategies should probably be directed at helping her achieve and maintain abstinence, if these are unsuccessful the approach may have to change. Planned supported withdrawal, augmented with lofexidine and diazepam, is probably the first option. If this is unsuccessful, conversion to methadone then gradual reduction – perhaps again with lofexidine augmentation in the latter stages – is the next strategy. However, if both these fail, maintenance on a 'low' dose of methadone (40 mg or less daily) may have a place within a harm minimisation philosophy (it will decriminalise her opiate use and lessen immediate financial pressures).

Some purists would argue that on the basis of published evidence there is little justification for prescribing less than 60 mg of methadone daily – doses below this are unlikely to 'block' additional opiate use and a person physically addicted to opiates should tolerate at least 60 mg of methadone without incapacitating intoxication. This is a 'grey area'. Experience suggests that many users, particularly young ones, subjectively and objectively appear physically addicted to opiates, yet are incapacitated by 'therapeutic' daily doses of methadone. In this case, it seems most appropriate to prescribe lower doses. These prescriptions are also possibly best viewed as short-term, although it may not always be useful to specify the term exactly.

In Fawzia's case, if community detoxification is unsuccessful, it would be appropriate to prescribe her a low maintenance dose of methadone, with a view to attempting residential detoxification. The waiting list for such services on the NHS is likely to be long. If her parents were able to fund private treatment (at a cost of several thousand pounds), this might be the best option for Fawzia. Assuming she successfully completes an in-patient detoxification programme, Fawzia is likely to attend some form of post-discharge relapse-prevention programme, involving group or individual work. Most residential clinics run these. Therapy may also include use of opiate antagonists such as naltrexone.

Narcotics Anonymous is oriented around the same 12-step 'Minnesota Model' as Alcoholics Anonymous and has groups in most large towns in the UK. Many people find NA very useful in providing support, although their style does not suit everybody.

Fawzia's other health issues include her sexual health. She needs effective contraception. She can discuss this with you or with the person in the primary health care team who is designated as having a particular interest in family planning. She has also been at risk of contracting a sexually transmissible infection – including a small, though not insignificant, risk of contracting HIV infection. Counselling and testing around all STIs can be undertaken within the primary health care team. Alternatively, she can be seen at a local genito-urinary medicine clinic.

Arguably there are also issues around Fawzia's self-esteem and self-image, which relate to her developing problematic drug use. These issues will probably be broached within her residential rehabilitation programme. If they seem particularly prominent, they may also be explored, either within the PHCT or through referral to local community mental health services. Conversely, you may feel that these issues of identity are a normal part of adolescence and that Fawzia has simply been unlucky in that they facilitated the development of problem drug use.

The same is probably true of many problem drug users – quite trivial, circumstantial factors may initiate drug use, which, in turn, becomes sustained and problematic through other factors. Most young people use drugs yet most do not become problem drug users. Certain personal and situational factors tend to distinguish controlled drug use from uncontrolled drug use (Zinberg, 1984).

FINAL THOUGHTS

The case studies describe simplified, and often idealised, representations of real practice. They also assume an enthusiasm on the part of the PHCT to work with problem drug users. Despite exhortations (sometimes with a hint of sanctions associated with non-compliance) from both professional bodies and the government (Department of Health, 1999a; Keen, 1999), many primary health care professionals seem less than enthusiastic about working with drug users. Mike Linnell of Manchester's Lifeline project memorably encapsulated these attitudes in a cartoon. A young drug user approaching his local health centre is met by a confusing array of doors, variously designated 'private patients', 'NHS patients', 'normal patients' and 'drug users'. He chooses the final door, only to discover that it is, in fact, the exit.

Some negative attitudes are probably related to simple ignorance and prejudice, but others may have a more complex basis. Some health workers may feel that they are being asked to collude in the inappropriate medicalisation of what is primarily a social problem. If 'substitute prescribing' principally achieves its effects through decriminalising drug use, might there not be more efficient and rational ways to achieve this? Unfortunately, the reality is that there is very little political will in favour of alternative approaches. As a result, in the present circumstances, substitute prescribing is perhaps the only pragmatic response.

There is a serious issue relating to collaborative practice within current service realities. Tables 11.1 and 11.2 (*see* page 161) indicate a possible range of collaborating professionals that may be involved in the community-based care of a person who misuses illegal drugs. These lists are not exhaustive, and they also indicate some overlap of service provision; as long as 'overlap' does not imply wasteful duplication, it can be a good thing. The tables also reflect another anomaly: in theory, 'care in the community' for substance misusers is primarily the responsibility of social services. The extent of the lead role social services are prepared to take in this regard is likely to vary, both between and within regions. Furthermore, where social workers do assume a major role, this may present challenges to what some GPs view as their clinical authority.

The gap between private and state provision is as wide in the field of substance misuse as in many other sectors of the NHS. Residential detoxification/rehabilitation typically involves waiting lists of over a year for a state-funded programme. In many cases, the primary care professional will be involved in protracted negotiations in order to secure funding for a patient. Conversely, if a person can pay, they can generally be seen within a week. Given the association between social disadvantage and problem drug use, private care is not a realistic option for most problem drug users.

Collaborative care for problem substance users involves potential difficulties in addition to those related to lack of resources. Health professionals may find themselves being advised by people whose advice they might not normally expect to take. Advocates from non-statutory agencies are the obvious example. Some professionals may doubt the expertise of such advocates, or may simply find the thought of taking any sort of apparently subsidiary role threatening. The other challenge in this area is for researchers to develop the evidence base informing care beyond its current meagre state. It is still depressing that, beyond decriminalisation, and a few adjuncts to short-term detoxification, very few interventions of any real effectiveness exist in this area. In particular, there is still a lack of reliably effective means to help people who want to stop using drugs, but have not succeeded themselves, to sustain abstinence in the long term.

> *Clearly, many GPs are unaided in caring for substance abusers and have to rely on their own judgement, experience and knowledge to do the best they can. People who abuse drugs have multiple and complex problems and frequently have to endure the stigma of being criminalised. Collaborative care in the area of substance abuse seems to be the exception rather than the norm. This lack of collaboration may be attributed to a number of factors. First, the problem of drug abuse does not feature as prominently on the government's agenda as it did some years ago. Second, health and social care professionals are not immune from the prejudices of the general public and some do not see care of substance abusers as a high priority for service input. Third, clients do not want to work with a variety of agencies, preferring to relate to one person whom they feel they can trust. The GP is central to the care of the client; 'drug services' may be more accurately described as 'prescribing services'. This chapter strongly demonstrates how to move beyond the clinical presentation towards an understanding of the person in his or her social context and how to establish a helping relationship with the client. Macleod notes that it can be difficult to find someone with whom to collaborate; because clients want help immediately, the promise of a consultation weeks or months later is not appropriate. This chapter contributes to the overall theme of collaboration in examining how collaboration does not, and perhaps cannot, occur in all areas. Readers may like to reflect on the fact that the chapter that illustrates the most considerable obstacles to collaboration is also the one that focuses on a highly stigmatised group of clients. (Editors' summary)*

REFERENCES

Beaumont, B. (ed.) (1997) *Care of Drug Users in General Practice: A harm minimisation approach*, Radcliffe Medical Press, Abingdon

Department of Health (1999a) *National Service Framework for Mental Health*, Department of Health, London

Department of Health (1999b) *Drug Misuse and Dependence: Guidelines on clinical management*, The Stationery Office, London

Keen, J. (1999) Managing drug misuse in general practice, *British Medical Journal*, **318**, 1503–1504

Prochaska, J.O. and DiClemente, C.C. (1986) Towards a comprehensive model of change. In Miller, W.R. and Heather, N. (eds.) *Treating Addictive Behaviours: Processes of change*, Plenum Press, New York

Ramsay, M., Baker, P., Goulden, C., Sharp, C. and Sondhi, A. (2001) *Drug Misuse Declared in 2000: Results from the British Crime Survey*, Home Office, London

Robertson, R. (ed.) (1998) *Management of Drug Users in the Community: A practical handbook*, Edward Arnold, London

Royal College of Psychiatrists and Royal College of Physicians (2000) *Drugs: Dilemmas and choices* [report of a working party], Gaskell, London

Stimson, G.V., Hickman, M. and Turnbull, P.J. (1998) Statistics on misuse of drugs have been misused, *British Medical Journal*, **317**, 1388

Zinberg, N. (1984) *Drug, Set and Setting: The basis for controlled intoxicant use*, Yale University Press, New Haven

12 SHARED ASSESSMENT, INTERVENTION AND CARE FOR PEOPLE WITH DEPRESSION

Jan R. Oyebode

Depression can occur in any age group. This chapter focuses on the care of an elderly person with depression. Depression in the elderly may be particularly hard to diagnose. Depression and grief following a bereavement have the potential to affect people in similar ways, and it may be hard to assess whether a person experiencing difficulties getting over a loss requires extra professional help. Both grief and depression are surrounded by ignorance and embarrassment and depression in the older adult may be poorly addressed. Current Department of Health guidance recommends that psychological therapy should be routinely considered an option when assessing mental health problems and this chapter illustrates a case in which clinical psychology was the main input. Although the author discusses accessing other agencies, the client acted as her own key worker, contacting the agencies herself, and there was no face-to-face contact between any of the service providers. The approach to collaboration taken here expresses the reality of many practitioners, who may neither have the time for it, nor the appropriate personnel with whom to collaborate. (Editors' note)

DEPRESSION: A MAJOR YET UNDER-DETECTED PROBLEM

Depression is a major problem, which has a significant negative impact on the life of the sufferer, and often also on the life of his or her family. The World Bank (Murray and Lopez, 1997) has found depression to be the tenth-highest cause of mortality, and it is projected that it will become the fourth-highest cause by the year 2020. Accurate identification of depression and effective treatment could therefore have a huge impact on general health and wellbeing in the population.

'Depression' is the term used for those mental health problems referred to by psychiatrists as 'depressive disorders' or 'depressive syndromes'. Depressed mood is usually the central feature but there are a range of other symptoms, a number of which would be expected to be present in order for a person to be identified as having depression. These include loss of enjoyment, interest and energy; disturbed, usually lessened, appetite, sleep and libido; agitation or slowing of movement; poor concentration and mental slowing; negative thinking or hopelessness; feelings of guilt or worthlessness; and thoughts of death or suicide. Depression is more far-reaching than the low moods that most people, understandably, experience in relation to adverse life events. It is more long-standing than a patch of 'the blues'. It can jeopardise a person's relationships, their job and their usual activities. In extreme cases, it can put physical health at risk and, through suicide, can endanger life itself.

Depression is very common. It has been estimated that one patient with mild depression or worse presents at each and every GP surgery session, and that for 50% of these people the depression will not be recognised (Paykel and Priest, 1992). The reasons for under-diagnosis are not clear. A proportion of those attending primary care with depression present with somatic complaints. Because of stigma and self-consciousness, it would probably take more than one standard GP consultation for others to disclose their true reason for attending. Depression may remain undetected in busy generic health-care settings, particularly when staff do not have special training in mental health issues.

It is particularly important to try to improve detection rates. Where depression is diagnosed, there are effective treatments available. There is evidence for the effectiveness of psychological approaches, such as cognitive behaviour therapy and interpersonal therapy (Department of Health, 2001a), and of pharmacological treatment with antidepressant drugs (Bernadt, 1998). Given these effective treatment methods, it is important to ensure that there is good liaison between mental health specialists and those in primary care.

Depression in adults can be a problem for all age groups, from early adulthood to old age. However, there are some issues that make this a particularly challenging area for those working with older people. They are more likely than younger adults to have physical complaints, with symptoms that overlap with those of depression, including slowing or loss of appetite. They are also likely to experience physical disability, which may lead professionals to think that depressed mood is only to be expected in the circumstances. What is more, bereavement of spouse, siblings and friends becomes more common with age and it may be hard for the practitioner to distinguish grief from depression. All these factors mean that a skilled, holistic assessment of physical state, mental state, coping style and life circumstances is necessary to gain an understanding. In this respect, a multidisciplinary input is often beneficial.

As a clinical psychologist, I have specialised in work with older adults for many years. In very many ways, older people are the same as younger people. The emotional, cognitive, behavioural and somatic aspects of depression are all present across the age range. The impact of depression on ability to carry on with activities of daily living and to sustain relationships is present, whether the sufferer is younger or older. However, the life stage and cohort of those over 65 years of age present differences that need to be taken into account in engaging, understanding and working with older clients. The example that follows has some features that are typical of depression in older people, and illustrates some of the contextual factors that are typical in later life. However, because of our common humanity and common experience of depression, it is also of relevance to work with people at all ages.

The following case is based on practice in the late 1990s and the context is changing rapidly. Previously, the specialist Mental Health Trust where I work concentrated on severe mental illness, but the advent of the *National Service Framework for Mental Health* (DoH, 1999) has led to the development of a primary mental health care service. Today, such a referral might come to this service. I have therefore referred throughout to 'primary mental health services' rather than to 'primary care psychology services'.

CASE STUDY   MRS G

Mrs G is a 75-year-old woman living on her own in a modern bungalow in a suburban residential area. Her bungalow is five minutes' walk from the bus stop and about a mile from local shops. Mrs G's husband died about nine months ago. She has one married daughter, with children, who lives locally. This daughter lives a busy life, with commitments to her family and her job, and regular, albeit brief, contact with her mother.

Mrs G has good physical health, except for her eyesight, which is very poor. She is registered as partially sighted; she is able to read, with a powerful magnifier, and to find her way around in familiar places. Her eyesight has deteriorated gradually, and has been very poor for about the past three years.

Mrs G had a happy childhood in a farming family in Holland and came to the UK soon after the Second World War, having met and married a British serviceman. He taught in a secondary school and Mrs G looked after the family and the home. Although she had a very happy marriage, Mrs G did not find it easy to settle into the UK, feeling that she was not accepted here. She coped by growing a thick skin and getting on with her own life to the best of her ability. She was a keen swimmer, encouraging her grandchildren to swim well too. After Mr G's retirement, the couple travelled to a number of places in Europe on holiday and they also visited Holland to see Mrs G's brother and his wife. Mrs G coped well with the loss of her eyesight, particularly with the help and support of her husband. However, she refused to learn to use a white stick when out and had given up going out alone.

Mr G died unexpectedly in his sleep. Since his death, Mrs G has hardly been out of the house. She has not found it worth cooking for one, and has lost her appetite and quite a lot of weight, although she is finding that a glass of sherry seems to help her to feel more settled. She finds it hard to get to sleep at night but has no energy during the day. She is neglecting her house and recently she cannot bring herself to bathe or wash her hair. She spends much of the day sitting on the sofa, with daytime TV on in the background. She tends to feel flat and empty, but sometimes finds herself sobbing uncontrollably, often in response to something trivial such as a sad item on the news. Mrs G is aware that she is not coping and berates herself for being stupid, telling herself that she is useless and always has been. She does not want to face other people and has been giving excuses to stop visitors coming to see her.

Mrs G has not actively sought help. Until recently, her daughter thought that her mother was reacting to the death of her husband and that she would soon pull herself together. However, when she discovered that Mrs G had missed her eye appointment, she decided to approach the GP regarding her mother's health. This is what led to Mrs G being referred to clinical psychology by her GP.

INITIAL RESPONSE

The information in the case study was gathered in the assessment, and during subsequent appointments with Mrs G. As is commonly the case, the referral letter received from the GP passed on the essentials, but did not include much additional information. The letter was brief and along the lines of: 'I would be grateful if you would see and treat this 75-year-old woman who has become depressed following the death of her husband nine months ago.'

In common with most other health professionals, any referral sets me thinking about the client. I anticipate what the issues might be and note aspects that I think I should concentrate on at the first appointment, although I might not always unravel these reactions and thoughts explicitly.

There were a number of issues involved in this particular referral. First, there were implications in the fact that the GP had chosen to refer to primary care psychology (as it was then), rather than to the psychiatrist or CPN at the local community mental health team. There is not, at present, any mutually agreed protocol for deciding who should be referred to primary care mental health services and who should be referred to secondary mental health care. GPs refer directly to primary care mental health services where the problem can be treated at a primary care level, without the need for specialist secondary mental health services. In other words, the problem would not normally be diagnosed as severe mental illness. Referrals are often for depression or anxiety linked to life events, relationship problems or physical ill health. If the problem requires a full mental health assessment, and a complex treatment programme or package of care, the GP would normally refer to the adult or older adult community mental health team, which has traditionally specialised in severe mental illness. Presumably, then, the GP had not assessed Mrs G as being at significant risk of suicide, and thought that psychological therapy would be the only intervention needed.

A second factor in my initial reaction to the referral came from my knowledge of the referrer. This practice and this GP referred quite regularly to psychology and tended to send appropriate referrals, so there was a level of trust in the GP's judgement. There might have been more scepticism with a GP who referred very rarely, or one who referred clients who were often not amenable to psychological therapy. In such a situation, I might want to pay more attention both to the level of risk, not knowing whether this would have been assessed in primary care, and to the diagnosis – whether the problem was indeed depression, and not simply within the range of a normal reaction to bereavement.

This issue highlights the communication gap that can exist between primary care and specialist psychological therapy or mental health services. Professionals are trying to read the mind of the referrer, using guesswork. Of course, it is always possible to pick up the phone and find out a little more from the GP. In Mrs G's situation, for example, a direct conversation would have revealed that a home visit would have been more suitable than an appointment to come to me.

A couple of factors combined to militate against me picking up the phone. There is the disadvantage of covering a large patch with a small number of specialist professionals. Some crude calculations indicate that, in my area, each older adult CPN relates to about 15 GPs and each psychologist to 40–50 GPs; the ratio is about the same for psychiatrists. Thus, with some exceptions, GPs and specialist mental health professionals, including psychologists, are relative strangers. This makes me hesitate to phone, in case my call is seen as intrusive or unnecessary. In addition, we are both so busy that it makes it hard for us to catch each other.

Already, even before seeing the person referred, there are questions about the communication and collaboration across boundaries, with three players involved: the GP/primary care team, the primary care psychology/mental health service and the secondary mental health services, including the psychiatrist and local community mental health team.

The referral letter led me to consider a number of other issues prior to my first appointment with Mrs G. First, what was the nature, severity and impact of her depression? Was there any element of risk of self-harm? Second, how was the depression linked to the bereavement of her husband? Third, could I find out from Mrs G whether psychological therapy might be helpful?

APPOINTMENTS

Making an appointment

Mrs G lived a single short bus journey from my office base. I was aware that this journey might be difficult for her, especially if her depression was severe or if she had mobility problems. On the other hand, the majority of 75-year-olds travel independently and I wanted to give her control over her attendance. I sent a letter inviting her to come for an appointment, but asking her to ring if this was inconvenient.

Mrs G failed to attend for that appointment, and for a subsequent one, so I wrote a final time to say that I would call to see her. This is in line with usual practice; three appointments are offered to a client referred directly from primary care, before concluding that they do not wish to use the service. This is another point at which direct communication with the primary care practice can be helpful, to determine whether or not to pursue a meeting with the client.

Most people ring if an appointment is inconvenient or if they need a home visit. It is rare for someone over 65 never to attend or to drop out of treatment. The high attendance rate among the older people referred may be a cohort effect and might be better labelled 'high compliance'. Older adults attend or permit home visits, even though many of them either have not been told or do not remember that they have been referred. Their compliance appears to be related to a generation who have high respect for and trust in professional people, particularly doctors. I did not know whether Mrs G had requested to be referred, whether she had been informed that she had been referred, or whether she was unaware of the referral. Her failure to attend could have been her way of saying that she no longer felt she needed to be seen. This might have been reasonable if she had recovered; alternatively, it would be very worrying if it was because she had become too depressed to come out. If she had not given her consent to the referral, it might indicate that she was unnerved by the notion of seeing a mental health professional, due to stigma and misleading public misconceptions.

Assessment appointments

I finally arrived at Mrs G's house three weeks after receiving the referral. Mrs G came to the door in her dressing gown despite the fact that it was 11.30am. She was clearly anxious about my visit; her manner was flustered and her breathing rapid. I could also smell alcohol on her breath. However, she invited me in and we went into the living room where we sat and talked about the referral, her feelings and her current situation.

It turned out that her failure to attend the first two appointments was due to a combination of reasons. Her GP had decided to refer after talking to her daughter and the daughter had agreed to discuss this with her mother, and indeed had. However, Mrs G was annoyed that her daughter had taken this step. She therefore felt ambivalent, not only about seeing me, but also about her daughter continuing to 'intrude'. She had not wanted to let her daughter know that the appointment letter had arrived, but felt she could only attend if she relied on her daughter for transport. She therefore let her annoyance with her daughter and her mixed feelings about seeing a mental health professional 'prevent' her from attending.

The first two visits to Mrs G served as the basis of an assessment. They were also important in establishing rapport and in giving an opportunity for me to convey to Mrs G the nature of psychological therapy. The appointments lasted approximately an hour each. They provided an opportunity to explore depression, bereavement and potential for psychological intervention; these were the three themes I had planned to address. They also provided me with unanticipated information, for example, about Mrs G's eyesight and about her high levels of anxiety.

The initial interviews confirmed a picture of depression. The clinical picture was supplemented with the use of a 14-item questionnaire, the HADS (Zigmond and Snaith, 1983), the scores indicating 'moderate/high' depression and 'moderate' anxiety. Asking about factors associated with a risk of suicide revealed that Mrs G had never made an attempt to end her life, nor had she any active plans at the present time. However, she did wonder whether life was worth living and talked about being reunited with her husband when she died. Mrs G felt quite hopeless about the future. However, she acknowledged that, although she had not asked to see a mental health professional, the fact that her doctor thought it might help had given her a ray of hope. My opinion was that there was a slight risk of suicide, which needed to be monitored. I would need to refer on to a psychiatric colleague in the mental health service if there was increasing hopelessness or an increased wish to die. This would be facilitated by easy communication between primary and secondary mental health care.

In discussing bereavement with Mrs G, my intention was to establish how she was adapting to being without Mr G, and to being on her own. I was interested to know how she was coming through the first three of William Worden's four tasks of grief work (Worden, 1991): understanding that the death is real, experiencing the pain and grief of loss, and learning to deal with the practical facets of life without her husband. I was also interested in a variation of Worden's fourth task of 'letting go'. I wanted to know how Mrs G's husband still featured in her life – the nature and strength of what is known as the 'continuing bond'.

It had taken some time for Mrs G to comprehend that her husband was really dead. However, over time, the permanent nature of the separation had sunk in, and she stopped believing that he would come back. This first task appeared to have been accomplished. In terms of experience of grief, again Mrs G's feelings in relation to her husband appeared, at least during the first six months or so, to be within the range that might be regarded as normal. She had felt intense pangs of loss and had often cried and sobbed when alone at home. She had felt some remorse and guilt at not taking more care of him and at not being with him when he died. She also felt abandoned by him at a time of need and had felt anger towards him. However, the guilt and anger had not dominated the picture, and the extreme feelings had subsided somewhat over time.

The third task appeared more problematic. Mrs G seemed to have found it very hard to tackle the practical tasks of living without her husband. As her eyesight had deteriorated, Mr G had had to help her more and more. She had continued to carry out most aspects of life as before, but he guided her, found things for her, wrote for her, chose matching clothes for her, and so on. When he died, she not only had to adapt to the loss of the relationship, but also, for the first time, to the loss of her eyesight.

Without her husband, Mrs G felt unable to go out. She had always prided herself on appearing self-sufficient to others and she refused to ask for help, even from her daughter. She found day-to-day life at home frustrating, and she would become very anxious and tense when she could not find things or when she made mistakes. She recounted an occasion when she had decided to bake a cake. She not only had difficulty finding the ingredients, but she found it very hard to see the scales to weigh the right amounts. The finished product was not edible and she had not attempted to bake a cake since. Over time, Mrs G had gradually given up activities because of the degree of frustration involved. This led to a decline in her self-esteem, and to a spiralling of anger and rejection towards Mr G for deserting her. She had given up so much and now thought of herself as totally hopeless. It all seemed to fit the paradigm of learned helplessness, later modified to learned hopelessness, in which a person fails to gain positive reinforcement for anything they do and so gives up attempting anything at all.

There were factors in Mrs G's past life that may have made her vulnerable at this time. She had experienced a lot of jibes about her Dutch accent, particularly in the 1940s and 50s, when many British people assumed she must be German. This had undermined her confidence in social settings, and given her a lasting feeling that, if she attracted attention to herself, this attention would be negative. She was therefore perhaps more sensitive than most when her eyesight failed, as she felt very uncomfortable with the idea of being conspicuous. She had been embarrassed at the idea of using a white stick in public and had adapted to her near-blindness, not by finding new ways of being independent, but by relying on her husband to keep her safe. When he died she felt her safety buffer against public ridicule had been removed.

Mrs G revealed that her daughter had been on the receiving end of bullying at school, where other children had called her a Nazi. This had caused a distance between mother and daughter, as her daughter seemed to have become ashamed of having Mrs G as her mother. Mrs G said her daughter had been close to her father and missed him keenly, but the relationship between the two women remained somewhat cool.

Mrs G had had a Protestant upbringing, which instilled a strong work ethic in her. She had fallen back on this when she felt excluded by her neighbours, feeling that she could at least take pride in the management of her home, showing them that she was able to manage perfectly well without their friendship. She felt that it was completely unacceptable for her not to be self-sufficient, competent and busy. This exacerbated her feelings of guilt and shame at not being able to cope easily. In talking about this she used 'should' and 'ought' a lot, further underlining her lack of self-worth.

So, would psychological intervention be suitable for Mrs G? In brief, I thought it would be appropriate. Mrs G had not sought psychological therapy but, after her initial uncertainty, seemed to regard it as just possible that her situation might not be hopeless and that psychology might have something to offer. She was able to talk about her situation and her feelings in a reflective manner and was willing for me to continue to come and see her. It also seemed possible to make sense of her depression using a psychological framework that could be used as a basis for therapy.

PSYCHOLOGICAL FORMULATION AND INTERVENTION

Overall, my opinion was that Mrs G was vulnerable because of her past experience. She had been led to believe that she was unwelcome in the UK ('I am not wanted here because of my accent' and 'I cannot rely on anyone here for any sort of help or friendship'). She had coped with this by putting her energies and pride into managing her home ('People may not accept me, but I know I am doing things well'), and by relying on her husband for a sense of safety ('When I am with my husband I am accepted by others'). Her reliance on her husband had increased in recent years as her eyesight had deteriorated.

Mr G's death had not only caused grief and sorrow, as might be expected, but was also a critical event that had removed Mrs G's sense of safety. Her original fears – 'I am not wanted in this country', 'I am not safe' – resurfaced. In addition, she developed a sense of anger towards her husband for leaving her in this position. Her loss of eyesight also meant that she could not fall back on her former coping strategy of taking pride in her house, leading to thoughts such as 'I am hopeless' and 'I cannot do anything properly'. Her attempts at coping included the use of alcohol, but more generally she had become bogged down in helplessness and depression.

In terms of intervention, the aim agreed with Mrs G was for her successfully to establish an independent and satisfying life, despite the death of her husband. Moving towards this outcome involved a number of subsidiary goals for which Mrs G could aim. These included:

- feeling pride in herself again rather than continuing to condemn herself as useless;
- regaining confidence and the ability to manage independently at home;
- being able to go out independently;
- accepting her husband's death and no longer feeling as angry with him;
- feeling she could trust others in order to establish social contacts, rather than being confined to an isolated way of life.

At this stage, the other professionals involved with Mrs G were the GP and the eye consultant. In addition, it was Mrs G's daughter who had instigated the referral. However, Mrs G and I established the goals of psychological intervention entirely independently, and without reference to medical colleagues or family members. At this juncture, I wrote back to Mrs G's GP to say that I had now seen her for assessment and to give him my formulation and our goals.

It might be reasonable to expect that the intervention would involve the respective contributions of various members of a multidisciplinary team. However, although a number of agencies and disciplines became involved in supporting Mrs G, there was no 'team' approach. This is not to say that the workers and agencies involved did not pull in the same direction, but there was no direct contact between them. The input from various sources of help is therefore described at second hand, giving a perspective that is necessarily limited. It is quite possible that each individual viewed his or her role, and that of others, completely differently.

In essence, throughout this intervention, Mrs G acted as her own key worker and care co-ordinator. My role was to provide understanding, encouragement and support. This was backed up by knowledge of the psychological factors that might hinder Mrs G from making progress, and my use of psychological approaches to release Mrs G from these blocks. Like most mental health professionals, I was also able to draw on my knowledge of the different ways into the web of services that are available.

The first goal was for Mrs G to regain some self-esteem. This was addressed through looking at aspects of herself both in the past and the present. Reviewing her past life was a means for Mrs G to acknowledge her capacity for strength in the face of adversity, boosting her view of herself as a person (Coleman, 1999). The application of a cognitive therapy approach was then employed to help her to tackle negative thoughts linked to current everyday life (Beck *et al.*, 1979, Dick et al., 1999). This encouraged Mrs G to challenge her belief that a person who is not totally competent is not worthwhile. This was done first through raising Mrs G's awareness of this habit of negative thinking, and second through helping her systematically to challenge her self-condemnation. In order to do this, Mrs G worked on transferring some of the tolerance she felt towards other people to herself.

The second goal – regaining independence within the home – was partly outside my own area of expertise. Mrs G had not adapted her home to help her cope with her failing eyesight because her husband had been there as her eyes. A source of specialist help was sought. Colleagues provided information about possible resources and Mrs G then contacted the Birmingham Royal Institute for the Blind (BRIB). This was not easy for Mrs G to do, and aspects of the fifth goal were tackled here as she prepared herself to make the phone call, which she imagined would lead to a cold reception and a probable rejection. She was pleasantly surprised by the response and received tremendous help, partly in the form of aids and adaptations to help in the house. For example, a pair of 'speaking scales' gave her back the confidence to try some cake-making again. But BRIB's input far exceeded the practical help; they also provided social contact. I never had any direct contact with the people at BRIB, although I did hear a lot about them from Mrs G.

In order for Mrs G to regain her confidence within the home, she also needed to set herself realistic, achievable goals. Her natural style was to set a high standard, expect a lot of herself and then be disappointed. Again, we were able to make use of psychological approaches to look at activities that might give her a sense of enjoyment and those that would give her a sense of achievement. These are often referred to as dimensions of pleasure and mastery, and a cognitive behavioural approach to depression suggests that it is helpful to try and reintroduce both of these. This led to a couple of goals, which were broken down into small graduated steps towards achievement, so that they became manageable.

For example, Mrs G wanted to send Christmas cards, but had felt defeated by the complexity of it. Doing the cards became a vehicle for addressing a number of our overall goals. The first goal was tackled again, as I helped Mrs G to challenge her tendency to put herself down for not having got this done. The fifth treatment goal of regaining trust in others was addressed, as Mrs G asked her daughter to buy her some cards. The fourth goal of adjustment to bereavement was also touched on, as she had to go through the desk looking for her husband's Christmas card list. In fact, she found an alphabetically ordered set of index cards with all the names and addresses. Discovering this, Mrs G was able to feel thankful to her husband for leaving her something so ordered, and lost a little bit of her anger with him. Mrs G asked her daughter for help in addressing the envelopes (the fifth goal again). In fact, Mrs G, her daughter and one of her granddaughters spent an unexpectedly enjoyable afternoon doing the cards together.

The third goal of the intervention was for Mrs G to be able to go out independently. She particularly wanted to be able to do her own shopping. BRIB got Mrs G started on this, as she joined a group of people all learning how to manage outside with very poor sight. I helped her to build further on her progress through pairing anxiety management techniques with graduated tasks, which we practised, initially together and later separately. For example, Mrs G and I would walk together to the bus stop. On the next occasion, Mrs G would come on her own to meet me there. This culminated in Mrs G being able to travel to the supermarket on her own on the bus and return home by taxi.

The fourth goal related to Mrs G's adjustment to bereavement and her anger at being abandoned by her husband. Initially, this was a source of serious distress. It is often hard to assess whether a person experiencing a difficult time getting over a loss requires professional help. Death is part of life, and essentially a person should be supported by their social network rather than through labelling (for example, 'abnormal grief reaction') and professionalising the help. However, in current British society, there is ignorance and embarrassment about death and grief. It is often assumed that the bereaved should come to terms with their loss within just a few months. In addition, there is often an awkwardness at talking of death, so that a daughter may not put into words her concern about her mother and vice versa.

Mrs G had some risk factors for difficult adjustment. She was experiencing a lot of anger and distress and, at the time of referral, was becoming more entrenched in this rather than moving forward. It therefore felt appropriate to address bereavement issues. My own opinion was that, in view of the degree of depression, the referral to primary care mental health services was entirely appropriate. However, the anger started to dissipate as Mrs G built up her confidence and realised she could live life on her own. At a stage at which the depression and withdrawal from activity and contact had started to lift, it was felt that Mrs G might benefit from the services offered by CRUSE. I supplied the details and Mrs G rang to make contact – the second time she had approached an organisation herself for help. CRUSE sent a trained volunteer counsellor to visit, and also offered contact with a group of people who had all suffered bereavement. Mrs G turned the group idea down. She found the individual visitor to be a good listener and said it comforted her to know that there were people who would accept her warmly, despite her accent marking her out as different. Once again, I had no contact with the CRUSE counsellor, and do not know whether the counsellor was aware of my involvement.

The final goal of intervention was for Mrs G to establish social contacts, to avoid an isolated way of life. My role was to look at the possibilities with Mrs G, and to help her address her uncertainties and her avoidance. BRIB provided a helpful service here, too. Mrs G joined a group of people, all with fairly recently acquired sight problems, who organised trips out together every few weeks. Through this group, Mrs G reinforced her confidence and built social links, which have continued. Relations between Mrs G and her daughter were also a focus here. Mrs G was encouraged to talk a little more to her daughter about her feelings, and was surprised to realise that her daughter was also still grieving for her father. Their memories of him drew them together and their relationship improved. Her daughter was probably pleasantly surprised to find that her rather proudly independent mother was turning to her for some assistance. We also touched on the complexities of being an immigrant to this country and having family in the country of origin. Mrs G was able to reframe her situation and consider that maybe she had a home in two countries and cultures, rather than belonging to neither.

I had approximately 20 appointments with Mrs G; older adults often need a lengthier period of therapy than most younger adults. There were many ways in which her symptoms of depression had lifted. The HADS (Zigmond and Snaith, 1983) repeated towards the end of treatment showed improved scores, with Mrs G having a depression score within the 'normal' range and an anxiety score within the 'mild' range. Towards the end of the intervention Mrs G was due to fly on holiday with her daughter and her family to Spain. On her return, she told me an anecdote that has given me a lasting memory of her successful recovery from this period of depression. The family had rented a villa with a pool. Mrs G donned her costume and dived in, and was surprised when she came up out of the water to see anxious faces staring into the pool. She told me with a laugh, 'How ridiculous! Just because I am 75 and have poor eyesight, they thought I would have forgotten how to swim!'

I was then able to write to her GP, giving a brief account of Mrs G's progress, discharging her and inviting him to contact me if he had any queries.

PROBLEMS WITH THE CURRENT APPROACH

At the time that I saw Mrs G, I thought this an appropriate referral. I was content to be the only mental health professional seeing her and was happy to communicate with her GP in writing. I did not think it strange that I had no contact with the two voluntary organisations that Mrs G contacted as a result of psychological intervention. The thought of speaking to the eye specialist did not occur to me at all.

Overall, in this case, I thought of the GP, myself, BRIB and CRUSE as pulling in the same direction, but with different and particular goals, to enable Mrs G to re-establish a satisfying life. The only person with whom I thought of myself as truly collaborating was Mrs G. However, in writing about my work with her, I have questioned how my lack of contact with others involved in her care may have impacted upon the management of her case, and may impact on others like it.

There are a number of stages at which greater communication or collaboration might be possible – within the processes of referral, formulation and planning for intervention, and during the carrying out of intervention and discharge. In addition, would better collaboration on health promotion issues prevent problems building up, and increased numbers of referrals having to be made?

Referral

Two issues occur at the point of referral. First, there is the matter of who is referred where; second, there is the matter of what information is passed on with the referral. The GP might have referred Mrs G to a psychiatrist, a secondary mental health team, a voluntary organisation or, as he did, to primary mental health care.

He might also have decided to treat her himself, decided she did not need treatment or, if not well informed about NHS services, he might have suggested she seek private counselling or psychological therapy.

Opinions on which route to follow undoubtedly vary from one primary care practice to another. They are influenced by a range of factors, including GPs' knowledge about mental illness and therapies, and about the local services available, as well as their past experiences of those services, waiting lists, effectiveness, accessibility to patients, and so on. In the case of depression, there may be particular difficulties because of the apparent overlap between primary, secondary and voluntary sector services, who may all appear to offer psychological therapies applicable to depression. In fact, these services will offer differing types of therapy to differing levels of competence.

This decision about where to refer may have become more complex with the development of primary mental health services. Prior to their development, Mental Health Trusts focused largely on the severely mentally ill, and psychology services and counsellors provided therapies for those with psychological crises or distress, who did not meet criteria for severe mental illness. An expansion and more coherence among these services are important to meet demand and to ensure quality. The reasons for the development of primary mental health care services appear fairly sound and the distinctions between them are apparent on paper. Primary mental health services should enable health services to fulfill Standard Two of the *National Service Framework for Mental Health* (Department of Health, 1999), which calls for all those attending primary care with depression or anxiety to have access to appropriate psychological therapies. They will also address requirements laid down in Standard Seven of the *National Service Framework for Older People* (Department of Health, 2001b), which focuses on mental health. The standard calls for early recognition and management of mental health problems, in primary care, with the support of specialist old-age mental health teams.

Alongside the issue of the GP knowing where to refer, there is a parallel issue of communication between primary and secondary mental health services. Primary and secondary mental health services need to have clear mutual understanding of respective roles and channels of communication. These come into play if a person is referred to one and their needs turn out to be more suitably met by the other. There should be a swift and easy transfer rather than a 'ping-ponging' to and fro between services. This was not an issue in working with Mrs G, but could easily have been so, if, for example, she had started to think seriously of taking her own life.

In ensuring referral to the right place, it is clearly not possible for a GP or practice nurse to ring and discuss the appropriateness of each and every case. There are a couple of alternatives. A primary care/mental health liaison worker may perform a triage function, providing an initial assessment and advising on the best referral route. Or there may be an agreed protocol that those in primary care can use to determine where best to refer patients, given the characteristics of their presenting problems. Apart from the resource implications, one hazard of a liaison worker model may be that it simply adds another layer into the system. A good protocol devised in a collaborative manner, involving GPs, counsellors, primary mental health workers (including psychologists), and secondary mental health services (including psychiatrists), could lead to more efficient services. In Mrs G's case, I would not then have had to worry about whether the GP was someone who knew our service and what we offered, because I would have been able to assume he was using the agreed protocols. The guidelines issued recently by the Department of Health on treatment choice in psychological therapies and counselling (Department of Health, 2001a) may be of help to services in developing sound protocols.

The referral letter for Mrs G was brief, with the GP passing on only the essentials. Perhaps because of the way mental health is separated in services from physical health, he did not mention the eyesight problems, which turned out to be quite central to Mrs G's depression. Some services have developed referral forms that ask for information that would be useful prior to assessment. However, many referrers prefer to write their own letters. The computer print-outs of recent visits to the surgery are often useful in alerting the psychologist to pertinent health issues; these would have been useful in Mrs G's case.

There is scope for improving referral information. Electronic health records with brief GP notes would be useful. With access to these records, I would have known that Mrs G had been referred as a result of her daughter contacting the GP, whether Mrs G had consented to it, and would have had more information about her physical health problems. And it would have required no extra work on the part of the GP. On the down side, clients may feel uncomfortable with this, expecting their consultations with their GP to remain entirely confidential.

An intermediate step towards easier communication might be the establishment of the use of e-mail through the NHS intranet. This would allow queries about referrals to be quick and easy, without interrupting busy professionals.

Intervention

During Mrs G's therapy, would direct contact with the GP, CRUSE and BRIB have been helpful? Would better or more collaborative care have been provided if we had been directly in touch with each other? It seems that there is less direct contact in adult services than in those working with children. In a case involving a child there might have been a case conference at the point of formulation. In Mrs G's case, this would have allowed those involved to share perspectives and ensure co-ordination. For example, BRIB and I could have ensured that the work being done to build up Mrs G's confidence proceeded in a logical and integrated manner. We could also have shared strategies. It seems likely that we would have shared learning in this process: I would have learned from their expertise on dealing with failing sight and they would have learned from mine on the psychology of depression. The same benefits could have been drawn from contact with CRUSE. In Mrs G's case, our different services seemed to dovetail well, but this is not always the case. For example, a primary mental health worker may be trying to build up a person's independence, while a home warden is discouraging the person from taking any risks. In such a case, collaborative working would be essential in order to avoid services working against each other and confusing the client.

It did not occur to me to seek contact with Mrs G's eye specialist. Mental and physical health do not operate separately, but the services tend to. In Mrs G's case, it would have been useful for me to know the prognosis for her eyesight. In addition, it may have been helpful for the consultant to know of the psychological programme, in order to encourage it. Of all the services involved, it would seem that the eye specialist would be the most likely to remain involved, since this was a progressive health problem. The specialist might then be able to play a role with the GP in continuing to encourage independence.

I had no further communication from the GP after the referral letter. I did not know if he had seen an improvement in Mrs G or whether he had remained concerned about her. I did not know if he had read my letters, had found them informative, or too long or too short. I had no idea whether he would be keeping a special eye on Mrs G following this period of depression. A dialogue could have ensured that Mrs G received the same messages from her GP and from me. It would surely give patients greater confidence to know that the health professionals involved in their care are in proper contact with each other.

Shared records would only have allowed the GP and myself to be informed about each other's appointments and decisions. E-mail correspondence could have allowed an exchange of information that would have led to better collaboration, without imposing a significant extra demand on time. For example, we could have agreed on the best time for me to discharge Mrs G.

There may be legal implications in the use of e-mails – if they have to be treated as a part of the official patient record, they take on a formality that would prevent them from being used informally in respect of smallish matters in clinical care.

E-mail has the advantage of being quick, which is often of key importance in providing a co-ordinated response to client needs. It is also efficient and inexpensive. However, there may be limitations because of concerns about confidentiality and trustworthiness. E-mail may be more open than conventional mail to a trespass on confidentiality, through 'hacking', and more easy to forge than a phone call, because the sender can disguise their identity. For some purposes, this is recognised in Trusts. For example, in our Trust, references must be supplied on an original letterhead and with a signature, ruling out faxed and e-mailed references as acceptable. Because this is such a new area, our Trust Caldicott guardian has not been able to give a clear-cut answer about whether e-mail is an acceptable way of sending/receiving a referral. Perhaps the best approach is to try to find ways of harnessing the new technology in order to bridge communication gaps, while being aware of gaps in security that need to be addressed.

Health promotion

As with many health problems, the public is ill informed on the subject of depression. Mrs G's daughter thought that her mother's depression was to be expected after bereavement and that she would 'pull herself together'. Neither Mrs G nor her daughter seemed to know about the range of normal reactions to bereavement. Mrs G herself had not heard of ideas of negative thinking and certainly had not heard of cognitive therapy.

Perhaps one of the most effective ways of collaborating to improve mental health would be for mental health professionals to become, once again, more involved in health promotion. This would involve liaison with GPs about which mental health areas to tackle and, with the voluntary sector, providing information and preventative services at health centres. According to the findings of a Kings Fund project on mental health priorities in primary care, users identified as a priority the provision of clear written material on mental health in waiting rooms (Greatly and Peck, 1999). Mrs G might well have picked up a large-print leaflet on depression or bereavement at her GP's surgery. Realising that depression is a recognised problem with effective treatment, she might not have felt the stigma so great that she had to withdraw and hide away.

CONCLUSION

Depression is common, but it is under-recognised and under-treated. Psychological treatment is one of the most effective interventions. For those who are not at risk of suicide and who are able to relate to a therapist, psychological treatment in primary mental health care may be the treatment of choice. In the case of Mrs G, an appropriate referral was made and psychological therapy was carried out effectively. However, there was no true collaboration between primary mental health care, the GP and the voluntary sector services involved. It was possibly as much by luck as by judgement that the referral came to the correct service and that the support Mrs G received was well co-ordinated.

Four main improvements would make care more truly collaborative:

1 A mutually agreed referral protocol;
2 E-mail communication;
3 A meeting of the different parties involved, preferably at the stage of drawing up the treatment plan; and
4 Greater collaboration in preventative psychoeducation.

Having written this chapter in isolation, I would be interested to know what the GP, the BRIB and CRUSE workers and the eye specialist would recommend, in order to improve the quality of care provided for Mrs G. Above all, it would be useful to know her views and the views of other people who have had episodes of care for depression.

This chapter demonstrates why some older adults can find it difficult to get their needs identified and met. It brings out the additional problems that immigrants might have in terms of their identity, how they believe themselves to be perceived by others and how confident they are in requesting help. The fact that individuals can have multiple problems, do not know which services are most appropriate, and may have relatives making arrangements without consultation, confounds their problems. This is made worse because practitioners in busy settings do not have the required time to spend with people like Mrs G. Where poor communication exists, it is not just that people do not get adequate services. In fact, health-care personnel often do not know where to turn for help. In Mrs G's case, the author persisted in making contact with the client and undertook a thorough assessment during a few home visits. As the relationship developed so too did the identification of needs; as these were met, so the confidence of the client rose. The imaginative way in which the author enabled Mrs G to act as her own key worker is a model of practice worth considering for other types of clients. Although the author reflects on the lack of quality face-to-face contact with other professionals and agencies, it is clear that the collaboration between client and therapist is by far the most important.

This chapter provides a thoughtful framework in which to reflect on the way the care of clients is shared with that of others, regardless of whether they are known to the therapist or not. (Editors' summary)

REFERENCES

Beck, A.T., Rush, A.J., Shaw, B.F. and Emery, G. (1979) *Cognitive Therapy of Depression*, Guilford, New York

Bernadt, M. (1998) Drug treatment of depression. In Stein, G. and Wilkinson, G. (eds.) *General Adult Psychiatry, Volume 1*, The Royal College of Psychiatrists, London

Coleman, P.G. (1999) Identity management in later life. In Woods, R.T. (ed.) *Psychological Problems of Ageing: Assessment, treatment and care*, Wiley, Chichester

Department of Health [DoH] (1999) *National Service Framework for Mental Health*, Department of Health, London

Department of Health (2001a) *Treatment Choice in Psychological Therapies and Counselling*, Department of Health, London

Department of Health (2001b) *National Service Framework for Older People*, Department of Health, London

Dick, L., Gallagher-Thompson, D. and Thompson, L. (1999) Cognitive behavioural therapy. In Woods, R.T. (ed.) *Psychological Problems of Ageing: Assessment, treatment and care*, Wiley, Chichester

Greatly, A. and Peck, E. (1999) *Mental Health Priorities for Primary Care: Essential steps for practices and primary care groups*, Kings Fund, London

Murray, C.J. and Lopez, A.D. (1997) Alternative projections of mortality and disability by cause, 1990–2020: global burden of disease study, *The Lancet*, **349**, 1498–1504

Paykel, E. and Priest, R. (1992) Recognition and management of depression in general practice: consensus statement, *British Medical Journal*, **305**, 1198–1202

Worden, W. (1991) *Grief Counselling and Grief Therapy*, Routledge, London

Zigmond, A.S. and Snaith, R.P. (1983) The hospital anxiety and depression scale, *Acta Psychiatrica Scandinavica*, **67**, 361–370

13 COLLABORATIVE CARE IN SUICIDE AND PARASUICIDE

Abid Kahn, Derrett Watts and Marie Holland

This chapter acknowledges the difficulties that practitioners face in managing the problem of deliberate self-harm. The authors suggest that professionals are often unwilling to take on such challenging patients. Shared responsibility between primary and secondary services is an effective way of providing care and treatment, and of assisting staff to cope with the feelings these clients generate. The authors emphasise the importance of teambuilding and describe how workshops, social events and meetings, where staff from both primary care and secondary services can reflect on their management of individual cases, can promote collaboration, mutual respect and an ongoing desire to work together. However, the authors are adamant that collaborative working should not be seen as a substitute for adequate resources to support the optimum management of DSH patients. (Editors' note)

INTRODUCTION

Suicide generates mixed reactions in health-care professionals. Recent studies have indicated that many professionals either avoid caring for those who attempt to kill themselves or elect to provide inferior services for them. However, it must also be acknowledged that there are some health-care personnel who are striving to improve services for this client group.

It is important to have a broad introduction to the subject of suicide and how professionals can work towards service improvement. All health-care practitioners need to have a good understanding of those who are likely to commit suicide, to be able to identify them during the course of assessments, and to be familiar with a range of strategies for dealing with them. Self-harm and suicide can be two of the saddest problems with which professionals have to cope, causing untold misery for those left to mourn.

The term 'deliberate self-harm' (DSH) is used to describe all forms of intentional harm to oneself, whatever the purpose. The term 'suicidal behaviour' refers to DSH where there is the intention to die, whereas the term 'parasuicidal behaviour' refers to situations where this is absent. Both forms of behaviour generate concern and most will come to the attention of health professionals. Whatever the intention, both forms may prove fatal. Generally, psychiatric services are not the initial source of help for survivors of DSH. If assistance is sought in the community, it is usually from the general practitioner. Alternatively, many survivors attend general hospitals, and usually receive attention in the accident and emergency (A&E) department or, if the condition is deemed to be life-threatening, are admitted to a medical unit.

Following a serious suicide attempt, where the intention is to die, patients tend to be referred to psychiatric services. These services can initiate appropriate treatment, as well as exploring the root cause of the problem. Patients who engage in parasuicidal behaviour may also be referred to psychiatric services, but this is not necessarily the case. Physicians and GPs see such patients as engaging in pathological behaviour that needs specialist review. It is therefore imperative that any work done with them involves collaboration, primarily with the GP and primary health care team, who will provide long-term care in the community, and in some cases with the general hospital. Collaboration between services can lead to prompt and appropriate services being provided, as well as long-term follow-up support.

BACKGROUND TO DSH AND SUICIDE

How common is it?

Precise figures for the frequency of DSH are not known. Not all episodes will be reported to health professionals, and not all of those who do have contact may be identified. However, it appears that the incidence of self-harm in the UK has increased during the second half of the twentieth century. A marked increase occurred from the early 1960s until the late 1970s. There was then a slight decrease until the mid-1980s, after which the rate has continued to rise (Hawton et al., 1996). Figures from the only UK centre with a continuous monitoring system, based in Oxford, estimate an incidence of 400 per 100 000 (Hawton et al.,1997). For a GP with a list of 2000 patients, this would equate to eight acts of self-harm annually; an average practice could expect to see about 35 cases a year.

The rate of suicide throughout most of the twentieth century remained static, although there were periods of fluctuation. The rate reduced during the First and Second World Wars, but increased during the economic depression of the 1920s and 30s. More recently, between 1982 and 1996, there was a 12% reduction in the suicide rate in England and Wales (Kelly and Bunting, 1994), resulting in around 6500 suicides each year, which accounts for nearly 1% of all deaths annually in the UK. This means that a primary care group with a population of 100 000 could expect 10 suicides annually; two or three of these people would have had contact with mental health services during the previous year (Department of Health, 1999).

What methods are used?

The wide variety of methods of DSH and suicide is reflected in the International Classification of Diseases (WHO, 1992), which has 25 different categories for intentional self-harm. In the UK, the most commonly used method is self-poisoning (88% of cases), followed by cutting. Alcohol also plays a significant role and has been deemed to be associated with 45% of cases (Ramierez and House, 1997). For completed suicide the likelihood of a more violent method of self-harm being used, particularly by men, is increasing. A study of suicide within 12 months of contact with mental health services in England and Wales (Appleby et al., 1999) found that the methods most commonly used by men were hanging (37%), self-poisoning (25%), jumping or multiple injuries (14%) and carbon monoxide poisoning (10%). For women, self-poisoning was most common (45%), followed by hanging (22%), jumping or multiple injuries (13%) and drowning (6%).

Who self-harms?

The most significant risk factors for self-harm appear to be previous episodes of DSH, a diagnosis of psychiatric illness, or the presence of social difficulties. A review of studies examining the rates of further self-harm in the first year after an attempt showed a suicide rate of 1%, which is 100 times the risk for the general population, and a range for rates of parasuicide from 6% to 30%, or 15–75 times the risk for the general population (NHS Centre for Reviews and Dissemination, 1998). One literature review of psychiatric illness and completed suicide revealed that, from a sample of 342 completed suicides, 96% had a psychiatric diagnosis, 48% suffered from an affective disorder, 23% from alcoholism, and 6% from schizophrenia (Hawton, 1987). In-patients on acute psychiatric units had a risk of suicide 50 times greater than the general population; the risk was highest during the early stages of recovery, whether as an in-patient or following discharge. The most vulnerable groups were young or middle-aged males with affective disorders or schizophrenia, and young females with affective disorders or personality disorders.

For parasuicide, however, only 30–40% of those who attend a general hospital receive a psychiatric diagnosis (NHS Centre for Reviews and Dissemination, 1998), and only a minority have severe mental illness. Most episodes are in response to social pressures, related to work (or unemployment, with the rate increasing with the length of time out of work), housing and difficulty with relationships (increased if single or divorced) (Ramierez and House, 1997). Women were previously two to three times more likely to self-harm than men, but, although self-harming behaviour in women remains high, there are signs that such behaviour is beginning to even out with regard to gender.

Although the last two decades have seen an overall decrease in suicide rates, among young men the rate has increased significantly (NHS Centre for Reviews and Dissemination, 1998).

Who repeats self-harm?

Identifying those who are likely to repeat self-harm is obviously an important part of any assessment. Table 13.1 lists features that can help in the assessment.

Table 13.1   Features that predict non-fatal repetition of deliberate self-harm or eventual suicide

	For non-fatal repetition	For suicide
Specific factors	Lower social class Alcohol or drug-related problems Criminal record Antisocial personality Lack of co-operation with general hospital treatment Hopelessness High suicidal intent	Older age Male Poor physical health Living alone
Common factors		A history of previous self-harm Psychiatric history Unemployment

Adapted from NHS Centre for Reviews and Dissemination (1998)

Government concern

The extent of government concern over this issue is evident from the *National Service Framework for Mental Health* (Department of Health, 1999), which refers to the target in 'Saving lives: our healthier nation' to reduce the suicide rate by at least one-fifth by 2010. The suggested means include the following:

- mental health promotion;
- high-quality primary mental health care;
- easy access to services for those with mental health problems;
- care planning for those with severe and enduring mental illness;
- safe hospital accommodation for those who need it; and
- support for the carers of those with severe mental illness.

CASE STUDY LENNY

Lenny, a 26-year-old man, living with his brother, had frequent admissions to hospital at weekends, after taking overdoses and then calling ambulances to transport him to A&E. During one such episode he presented in an intoxicated state saying he had taken an overdose of anti-epileptic medication and other drugs. He was admitted to a medical ward, and referred for psychiatric assessment. We noted his past history of repeated overdoses, and transferred him to our in-patient facility for a comprehensive review. Generally, he appeared to cope reasonably well, but following arguments with members of his family, especially after drinking alcohol, would resort to taking overdoses, raising anxieties and leading to hospitalisation.

A comprehensive assessment took place during his in-patient hospital stay, with the full participation of different members of the multidisciplinary team (doctors, nurses, social workers and day hospital staff). No evidence of depressive disorder was apparent, as he was reasonably cheerful in the ward, relating well to other patients and socialising easily. We formulated the opinion that he had developed a maladaptive behaviour (taking an overdose and getting admitted to hospital) in order to escape the stresses of his personal life. He had done this more than two dozen times, and on each occasion his family adopted a more sympathetic attitude towards him once he was admitted. A strategy was needed to change this behaviour. One major concern was his accommodation; sharing a house with his brother seemed to lead to frequent arguments and overdoses.

After completing our assessment, we discussed with Lenny the fact that we did not believe he suffered from a depressive illness. Although we very much wanted to support him, we told him that we did not feel hospital admission was helpful to him and would not be offered in future. He was also informed that if he were admitted inappropriately in the evening or over the weekend, he would be discharged on the next working day. We offered support through the day hospital, which he could attend five days a week, appointing a key worker from there, whom he could see regularly. As nurses were the predominant resource in the day hospital, and one of the staff nurses from there was part of his multidisciplinary team, it was suggested that she should be the key worker. She was keen and willing to undertake the role.

When this plan was implemented, initially he did not agree with the limits set and repeatedly tested them, by taking overdoses and asking for admission. On one occasion it was recorded that he had been discharged one day, and was then found to have taken another overdose the next day. Part of our strategy was to educate others involved in his care, including the GP, physicians and the A&E staff, so that alternative strategies to admission could be found. Fortunately, the key worker was not only willing to work with the patient but also had compassion and a liking for Lenny. She developed a relationship with him, and was not always dejected by his non-attendance. However, each time he took an overdose when medically fit, he would be discharged to the day hospital, to see her to talk through it.

As Lenny received progressively less attention following acts of self-harm, he began to realise that the best way to cope with his problems was to talk them through with his key worker. Relating to one compassionate and non-judgemental key worker was a major issue in helping him to give up the inappropriate dependency he had developed on the in-patient facility. All concerned, including his GP and staff at the local general hospital, were happy to manage Lenny by directing him to his key worker if problems arose. Gradually his attendance at day hospital decreased and he now attends there on a weekly basis while also attending the outpatient clinic for follow-ups.

Despite threats to self-harm, Lenny has not carried them through, and has not required admission for over four years.

THE STAFFORD LOCALITY

Collaboration between the general and psychiatric hospitals

In our local general hospital, covering Stafford and surrounding areas, about 500 patients a year are admitted to the acute medical unit after acts of self-harm, mostly overdoses, while at least the same number are discharged directly from A&E.

Historically, the only collaboration between the general and psychiatric hospitals, which are on different sites a mile apart, had been through medical staff. The attitude of general hospital staff towards psychiatric patients seemed to indicate that they were seen as an inconvenience, inappropriately placed, especially because of pressure on beds. As soon as a patient became physically well, they were referred to the psychiatric services for assessment. Historically, medical staff dealt with this function. The Royal College of Psychiatrists has highlighted the fact that trainees in psychiatry should gain experience in the assessment of overdoses and liaison referral.

The geographical split meant that it was not possible for psychiatric trainees to attend Stafford General Hospital in the evenings or at night. It was, therefore, imperative to develop a different form of collaborative working. Initially, this took the form of asking the general hospital to refer people who had self-harmed by 10am the next morning. This gave trainees time to assess patients during the working day. Patients who deliberately self-harmed in the evening would stay in the general hospital until the following day. Despite this 'next-day service', the psychiatric patient in the general hospital remained alienated, with physicians continuing to feel that they needed more support.

Nationally, the aim that all DSH patients discharged directly from A&E should receive a psychosocial assessment remains an ideal rather than common practice (NHS Centre for Reviews and Dissemination, 1998). Locally, these patients are directed back to the care of their GP, from whom they may or may not seek help; only very rarely are they referred for psychiatric outpatient assessment. In our personal experience, this 'ideal target' can only be achieved by further investment and allocation of resources. The mental health services in our area are stretched. Social services are unable to contribute to these assessments; they focus their attention on people suffering from severe mental illness, and question whether people who engage in DSH come into this category. In this way, this large group of vulnerable patients is disowned, although some certainly do have severe mental illness. In the face of a lack of investment in the mental health services to cater for this group, our approach has been to promote collaboration with Stafford General Hospital. This has been done through the development of a liaison service to assess in-patients, and a crisis response service (which the A&E department can call upon for advice).

Who should perform assessments after DSH? Until the 1990s, across the country, the answer to this question would generally be a doctor (Johnson and Thornicroft, 1991). In Stafford, in keeping with national trends, this has altered over the last decade, with an increased role for nurses. Sadly, research findings often fail to change practice; in 1984, DHSS guidelines concluded that there was evidence that professionals other than psychiatrists could carry out competent assessments in DSH situations (DHSS, 1984). The conclusion was presented with the proviso that there should be adequate supervision and support from more experienced colleagues.

The development of the liaison service in Stafford was given impetus by our chief nurse (mental health) having a particular interest in liaison psychiatry, having taken a Masters Degree in this subject. Two nurses were appointed, to be based in the medical unit, with a remit to liaise closely with nursing and medical staff, providing regular assessment and support for patients admitted there. Interestingly, although these nurses were funded by the psychiatric Trust, the general hospital wanted to declare ownership of them by providing them with offices and their Trust badges, perhaps indicating how they valued them. This development resulted in some improvement of the services for DSH, but minimal resources mean that there is still a long way to go. Not only has the liaison helped with service provision, it has also been an extremely important resource for training junior doctors, especially those with no previous psychiatric experience. Trainees usually conduct their first assessment for DSH with a liaison nurse present, giving supervision. Once the patient is medically fit, he or she is assessed by either a junior doctor or a liaison nurse. This assessment involves a detailed psychiatric history, and an enquiry into the circumstances of the DSH, the social situation and the various stresses in the patient's life. Once this has been completed, future care provision can be formulated. Its scope may range from counselling by a community mental health nurse (CMHN) in primary care to outpatient follow-up and even admission to a psychiatric bed.

The crisis response service has developed over the last two years, with the aim of improving access to psychiatric services for the community. It is led by an 'H' grade mental health nurse, with a team of four mental health nurses, providing a 24-hour service, so that patients can be assessed at home before admission. It aims to support GPs and also to prevent inappropriate admissions to Staffordshire's very limited number of psychiatric beds. (Stafford is at the extremely low end of national in-patient bed provision and Staffordshire Health Authority's spending on mental health is the second-lowest in England.)

The crisis response service is also intended to support the A&E department. Initially, it was hoped that the service would provide assessments for mentally ill people who attended the department, but a lack of funding means that this has to stop at 9pm, although the A&E department can obtain advice from the duty consultant psychiatrist throughout the night. Another aim of collaboration with A&E was to increase the confidence of A&E staff to cope with psychiatric emergencies. Tutorials for A&E doctors and nurses were held in the A&E department every few months. These were well attended and it quickly became obvious that, when both teams were keen to improve services, staff were willing to learn together and from each other. These collaborative activities led to an A&E specialist registrar spending a six-week secondment in the psychiatric unit. Such collaborations have led to better relationships between our hospitals.

Development of community mental health services

In the community, care for this group of patients is imperative, as there is an increased likelihood of DSH being repeated and the likelihood of death by suicide is increased. In response to this, a shared care module with primary care has been established in Staffordshire.

Around 15–18 years ago, there was a drive to develop community mental health services in Stafford, relying on experienced psychiatric nurses working in the community. Typically, they were the more experienced, confident and motivated nurses, who felt able to work independently. They were based in primary care and quickly became well integrated in the primary care teams. They did an excellent job, maintaining little contact with the hospital and, in fact, no longer worked in secondary care. When I (AK) arrived in Stafford as a consultant and tried to involve the nurses in the development of catchment area services, these approaches were not welcomed by the GPs, who felt that their territory was being invaded; the CMHNs were part of the primary mental health team. One of the GPs, now a close collaborator, even stated that any communication with the CMHN at his practice should be through him. The GPs felt protective about the CMHNs, but this reaction also reflected the significant division between primary and secondary mental health care.

Our team did not believe in this division, desiring instead a seamless service. We anchored on to these CMHNs in primary care, and they became the main focus for developing psychiatric services in primary care, and promoting closer links between primary and secondary care. Indeed, partnerships have progressed so that CMHNs based in primary care are now part of both mental health and primary care teams. The responsibility for providing care for mentally ill people does not rest solely with psychiatric services, but is shared between primary and secondary services, working together.

Promoting collaboration should not be dependent upon one discipline or one motivated person, but must be seen as a team effort. There is no one individual with whom primary care or Stafford General Hospital has to collaborate. Instead, it is a shared responsibility for the whole team, who work following a multidisciplinary philosophy. Developing collaboration is not an easy process – indeed, it may be quite stressful – and it is essential first of all that professionals are willing to work together as a team. Links must then be built up with professionals in the community; this demands intensive time and work from the team. Collaboration does not develop itself; it requires constant attention.

The mature, friendly people within our team all try to help each other, but we still regularly look at our own practice. To this end, we have developed 'monthly practice review days' as part of our teambuilding effort. They involve either an afternoon or whole day away from the hospital, with all the team getting together and discussing the issues we face. During the team's absence, another team within the hospital gives vital support to the practice by providing cover. All disciplines from within the mental health team attend the days, including our ward staff, whom we see as a dynamic ingredient of the multidisciplinary team. Without their back-up, community-based staff would not be able to function as effectively.

The practice review days are usually divided into two sessions. The first deals with problems faced in the preceding six months and the difficulties encountered. Following a lunch break, the subsequent session looks at defining a way forward and formulating a plan for the next six to eight months. This may raise concerns over resources and, subsequently, a letter is compiled by one of the team members, usually the consultant psychiatrist, and sent to management, highlighting the resource deficiencies identified.

The second component of teambuilding is frequent social events, which are not restricted to Christmas or New Year celebrations! Although there is no formal conversation about work issues, social events are an imperative part of building the team together. We usually go out at least once every three months for dinner, as well as on other occasions, such as when someone joins or leaves. This social activity promotes friendship and informality in a relaxed atmosphere and has been a great source of strength and cohesion for the team.

IMPROVING COLLABORATIVE CARE

The following factors could be helpful in developing better collaborative working with primary care:

- developing regular outpatient clinics in general practices;
- being available when needed, so that GPs can discuss individual patients and receive advice on their management;
- having joint educational meetings;
- developing protocols for disease management;
- embarking on education about patient management by conducting workshops for GPs in our area. These workshops sometimes take the form of role play, which allows education to be fun.

The development of clinics in primary care has been greatly appreciated by the GPs. At a stroke it has conveyed the message that we do not see ourselves as confined to the hospital, but would rather be out there sharing care of mentally ill patients with them. It has brought us into contact with other members of primary care, including district nurses and practice nurses. Most importantly, the GPs are no longer just names, and this makes it easier to relate to them on a personal basis. We have also been able to form a bridge between the hospital, primary care and our CMHNs. In the past, they had been part of primary care but now they could relate to us, seek our advice, and start to become involved in the care of severely mentally ill people. With the development of the care programme approach, they were willing to become key workers, not just for people with minor mental illnesses but also for people with schizophrenia or other major mental disorders, working extremely well in helping the families of such individuals. For example, a patient was recently admitted with a severe and treatment-resistant depressive illness. It had been extremely difficult for his wife to cope with this over a number of years, and she had become depressed. The CMHN, based in primary care, provided his wife with an alternative support, so that she felt better able to cope.

It is imperative to be available when our GPs need us, so we have always promoted personal contact between the hospital and primary care. We encourage GPs to contact us directly for advice about the management of patients, should they encounter difficulties. This support has been particularly important in reducing inappropriate admissions to the hospital. A level of trust has developed, with a belief that urgent referrals will be responded to quickly, and that problems will not be left in the lap of GPs and CMHNs. It is no longer necessary for *every* referral to be marked 'urgent'!

Having felt secure as a team, we then embarked upon sponsored teambuilding dinners with primary care teams. The primary aim was for our team to meet the individuals who comprise the primary care team. Brief introductory talks were given about the individuals in both teams. We then mixed in small groups and, at the suggestion of our psychologist, changed places after every course, thereby meeting as many people as possible. In this relaxed atmosphere, it was very easy to find out about the different disciplines of each team. These dinners, one for each of the four big practices that our team covered, broke down many of the barriers between primary and secondary care.

Subsequently, as the primary care clinics developed, we looked at enhancing our practice and developed protocols for disease management, in particular for depressive illness. These were welcomed, especially by the CMHNs based in primary care. It transpired that a high proportion of patients with psychological issues were being sent to them, creating heavy caseloads. In conjunction with the GP and the CMHN, we tried to develop protocols to give the GPs confidence in treating a significant group of depressive patients themselves, without referral. These protocols helped to identify patients who would benefit from antidepressants, and those who needed referral, whether to their CMHN or a psychiatrist.

It is vital to understand that collaboration is not a one-day project. It is an ongoing process and all members of the multidisciplinary team have to be involved. Collaboration helps us to know other members of the primary care team – district nurses, health visitors and practice nurses – each of whom has valuable skills that can help in the care of mentally ill people. A practice nurse, for example, can be involved in administering depot injections and a district nurse or health visitor can support mothers with post-natal depression.

To continue and improve regular contact with GPs in primary care, we organise disease management workshops for GPs across Stafford. The workshops are fun projects, done as a team. One concerned the management of depression and use of secondary care services. Various members of our team took part in role play, pretending to be patients with particular problems, all in relation to depression. GPs were divided into small groups with one member of our team to interview, after which they presented a formulation and a treatment plan. We and the audience, which included a number of GPs, then commented on the findings. This kind of workshop provides an opportunity for two-way learning, allowing GPs and secondary care to see each other's point of view and working conditions, facilitating discussion of new developments within services, and promoting partnership, collaborative working and friendship. The workshops usually end with a dinner.

THE ASSESSMENT – WHAT TO DO

The value of mental health assessment following DSH was illustrated by a study in London, which showed that patients who attended an A&E department after self-harming, but then discharged themselves before an assessment took place, were two to three times more likely to self-harm again over an 18-month period. This was in comparison with a group who had had an assessment (by a psychiatrist or specialist nurse) before going home (Crawford and Wessely, 1998).

In Stafford, DSH patients who are admitted to a medical ward are referred to a trainee psychiatrist or liaison nurse on the following day for assessment. After this, further management can be arranged by the psychiatric team covering the patient's geographical area or, if this is felt not to be necessary, or it is refused, patients can be referred back to their GP, who may involve an attached CMHN. Patients who are not admitted may be seen by a psychiatric nurse in A&E, although the assistance of the on-call consultant may occasionally be required. If patients have not attended A&E, or discharged themselves without a psychiatric assessment, they may be seen by their GP or CMHN, but have support from the secondary services to provide rapid assistance, such as hospital admission or urgent outpatient appointments when requested.

When consulting individuals who have deliberately self-harmed, it is important to make a full assessment of the episode of self-harm itself, and to look for factors that may have precipitated it, or may increase the risk of repetition.

With respect to the event itself, it is important to establish the time and place it occurred, who else was present (or if alone, what time someone was expected to visit them), its exact nature (for instance, if an overdose, how many tablets of each different sort had been taken, and from where they were obtained), what medical intervention had been required for the self-harm, how much planning had been involved (was it on the spur of the moment or had a note been written), and how the patient had been discovered and brought for professional help. Having survived the episode, is there any remorse expressed about the actions, or is there the desire to self-harm further? It is also helpful to understand the circumstances that precipitated the self-harm, and whether they have been resolved, or could recur.

Further enquiry would seek to identify risk factors for repetition. This would include discussing previous episodes of self-harm, and detecting past or current psychiatric disorder (including substance misuse), untreated physical illness, social isolation, unemployment, and any family history of self-harm or psychiatric illness.

An individual's access to the more lethal methods of self-harm should also be noted. For example, we have a number of farmers locally in Staffordshire, so discussion about gun ownership is appropriate.

Interviews with nearest relatives or close friends should also be common practice. This can help to establish exact details concerning the episode, and also assist in the decision about whether in-patient treatment is necessary or not. If a patient is not admitted, their partner or carer needs to be helped to understand the nature of risks present, what actions should be taken if the situation changes, and where advice could be obtained if required, at any time of day or night.

Following such assessments, we aim to devise plans that enable patients, their carers and all involved health professionals to be clear about the future help that is available and being offered. Communications by telephone and letter are both used routinely.

One particular area of difficulty is that of patients who, often after using considerable amounts of alcohol, say they have harmed themselves, but do not want any medical intervention. Such situations demand effective collaboration between A&E, the police, GPs and psychiatrists. If intoxication is present, often the best course of action is to re-examine the patient after a 'sobering-up period'. However, this may not always be applicable or possible, and may not alter the patient's attitude. Where an overdose of tablets is believed to have been taken, it is appropriate to undertake blood tests using common law (*see below*). Our experience suggests that this is the preferable course of action in such circumstances, given the risk of permanent damage if significant overdoses are left undetected and untreated.

It is important to draw a distinction between the provisions of statute law (meaning laws that are laid down in Acts of Parliament) and common law (laws developed by court judgments, but not enacted). Under common law, patients normally need to give valid consent before medical treatment can be commenced. The only exceptions to this are provided by statute law (as detailed for instance in Part IV of the Mental Health Act, Sections 57–63) and common law, which allow for treatment of those without the capacity to consent, if the treatment is:

> ... *necessary to save life or prevent a deterioration or ensure an improvement in the patient's physical or mental health; and in accordance with a practice accepted at the time by a reasonable body of medical opinion skilled in the particular form of treatment in question.*
>
> (Mental Health Act 1983, *Code of Practice* – DoH and Welsh Office, 1999)

The three case studies below illustrate some of the more difficult areas of management of DSH, and include descriptions of collaborative patterns of working in each background.

CASE STUDY MARY

This case study illustrates DSH as part of a factitious disorder (Munchausen's Syndrome), and how an assessment admission to a psychiatric ward can allow a collaborative plan to be devised, avoiding further admissions.

Mary is a young lady in her 30s who presented to us complaining of depression, lack of energy and suicidal ideation. She repeatedly made threats to self-harm and was admitted to hospital for assessment. This revealed she had suffered sexual abuse in the past and frequently complained of a variety of physical ailments. Investigation of these gave normal results, although she had undergone a colostomy, which caused her problems from time to time. During the course of her assessment, she became agitated at the prospect of being requested to attend Stafford General Hospital for further investigations. We felt she suffered from severe personality disorder and was set in a 'sick role'.

During her admission, her renal symptoms, bowel problems and consistent depression were further assessed. She started to complain of auditory hallucinations and would quickly pick up symptoms from other patients and then present with them herself. She would go dizzy from time to time and collapse, especially when around staff. She constantly expressed thoughts of self-harm, suggesting she had taken overdoses, but investigations would reveal no ingestion of paracetamol.

Efforts to discharge her from the hospital were strongly resisted, but eventually, after 10 months, she was discharged. It was felt that she suffered from a severe personality disorder and Munchausen's Syndrome (factitious disorder). It was imperative for us to involve Stafford General Hospital and her GP so she could be managed in the community. Our assessment was that her threats of self-harm were not serious and that, if she did self-harm, it would be unlikely to lead to suicide. This opinion was discussed with her GP, but Mary continued to make herself known to Stafford General Hospital and was investigated under various physicians for a variety of complaints. Her suicidal thoughts and threats to self-harm were ignored by her GP and the primary care team has worked effectively with us to prevent re-admission to hospital.

We feel the GP has been instrumental in keeping Mary in the community, and we have supported the GP's management by close discussion. Should there be anxieties about any threats Mary makes, we usually agree on an outcome, so that she has not had any emergency admissions for the last three years. However, we provide monthly outpatient appointments and she has had one seven-day respite admission to relieve the primary care team as she had started to cut herself.

We felt we would not have been able to work with Mary were it not for our close links with her GP. The most important aspects of her care were the comprehensive assessment, leading to a care plan, in which we involved the GP, who helped us implement the care plan in order to discourage inappropriate behaviour and admissions. Mary continues to make threats of self-harm and one day may attempt suicide, but we do not feel a need to respond to the threats of self-harm by encouraging the sick role and hospital admissions.

CASE STUDY ROSE

This case study illustrates the collaboration required to provide long-term management for an enduringly depressed widow who is unable to cope with loneliness, and self-harmed.

Rose, a 57-year-old lady, was taken to A&E after taking an overdose of approximately 14 tablets, a mixture of antidepressant and anxiolytic medication. The overdose had been revealed to her practice-based CMHN, who had arrived at her home for a scheduled appointment. She had expressed the desire to take all her tablets for many months, but on this occasion had only taken a relatively small amount, suggesting that she was not actually intending to end her life. The consultant psychiatrist was contacted and arranged admission to the psychiatric unit, with the CMHN conveying this information to the psychiatric liaison nurse and the GP.

Rose had been treated and supported by the mental health services intermittently for approximately 23 years. She had a diagnosis of enduring depression with mild schizoaffective features. Her past treatment had included psychotropic medication, ECT and two years' group support at the psychotherapeutic day centre. Although she had gained some insights into her difficulties, her main comfort was the transference process of becoming attached to the staff; indeed, she was seen to plunge into despair when one staff member took maternity leave.

Rose had a history of inadequate parenting (her mother having suffered a similar illness), and a loveless but dependent relationship with her husband. Since his death five years before, she had felt desperately lonely and isolated, with no close friends. She would spend weekends with either of her two grown-up daughters and grandchildren, whom she saw as the only good things in her life worth living for, and in whose company she felt and behaved normally. However, when back in her own flat, she reverted to her helpless and hopeless victim existence, which could be viewed as a resistance to coping alone. She was thoroughly preoccupied with her futile existence, felt no one understood or cared, and believed no one could feel worse than she did. She became more depressed and needed extra medication to enable her to go out if she had to.

On reflection, a planned short stay in hospital may have met her need to take drastic measures in order for someone to take notice of what she was feeling. Rose was given complex CPA status and the practice-based CMHN was the key worker. Review meetings took place during her in-patient stay, to plan and begin her rehabilitation process into the community. Part of this was designed to reduce the amount of time she spent in isolation, as this seemed to have precipitated her worsening depression.

On discharge, she agreed to attend the social services day centre four times a week for planned activities and could 'drop in' any time she wished. The mental health social worker and CMHN would visit fortnightly, on alternate weeks, and outpatient appointments to see the consultant psychiatrist (whom she regarded as the head of the team, taking comfort in his interest in her progress) were arranged. The GP was available for any physical problems and was aware of the need for a sensitive approach. Time spent with her daughters was also incorporated into the plan, while short periods of planned respite, if required, could be arranged, to be viewed as a positive part of long-term management.

This package of care, agreed by the CPA, allowed Rose to stay in her own home, with comprehensive support. Her pattern of maladaptive behaviour was known and amenable to change, with potential risk factors acknowledged and managed. The collaboration of primary and secondary care resources created a seamless selection of support, which Rose agreed would help her to cope on a long-term basis. It was acknowledged that, due to her dependency, she would require intensive support and supervision, probably for the rest of her life.

CASE STUDY STEPHEN

This case study illustrates the role of collaborative care following suicide.

Stephen, a single man in his early 30s, living with his parents, and working as a laboratory assistant, was referred by his GP for an urgent psychiatric assessment. He had felt low for two months, with decreased appetite, lethargy, poor concentration, anhedonia (an inability or decreased ability to experience pleasure, joy, intimacy and closeness) and disturbed sleep. A month previously, he had experienced palpitations and chest pain, resulting in a brief admission to the general hospital, with plans for further investigation on discharge. On the next day, he attempted suicide using the exhaust fumes from his car; before he became unconscious, he became agitated and sought help, leading to the police taking him to A&E. Following this, he was seen urgently by the duty consultant psychiatrist and commenced on sertraline 50 mg daily, along with support from a CMHN. Two weeks later, when seen by his GP, he was still low but not suicidal. His medication was increased to 100 mg daily and a referral was made to his locality psychiatric team.

His only contact with psychiatric services had been seven years previously following an overdose of paracetamol, which had not required hospital admission. He was diagnosed as suffering from depression, but responded to imipramine and was discharged the following year. His sister, who suffered from schizoaffective disorder, was the only other family member to have a psychiatric illness.

Eye contact was minimal and rapport was difficult to establish. Objectively and subjectively he appeared low, with ideas of worthlessness. No psychotic features were evident. Since his attempt at suicide the previous month, he had had some fleeting thoughts of self-harm, but no plans to act on them. The diagnosis of depression was confirmed, and his treatment plan of CMHN support and antidepressant medication continued, with the sertraline dose raised to 150 mg a day.

Initially, he did not engage easily with his CMHN, and his mood remained low. In view of the lack of response to sertraline, he was switched to lofepramine, while thioridazine was added as an anxiolytic. During the switch-over period, he was seen by a psychiatrist on a weekly basis and also agreed to CMHN involvement. He expressed concern that his physical investigations had not given an explanation for his lethargy. He continued to have occasional, brief thoughts of self-harm but did not plan to act on them. As he did not want admission to hospital, he was referred to the day hospital.

Fifteen days after commencing lofepramine, Stephen was admitted to the district general hospital with vomiting. He denied taking an overdose, but blood tests showed paracetamol to be present, along with liver damage. Subsequently he went into liver and kidney failure and died four days later.

Following his death, members of the community psychiatric team reviewed his history, and a family meeting was arranged, which his parents and brother attended. It was felt that Stephen was suffering from a depressive illness. He had received antidepressant medication and CMHN support, but had been opposed to hospital admission, and at no point appeared detainable under the Mental Health Act. Quick responses had been made to requests for assessment by the GP, who had continued to review progress even after specialist referral. This collaboration continued after the overdose, with communication in both directions. The GP also visited the family and helped to arrange the meeting with them.

Continuing to work together, even after suicide, is important, to help families with the grieving process and reduce difficulties they may experience if they need to approach their GP for physical health concerns or use psychiatric services in the future. Additionally, it strengthens the working relationship between primary and secondary services.

THE WAY FORWARD

These case studies demonstrate the essential place collaborative care has in the management of people who deliberately self-harm. This is also implicit in three of the recommendations in the National Health Service Framework (Department of Health, 1999) for reducing the suicide rate. These recognise the need for the following:

- high-quality primary mental health care;
- easy access to services for those with mental health problems; and
- care planning for those with severe and enduring mental illness.

Effective working in the primary care environment has a number of advantages. It provides easier geographical access for clients, and helps to reduce the stigma related to mental illness. Familiarity among colleagues produces goodwill and more time to share information in a mutually supportive fashion, whilst 'softening' professional barriers.

What is the future of collaborative care? What are the specific reasons why it should be embraced? First, we believe that it is *inevitable*, given the enhanced 'gatekeeper' role for access to specialists that GPs have been given, particularly with the advent of Primary Care Groups/Trusts. As more consideration is given to the effectiveness of services provided to meet the needs of primary care, closer working relationships can be developed, often beginning with those partners in a practice who have a special interest in this area.

Second, collaborative care gives the opportunity to *increase knowledge and skills*. Joint educational programmes allow GPs and other primary care workers to deal more confidently with mental health issues. This will also help the response to the demands of clinical governance, which requires regular review of practice against expected standards of care. Currently, much work is being done on care pathways, which provide clear and agreed processes to be followed by all practitioners involved with a particular client.

Risk assessment is important to consider in relation to DSH, and an area where further training is needed. This may be viewed on two levels:

1 Initial risk assessment of a new client, where established criteria, standardised questionnaires and protocols may be used by a variety of professional disciplines; and
2 Continued assessment and monitoring of the level of higher or lower risk, which will determine what action is required and by whom, according to the formal collaborative treatment plan.

A thorough risk assessment is vital to answer the key questions about whether an individual presents a risk to themselves, or to others, if they remain in the community, and whether professionals feel safe treating them in the community. This involves an understanding of the individual's current pattern of behaviour, whether it has happened before, and how it was managed in the past. It may be necessary to interview relatives or friends, and have discussions with other professionals involved. Concerns over risk must be clearly communicated to other professionals. It may be useful to identify a client at risk, and to put a summary of the plan of action on to the general practice computer system. Relapse plans must be regularly reviewed and submitted to crisis response teams, to ensure the current facts and care plan are in the right place, and facilitate continued effective interventions.

Advanced practitioners have inter-personal skills and professional intuition, developed through experience rather than via training. They often internalise their skill processes and describe them in terms of intuition or gut responses, which steer their actions. These processes need to be formally described, demonstrated and documented in terms of risk assessment and acted upon appropriately.

The third benefit of collaborative care is that it *improves morale*, giving professionals a greater sense of support and less sense of isolation. Collaboration emphasises the fact that workers have roles that are complementary, not interchangeable. This generates a culture of mutual respect, acknowledging varying skills and contributions, and allowing a greater understanding about the overlapping aspects of care. Joint training initiatives will facilitate this.

Supervision is essential for this process. Team members need an identified colleague with whom they can regularly meet, in order to discuss emotions and feelings generated by difficult situations, which may impact on performance and practice.

The organisation needs to provide opportunities for support. Practitioners have a personal professional responsibility to keep up to date, but many reports require action at management level, for example, the recent *Confidential Enquiry into Suicides and Homicides by People with Mental Illness* (NHS Executive, 2001). Primary care workers who feel assured of receiving adequate support from secondary care are better able to develop initiatives and treatment packages for people suffering from mental illness and DSH. This is an enormous resource and should be utilised effectively.

Finally, in view of the pivotal role PCGs have in the organisation of services, collaborative working can allow primary and secondary care input to *identify deficiencies* in services, and seek to remedy them. This often demands the allocation of more resources. The lack of crisis management teams, and the need to work intensively with some patients, can create difficulties for professionals in fulfilling their routine scheduled appointments with other patients when emergencies occur. These concerns must be addressed if all people who engage in self-harm behaviour are to receive psychosocial assessments.

Collaborative working should not be seen as a substitute for a lack of resources. Similarly, a duty on-call consultant should not be viewed as an answer to a 24-hour accessible service. Instead there needs to be a dedicated team of people available to provide this service. The target of the National Service Framework (DoH, 1999) in terms of providing a 24-hour accessible service is a blatant reminder that these services are not currently in existence and they will only come about if there are directives and requirements for managers to spend resources in order to establish them. Once they are established, it is imperative that they should be accessible not only to the community but also to the A&E department and medical wards within the hospital, as patients with DSH usually present to these settings.

CONCLUSION

Collaborative working is not an added extra to one aspect of the work of practitioners. Instead, it is embedded within the philosophy of care and runs throughout contact with users, carers and other disciplines and services. We and other colleagues are working collaboratively, not only with primary care practitioners, but also with staff at the local district general hospital to improve understanding and all aspects of services for people who attempt suicide or DSH. Collaboration in this area can be, quite literally, life-saving. In a perverse manner, lack of resources can provide a stimulus towards collaboration, which might otherwise never emerge, or take longer to emerge. Practitioners are now engaged in a range of effective collaborations, but these have taken time to develop. They have been nurtured over many years, through the provision of a diversity of opportunities for contact between practitioners – formal and informal, work-related and social, sometimes unidisciplinary, sometimes multidisciplinary. Two further vital elements of collaboration are the extension of the role of nurses, and the development of trust between practitioners from various parts of the service.

> The authors demonstrate in this chapter how their concern and care for clients who self-harm have led them to collaborate with a variety of services. Compassion for clients is seen to be a powerful driving force in seeking to improve collaborative working. The authors are clear that motivation and energy are essential, to ensure that all the relevant teams are involved and not just a few individuals. It is important to provide social opportunities for personnel to enjoy each other's company in a relaxed atmosphere, as it is difficult to get to know people during the course of a busy day, when attention is focused elsewhere. Respecting and valuing people, and impressing on them that they are special, are features of the literature on good practice in teambuilding. Access to high-quality information and research is insufficient if the work environment in which such knowledge must be applied is hostile to new ideas. The reader is urged to note the excellent practical ideas to assist collaboration that are contained in this chapter. *(Editors' summary)*

REFERENCES

Appleby, L., Shaw, J., Amos, T. *et al.* (1999) Suicide within 12 months of contact with mental health services: national clinical survey, *British Medical Journal*, **318**, 1235–1239

Crawford, M. and Wessely, S. (1998) Does initial management affect the rate of repetition of deliberate self-harm? [cohort study] *British Medical Journal*, **317**, 985–986

Department of Health (1999) *National Service Framework for Mental Health*, Department of Health, London

Department of Health and Social Security (1984) The management of deliberate self-harm, HN (84)25, HMSO, London

Department of Health and Welsh Office (1999) Mental Health Act 1983, *Code of Practice*, Chapter 15, The Stationery Office, London

Hawton, K. (1987) Assessment of suicide risk, *British Journal of Psychiatry*, **150**, 145–153

Hawton, K., Fagg, J. and Simkin, S., *et al.* (1996) *Deliberate self-harm in Oxford 1996*, Oxford University Department of Psychiatry, Oxford

Hawton, K., Fagg, J., Simkin, S., Bale, E. and Bond, A. (1997) Trends in deliberate self-harm in Oxford 1985–95: Implications for clinical services and the prevention of suicide, *British Journal of Psychiatry* **171**: 556–560

Johnson, S. and Thornicroft, G. (1991) Psychiatric Emergency Services in England and Wales, report of study commissioned by the Department of Health

Kelly, S. and Bunting, J. (1994) *Trends in suicide in England and Wales 1982 to 1996*, Population Trends, London

NHS Centre for Reviews and Dissemination (1998) Deliberate self-harm, *Effective Health Care*, December 1998, 4(6)

NHS Executive (2001) *Safety First: 5-year Report of the National Confidential Enquiry into Suicide and Homicide by People with Mental Illness*, Health Service Directorate, Mental Health, London

Ramierez, A. and House, A. (1997) Common mental health problems in hospital, *British Medical Journal*, 314, 1679–1681

World Health Organisation [WHO] (1992) *International Statistical Classification of Disease and Related Health Problems*, 10th edition, WHO, Geneva

14 COLLABORATION AND CARE OF OLDER ADULTS WITH DEMENTIA

Julie Marlow and Tracy Smith

The care of older people is likely to prove increasingly challenging as the number of people in later life rises steeply. The elderly tend to have multiple issues and require considerable input into their care.

The literature suggests that there are instances of good practice in the care of the elderly, but services are not available to all. Services for older people should be multidisciplinary; sufficient time to deliver interventions needs to be available, and interventions must be co-ordinated. These points are well illustrated in the case study reported in this chapter. The reader may wish to reflect on the number of assessments involved in the care of Edwina as a result of the involvement of a range of health professionals. Assessment may be a good way of getting to know a patient, but must every professional conduct a separate assessment? Collaboration means sharing each other's assessment data and avoiding duplication of effort. The CMHN authors of this chapter subject their work to critical enquiry and are aware of the shortcomings of their service. They describe their contact with Edwina and Tom in compassionate and professional terms, and are clearly endeavouring to do their best to raise the level of patient care by improving their relationships with other professionals and agencies. (Editors' note)

INTRODUCTION

People today are living longer. There has been an enormous increase over the past three decades in the population of the so-called 'oldest old', and these elderly people are among some of the most disadvantaged members of the society. Deprived of work and status, they are regarded as a burden by many people. Their care has been neglected for years (Rees *et al.*, 1997), but more recently issues of how best to provide for them have been very much to the fore.

Although the number of people under the age of 65 years suffering from dementing illnesses is small, dementia in the over-65 age group is much more common. On the other hand, 8 out of 10 people at the age of 80 do not have any problems of this nature (Burns and Levy, 1994).

When older people present with health problems, they frequently have a mix of social, medical and psychological problems that require special attention. They may also have multiple problems in each of these areas. Various forms of dementia have, at different times, been classed as social or medical problems (Wolff *et al.*, 1995). The reality in most cases is that the condition comprises both facets; it is rarely one or the other.

One of the biggest problems encountered in caring for older adults, in our experience, is the 'ageist' attitude held by many of the people – carers, relatives and professionals – who exert significant influence over the type and quality of care provided to them. Despite the amount of research undertaken and education provided in this area, people with dementia are more likely to suffer poor management and neglect at the hands of those who care for them than from people they do not know. Because of the variances in attitude on the part of those who provide services, and in the environment in which they care for people, levels of care nationally are far from satisfactory.

Best services are those where early referrals to specialist services are encouraged and where appropriate assessments, including physical health screening, are undertaken, in order to rule out any treatable causes of cognitive deterioration. Professionals need to be aware that many physical illnesses can both cause and exacerbate cognitive deficits. They also need to keep in mind the fact that some individuals with dementia may have enough insight to be able to make decisions about their future needs, financial affairs and care arrangements.

If there is early diagnosis, education and support can also assist carers to cope with the many problems, uncertainties and fears created by the illness. Repeated studies have confirmed that depression and stress among carers is much higher than in the general population. Access to emotional support and practical information can be invaluable in supporting them. Carers who are supported provide services that are as good as, if not better than, those provided by professionals; yet the number of carers who receive adequate support is minimal. As community mental health nurses (CMHNs) for older adults working in primary care, we are requested to carry out assessments and provide nursing interventions for a wide spectrum of people with mental health needs. Because we believe in the importance of our service, we are constantly endeavouring to seek ways in which it can be improved. We feel most challenged when asked to make an urgent assessment of an individual with dementia who has no formal support. There are many cases in which the carer of an individual with dementia states that they can take no more, overwhelmed by the desperation and isolation created by single-handedly attempting to cope.

CASE STUDY   EDWINA

Edwina's case was somewhat typical of our work, and had a favourable outcome. We have an open referral system and this particular referral started with a telephone call from a practice nurse at a local surgery, who asked us to see a 67-year-old lady patient. Once approval to visit the patient at home was agreed with the GP, we arranged to visit her.

The practice nurse reported to us that Edwina, on a recent visit to the surgery for a routine blood-pressure check, was evidently having difficulty retaining new information. She had forgotten a follow-up appointment between leaving the practice nurse's treatment room and getting to the reception area. During the initial CMHN assessment, it became apparent that Edwina had short-term memory loss, having difficulty recalling recent events. She also had some paranoid ideation relating to a neighbour. Unfortunately, her husband was in hospital at this time, so it was not possible to corroborate Edwina's information. A cognitive screen was done using the Mini Mental State Exam (MMSE). It gave a result of 20/30, which is not in keeping with normal ageing, but generally indicative of mild memory deficits, typically dementia.

In order to make a full assessment of Edwina's cognitive level, a request was made for the involvement of the team psychologist, who could provide a valid baseline assessment of her cognitive and psychological functioning. In addition, a referral to the team occupational therapist was made, to clarify her functioning abilities and to assess any practical safety concerns.

EARLY ASSESSMENT AND REFERRAL

Utilising other team members in the assessment phase ensures that all aspects of a patient's care – physical, psychological and safety dimensions – can be considered. Having continued access to other professionals (GPs, OTs, practice nurses, physiotherapists, psychologists, district nurses, and so on) means that patients can have their needs assessed by experts, and their care tailored to their particular needs. Access to both the mental health team and the primary care team is certainly beneficial to the patient as it allows a more thorough discussion and evaluation of a client's care. Time devoted to client assessment is time well spent, but it has to be acknowledged that such collaboration is costly and time-consuming and that those resources are not available for all clients. However, people with dementia frequently have multiple problems and require regular multidisciplinary reviews.

The route of Edwina's referral to our team was a fairly typical one. We have worked hard over the past few years to establish and build links with our primary care colleagues; the importance of this has been emphasised by recent government policies. The inauguration of GP fundholding seemed to raise awareness at a primary care level that mental health in surgeries was going to involve personnel who work there. The setting up in 1999 of Primary Care Groups (PCGs) continued this trend and many GP practices began to take a greater interest in secondary mental health community practitioners.

The links we have forged have led to much-improved communication networks and broken down many barriers. We are now on first-name terms with many practice staff, which is a great benefit when assistance is required. This has also had a knock-on effect with the practice nurses, many of whom now know who we are, and refer directly to us; this avoids the delay of the client having to wait to be seen by the GP at a later date. Obviously, practice protocols do vary and in some practices nurses still have to obtain GP approval first. In our experience, referring directly saves time and makes for a better working relationship with clients and their carers. In the case of Edwina, the practice nurse had not had to seek authorisation from the GP, but had to update him as to what was happening. At our end of the referral line, although we have an 'open referral' system (one that allows anyone – consultant psychiatrist, GP, social worker or relative – to refer to us), we still seek authorisation from the GP to confirm that our input is preferred. We also check whether a consultant psychiatrist is involved.

CASE STUDY   EDWINA'S VISIT TO THE SURGERY

Edwina had been visiting the practice on a regular three-monthly basis for her blood pressure to be checked by the practice nurse. She was hypertensive and her blood pressure with medication remained at the upper end of normal range. Her husband, who had always seemed very concerned and involved with her care, had always accompanied her to the surgery and into the consulting room. This visit was different; Edwina appeared quite unsure of herself and quite perplexed. She was alone and reported that her husband was currently in hospital with what she thought were prostate problems. Despite the practice nurse taking time to discuss her medication with her, she still appeared unsure and overly concerned about everything. Her behaviour prompted the practice nurse to arrange another visit sooner than usual and when she was seen again she was still perplexed and did not seem to process information normally. It was at this point that the practice nurse broached the subject of someone visiting her to see how she was getting on at home, and to see if there was any help that she might need. Edwina had no objections, so the referral was phoned through shortly afterwards.

Those who refer clients to CMHNs often do so in a friendly, conversational tone, always emphasising that it is another form of specialist help. Some older people harbour a fear of psychiatry or mental health services; any indication that they are about to be put in touch with them can further exacerbate distress, so great sensitivity has to be exercised by all parties when referrals are being made.

After receiving the referral and establishing basic details, a telephone call is made to the client, to set up a suitable time to visit. Making a phone call to the client also provides some information with regard to the client's cognitive functioning – are they able to understand simple instructions and write down messages? Do they know the day of the week? This all adds to the assessment process. It is also important to visit at a time suitable to the client, so that the client feels in charge as much as possible.

A telephone call was made to Edwina, an appointment was arranged for two days later, and confirmed in writing. Letters are a useful means of communication with people experiencing some cognitive impairment. A letter often consolidates partly retained information, especially for carers. A carer may ask, 'Has anyone called?', and receive the somewhat vague reply, 'I think so and I think they're coming to see me some time.' Having written confirmation can be a source of great comfort to a carer, who then knows what is going to happen.

ASSESSMENTS

Assessments may take many guises. Generally, as CMHNs, we tend to adopt a counselling approach, utilising both verbal and non-verbal communication. This not only elicits factual information, but also teases out and explores the person's perceived needs and feelings. This is then supplemented by assessment tools and formalised tests as necessary. Assessment is not a 'one-off' activity; every interaction undertaken with the client or carer contributes to it. With the majority of clients, it needs to fulfil a number of criteria. As early as possible on our first visit we try to do the following:

- formulate an idea of a working diagnosis;
- estimate levels of risk; and
- elicit what support and help may be needed. This may range from help at a practical domestic level, to day care facilities, home care, or psychosocial support.

With clients who have dementia, corroboration of information is important (keeping in mind the codes and practices relating to confidentiality; this can lead to conflict at times). Although assessment starts from the moment the referral is received, there are other times when greater emphasis is placed upon it. One such period is the initial assessment. No two assessments follow the same format, although the same information is elicited, albeit in different ways. Counselling-based assessments tend to follow the flow of the client's thoughts or agenda, and not those of the assessor. It is very rare that we lead the assessment, unless we are looking for specific details.

The initial assessment is mostly done within the home environment, unless the risks outweigh the benefits, or the client requests otherwise. Assessment in the home allows the client to be more relaxed, and provides the assessor with a better picture of coping abilities and, relevant in the case of dementia, of residual skills or deficits that may benefit from assistance. Home visits also allow the assessor to see if the house is basically clean. Is it warm enough? Is it safe? Are there basic facilities?

CASE STUDY EDWINA'S ASSESSMENT

Edwina lived in a first-floor maisonette. On our first home visit, she had lost track and was expecting us the following day. She had apparently received the letter but told us that she had put it away safe to show her husband when she next visited him in hospital, but was unable to find it. She thought it was still morning when in fact it was afternoon, and questioned why we were so early.

Edwina was initially quite defensive, but she made an effort to be welcoming and offered to make a cup of tea. We accompanied her and observed her in the kitchen, and it became evident that she had some sequencing problems, making a couple of attempts to ignite the gas cooker and to boil the kettle. It later became apparent that she was experiencing a degree of performance anxiety, rather than having unsafe abilities. She placed the teabags first in the sugar bowl, then in the cups, then in the teapot. She was easily distracted from the task in hand and frequently uttered, 'Now, what was I doing?'

The kitchen and the house were basically clean but there was evidence that no housework or cleaning had been done for a few days. Worktops had not been wiped down, and there were crumbs and tea stains on them, and there was a few days' worth of washing up in the sink. Edwina told us that her husband did most of the housework as 'he liked to keep busy'. Edwina was unsure about when she had last been shopping and agreed to let us check to make sure that she had essential provisions. There was plenty of food – the fridge was stocked with easy-to-cook foodstuffs – but there was evidence that it was only sandwiches, cakes, and so on, that had been eaten. She told us that she was missing her husband and that it was 'too much effort to cook'.

It is often worthwhile checking fridges and cupboards if the client is in agreement. This can reveal a lot. For many individuals experiencing dementia, especially those who live alone, the principles of basic food hygiene seem to go awry. They lose their understanding of what needs to be frozen or refrigerated; items in a cupboard may be lost or disordered; and they no longer recognise 'use-by' dates, so items may be long out of date. Shopping may not be undertaken on a need and want basis, but out of habit, with just certain items remembered each time. It is not uncommon to see someone with six dozen eggs and eight packets of biscuits, and little else!

CASE STUDY   TALKING WITH EDWINA

Edwina settled down with a cup of tea in her lounge, an environment where she felt relatively safe, and appeared to be relatively relaxed. The CMHN began by asking Edwina about herself and her life. This allowed for trust and a rapport to be established, and helped Edwina to relax. Her life had focused around her family, and she spoke a lot about her husband and their marriage. They had been childhood sweethearts who married young, and, although their marriage had had the usual ups and downs, it had been generally happy. This period while her husband was in hospital was the first time they had spent time apart since they had both retired. Edwina was aware that he was in hospital and that it was as a result of prostate problems, but she did not know which ward he was on or how long he would be there for. She was also quite vague as to when he had been admitted, and also if anyone had been in to see how she was getting on. There was an element of confabulation, with Edwina obviously covering up a forgotten date or name, along with some perseverance, with certain points, facts and incidents being repeated again and again.

The CMHN began to seek information about Edwina's support network while her husband was in hospital. Edwina voiced paranoid delusional ideas related to the man who lived in the ground-floor maisonette below her. She explained in great detail and at great length about how he managed to get electricity into her flat from his, via the walls, roof, plants, and so on. She reported that he had been very busy doing this since her husband had been admitted to hospital, but that it only happened occasionally when her husband was at home. These beliefs were absolutely concrete and, when asked about them, she stated that she did not feel unduly distressed, but had a feeling of frustration towards her neighbour for 'doing these things to her'.

Delusional ideas, along with hallucinations, often exist in conjunction with dementia, or as part of the clinical dementia picture. There may also be a pre-existing mental health problem such as schizophrenia or bi-polar disorder, which is further complicated by dementia.

The CMHN gradually elicited relevant information from Edwina to establish the basis for the ideas, and to attribute the causal factor. This involved open questioning, reassurance, with reflection and paraphrasing; acknowledging her feelings about the thoughts, taking great care not to collude with her delusions, or to dismiss them. Edwina was rather edgy about it. When she felt that she was not being believed, she became momentarily angry, and changes occurred in all aspects of her body and verbal language. She would suddenly become loud, her face and her voice tone would harden, she would move forward in her chair, her eye contact would become longer; these are all indicators of anger and, potentially, aggression and, therefore, risk. This needed to be both acknowledged and diffused, which with Edwina proved to be relatively easy by using the distraction technique of taking her back to previous comments.

When talking of the neighbour, Edwina mentioned that she did not know how long it had been going on, as she did not 'always remember' and 'forgot when things happened sometimes'. This provided the CMHN with a way into discussing her memory, at a point in the session that was natural, and at Edwina's pace. With gentle prompting and reassurance, Edwina spoke of how at times she felt unable to remember what was happening, what day it was, what she was supposed to be doing, and so on. She discussed the fact that her mother and her maternal grandmother had needed to be cared for in the local psychiatric hospital, due to memory deterioration. She did appear to make a connection between her own memory difficulties and those of her family; however, she did not appear to perceive the full implications of the potential impact upon her life. Edwina also disclosed feelings of loss and ineptitude, describing herself as always having been a 'doer' and the organiser of the household; as her husband had taken more control, she had felt less useful.

At this point, Edwina became quite tearful. She spoke of her loneliness, how worried she was about her husband and how she did not understand why he was in hospital or how long he would be there. Edwina was supported through her tears and positive reinforcement was provided. When she had stopped crying she was gently steered back to her disclosed memory problems. She agreed to take a fairly standard Mini Mental State Exam (MMSE), so that the CMHN could see which areas were most difficult for her to remember. Her score of 20/30 fitted in with how she presented, as mildly confused. The MMSE uses a series of questions and tasks to assess cognitive functioning and to provide an indicator as to where cognitive problems may lie.

Edwina had problems with her recall, and with sequencing. Although she had been disoriented on our arrival, she had retained the re-orientation information given. The basic MMSE provides a basis from which to measure improvement or deterioration in later tests. These brief tests are generally not complex or specific enough to be used as diagnostic tools, but are useful as a means of discerning areas where function may be deteriorating.

As in many cases, as Edwina relaxed in the company of the CMHN, and when she was not pressurised to recall specific information, her natural recall of facts and dates was quite good. In the middle of talking about how she had had one daughter, she remembered that she had read a note from her just before our arrival. She was able to get up and go straight to it. It was a request from her daughter asking us to contact her at work after our visit. Edwina appeared pleased with this request, had no concerns about us speaking with her daughter and gave permission for us to discuss her openly.

This was taken as a means of closing the visit, and a second visit was arranged for later on in the week, to see how she was faring. Edwina was given an appointment card with the next visit recorded on it, as well as the CMHN's name and a contact telephone number. The appointment was also written on her calendar in the kitchen, which she appeared to use as a reference point. It was felt that, although she had had a few problems making the cup of tea, and igniting the gas cooker, she was relatively safe and of no great risk to herself or others. It was felt that an occupational therapy assessment at a later date might assist in further assessing her functional abilities and safety in the home, but that this would best be discussed after a relationship had been established.

A phone call was later made to Edwina's daughter, Sue, who disclosed that she was feeling fraught and at a loss about what to do about her mother. She described how over the past year she had noted changes in her behaviour, functioning and memory. She had spoken a number of times with her father, who had either made excuses for Edwina ('she's tired', 'it's her blood pressure') or told Sue not to worry. A couple in an established relationship may have differing defined roles, with one individual within the relationship automatically compensating for the other if deficits begin to occur. Sue now realised with the benefit of hindsight that he had been compensating for Edwina. She had imagined that his helping out in the kitchen was out of helpfulness, whereas it was out of necessity, as Edwina's previous skills had diminished so much.

Sue's father, Tom, had been admitted to hospital as an emergency the previous week. He had phoned her and asked her to get a quite specific shopping list of easy meals, snacks, and so on, which she had delivered to her mother. A few days later, Sue realised that Edwina had not touched the meals, although all the crisps and snacks had gone. Since that time, Sue had been popping in on a daily basis to cook a meal for Edwina, who each time had refused to let her tidy the kitchen, saying she would do it herself later.

Tom was due out of hospital on the morning of the next planned visit. Sue felt that we should go ahead and visit as arranged. She had told Tom that the GP was sending out a nurse to see Edwina and he had seemed quite relieved, although he was a little uncertain as to how Edwina would respond. He had also told Sue that he had felt that they needed help, but that he was scared, both of Edwina being taken away, or of Edwina becoming angry with him. Apparently, she occasionally got aggressive with him, mainly about her delusions. Sue thought that her mother would be quite safe at home, with her own daily visits, until Tom came back. She did feel that further assessment regarding Edwina's functioning should be done at a later stage.

The next stage in the process for the CMHN is the completion of all the relevant paperwork, including care plans, CPA documentation, and so on. This is a means of systemising and processing the information, and of collating it in a logical and meaningful format, which not only identifies weaknesses and deficits, but also highlights strengths and residual skills. As a service we do not use a specified nursing model, although our documentation is loosely based on Roper, Logan and Tierney's 'Activities of Daily Living' (1981), alongside a mental status examination, with additional emphasis placed upon the social/environmental aspects. In common with the majority of nurses, our notes are based on the established nursing process of assessment, planning, intervention and evaluation. We also complete computer-generated records of contacts made and input given; this is used by the Trust for data collection and analysis, and is fed back to the PCGs. A letter is always sent back to the referrer regarding the initial assessment and any planned interventions; this is also copied to other professionals who may be involved. If the referrer is not a GP or consultant, our letter tends to go to them and we provide telephone feedback to the referrer. This was the case with Edwina.

COLLABORATION IN ACTION

CASE STUDY   **EDWINA'S SECOND ASSESSMENT VISIT**

The second assessment visit to Edwina, with her husband present, allowed for further elaboration of the situation and provided another facet to the assessment process. Edwina was quite insistent that I (JM) should speak with Tom alone first. He told me how her memory had been declining for the past year or so; initially, it had been the odd date that she forgot and now she was regularly forgetful, particularly in the evening. Over the last three months, she had become preoccupied with the downstairs neighbour. He could identify no causal event for this; when he told her 'not to be so daft', she had occasionally become very angry with him and tried to hit him. Tom had felt that he could cope no more and was on the point of discussing Edwina with his daughter and his GP when he was taken ill and went into hospital.

Edwina was waiting for us in the other room, so brief support was offered, as Tom had become quite tearful. Problem-solving approaches were discussed with him, to explore ways of attempting to diffuse Edwina's anger by distraction. He was also encouraged not to challenge or discount her delusions, yet at the same time not to reinforce them and collude with her.

Edwina was much more relaxed than at the start of the previous visit. However, whereas she had previously spoken quite freely about herself and her family, with Tom present she was quieter. When questioned, she would look to him in the first instance to answer. When she did try to answer, he had a tendency to talk over her.

At this visit, both Tom and Edwina agreed that her memory was perhaps not as good as it should be and a plan was discussed to provide some help for her. First, it was agreed that the CMHN would continue to visit to provide a number of interventions. The CMHN would monitor Edwina's memory and safety, the extent and intensity of the delusions, and provide her with the opportunity to talk through and explore the impact of her memory problems on her life. The CMHN would provide carer support, coping skills and education for Sue and Tom, and would act in an advocacy role with regard to benefits and services. It was also agreed that Edwina and Tom would benefit from an occupational therapy (OT) assessment. This would look at Edwina's functioning skills within the home, and determine whether Tom and Edwina might benefit from any home adaptations, such as a second stair rail.

During this visit it also came to light that Edwina was prone to urinary incontinence, especially at night. It was agreed that a urine specimen would be taken to the surgery for analysis, although it was unlikely that Edwina had an infection, as she had been having problems for some time. Neither of them reported an excessive urine smell, and Edwina could not describe any feelings of discomfort upon micturition, except urgency. However, incontinence provides the potential for infection and this needed to be ruled out as a causal, or worsening factor. We agreed that a district nurse should visit and undertake a continence assessment.

Discussions with the GP came to the conclusion that, as Edwina's memory appeared to fluctuate, the signs and symptoms pointed more to Alzheimer's Disease than to a vascular dementia (although she did suffer from elevated blood pressure). Once the OTs had completed their assessment with Edwina, she was referred to the psychologist, to establish a baseline measurement of specific cognitive functions.

Dementia syndromes present differently. Generally, people with a vascular dementia tend to deteriorate in a stepwise manner, as vascular accidents occur. Those with Alzheimer's-type dementia decline at a more regular and gradual rate.

Over the next week, Edwina was seen at home by the district nurse who undertook a holistic assessment, which included documenting her biographical details, previous medical history, current medication, and the domestic environment and Edwina's safety within it. The assessment focused on the current situation of short-term memory loss, disorientation and urinary incontinence. Edwina's ability to maintain independence in the 12 activities of daily living (Roper et al., 1981) was then assessed, with any actual or potential problems determining any nursing or social needs. A full continence assessment was undertaken, including urinalysis to rule out infection (this had already been sent off), hygiene and skin assessment. Tom was also assessed in respect of his perception of the help that he needed in order to look after Edwina. This included a limited financial assessment, to ascertain any need for application for benefits and/or social support and home care, all of which he declined at the time.

It was decided that Edwina would benefit from incontinence pads, mainly for night-time use, and these were ordered and subsequently delivered on a monthly basis.

Edwina had been finding it difficult to manage to bathe effectively, and the skin assessment highlighted this, so the nurse auxiliary from the district nursing team would visit weekly to bathe her. Tom decided to invest in a good-quality mattress cover and declined the plastic one offered. At regular intervals, a qualified member of the district nurse team reassessed the situation and informed those involved of any changes.

Over the next few months, Edwina and Tom were seen by the occupational therapist on a number of occasions. Again, the main thrust of the OT's assessment was based on the degree of Edwina's functioning within the 'activities of daily living'. Difficulties were identified, so that possible solutions might be sought, with the primary aim of maintaining Edwina's independence and also supporting Tom. For Edwina, three main areas of activity were assessed as being difficult:

1 Access to the first-floor maisonette: Edwina appeared to find the stairs quite difficult and pulled heavily at times on the single hand rail. The agreed solution was to apply for a second rail to be fitted. In the future, a stair-lift might need to be installed.
2 Bathing and personal care: Edwina was finding it difficult to bathe and had problems washing her bottom, especially after she had been incontinent. She was very reluctant to seek help from her husband and he felt that he could not insist that she let him help. By obtaining both a bath seat and rail, Edwina was able to bathe herself much more easily, and the equipment was also of assistance to the auxiliary district nurse on her visits. A commode was considered for during the night but Edwina declined this, as she was apparently incontinent prior to waking, not on, or post waking. Edwina was capable of dressing herself, although she did not always choose items that were congruent with the season or the day's activities. Tom was advised on the best way to maintain and maximise her skills and to help her adjust her choice so that it was more suitable.
3 Domestic skills: Edwina had lost the ability to make complex meals, but she had retained the skills to make drinks and snacks quite safely once she had relaxed in the OT's company. Occasionally, she had problems igniting the gas rings (usually when under pressure to perform) and her husband agreed that he could monitor this, as she normally only used the cooker when he was around. Edwina unfortunately had lost her ability to manage her finances, and Tom had taken over the shopping duties. As Edwina had expressed concern about her loss of roles, this was discussed. It was subsequently established that they would shop together and that Edwina would be involved in the planning and preparation of meals, especially those snacks that she could do alone, or with minimal assistance.

The main constraints experienced by OTs are the same as those inflicted upon most NHS staff – time and resources. In an ideal world, there would be regular follow-up assessments, providing and fitting equipment as soon as it is required. In this case, the CMHN arranged further OT intervention, as necessary.

CASE STUDY Edwina's referral

After discussion with the GP, Edwina was referred on to the psychologist, with a view to establishing the cause and extent of her memory problems. An initial assessment was undertaken during a meeting with both Edwina and Tom at home. This ascertained the onset, duration and cause of the problems. In addition, the assessment covered the subsequent impact of these problems on everyday living and mood, Edwina's personal history, family, education, occupation and physical health, and her current coping strategies. As both Edwina and Tom were willing, and it was deemed appropriate, Edwina then attended the hospital, to undertake some screening on her own. This involved the Camcog, part of Camdex (Cambridge Index of Mental Disorder in the Elderly) (Roth et al., 1986). This was followed up by a full and detailed neuropsychological assessment using a battery of specific tests that were prioritised to suit both Edwina and the purpose of the assessment, to establish a probable diagnosis and level of functioning.

The psychologist concluded that Edwina probably did have Alzheimer's Disease, and that her delusions were likely to be part of her dementia syndrome. These were already being treated by the GP with a small dose of risperidone (one of the newer and cleaner antipsychotics), and were becoming less intense, with Edwina experiencing few side-effects. Throughout all of these interventions by members of the primary and secondary teams, Edwina and Tom were still seen by the CMHN on a regular basis and by the practice nurse or GP at least quarterly.

Gradually, Edwina began to deteriorate further and her abilities declined, necessitating more support from her husband. As this happened, Tom took over the more physical aspects of her care, refusing assistance from social services. Alongside her cognitive decline, Edwina also declined physically and her mobility worsened. This obviously impacted on Tom's ability to care for her, so the physiotherapists became involved, to try to maximise and maintain her mobility. The physiotherapist completed a mobility assessment, which looked at both the potential reasons for loss of mobility (her physical health, neurological symptoms, etc.), and at her present level of mobility, taking into account safety and likelihood of falls. It was felt that Edwina would benefit from a Zimmer frame to provide both support and to aid her balance. Her husband was given advice with regards to safety and he decided to remove some rugs from the floor. They were also given some exercises to help strengthen her lower limbs, improve co-ordination and reduce any swelling. They both did the exercises with great commitment every day. Ideally, the physiotherapist would have liked to be able to see Edwina on a weekly basis, to monitor her progress, but had to make do with a time-limited intervention.

Edwina and Tom are still being seen by our service, and Edwina now needs help with even her most basic needs. Tom is still at the hub of her care, although he has now let social services be involved in part of the package, and Edwina has regular home care, day care and respite. In many situations of this type, social services have a vital role to play in supporting informal carers, assisting them to continue in their caring capacity. The CMHN still visits, as Edwina continues to display behaviour that can be interpreted by others to be problematic, but has been caused by the dementing process.

We continue to work with Tom, to enable him to cope with the changes in Edwina's mental health, and with the emotional impact they are having on him. The opportunity to acknowledge feelings of loss surrounding his expectations for the future has provided him with a safe and therapeutic outlet to express his innermost thoughts and feelings. He says that this has enabled him to care actively for Edwina for far longer than he expected. Continued informed support from everyone involved has allowed the collaborative care relationship to prosper.

IMPROVING ACCESS TO SERVICES

Currently, mental health services for older adults are accessed through a number of routes. If a person with dementia or their carer goes to the GP surgery with a problem, the GP can refer either to a consultant or to a CMHN, depending on how the GP perceives the problem at the time. If the referral is to the consultant, the consultant may then involve the CMHN if needed. The CMHN service operates an open referral system, in which individuals can self-refer or can be referred by any another agency. GPs are always kept informed of where patients are in the system and who is assuming responsibility for them. Although GPs have a 'gate-keeping' role, they cannot assume total responsibility for all patients with mental health problems (Gray *et al.*, 1999). Keady (1995) has remarked that it is by involving others, and working closely with them, that patients such as Edwina can receive early holistic assessment, care and treatment, characterised as being 'proactive rather than reactive'.

As secondary services are based in different localities, regular multidisciplinary meetings are held to review certain clients and explore how collaboration can be improved. Nurses, doctors, occupational therapists, physiotherapists and psychologists attend these meetings, as well as social workers from the local area offices. This model of collaboration within secondary care and its identified benefits can give an insight into how potential benefits could be obtained from maximising collaboration within primary care.

Although CMHNs are part of the secondary services, they have been linked in with primary care for a number of years. In the 1980s, there was a definite push for CMHNs to be offering counselling services in the GP surgeries (McFadyen and Farrington, 1996), but Trusts saw the role of CMHNs as focusing on the needs of those with serious and enduring mental illness (SEMI). However, some GPs, especially fundholding GPs, had a preference for CMHNs being involved in counselling with people with depression and anxiety. In the 1990s, care for individuals with SEMI was deemed a priority for CMHNs and this created some ambiguity and disharmony between GPs and CMHNs. The existing degree of collaboration suffered, and CMHNs were re-directed to focus on SEMI. Previous regular contact in surgeries was reduced as nurses withdrew from sessional counselling work to concentrate on the enduring mentally ill. The lesson is that collaboration is possible and can be successful, but all parties have to be in agreement. Imposing directives from outside may not always be the best way of meeting patients' needs; without the involvement of primary care staff, future collaboration is not guaranteed to succeed.

Over the past five years prior to the formation of PCGs, the CMHN service for older adults within our Trust attempted actively to offer a greater link with GPs. The success of this has been varied; some GP practices welcomed it, viewing a more active link with secondary mental health services as useful. The opportunity to provide care for older people with mental health needs in a much more sensitive and purposeful way than was hitherto the case is preferable to staff, and beneficial to patients and their carers. However, these ways of working, and even the invitation to attend monthly meetings, have sometimes been turned down, despite the enthus-iastic efforts of CMHNs. This reluctance to be more actively involved with CMHNs is surprising; it can take months for a GP to get a response from secondary services following the referral of a patient (Badger and Nolan, 1999). We aim to ensure that all communication with GPs is carried out immediately following any decision.

Our service has not been adopted widely, neither has it been seen as a success in all primary care areas; however, the set-up allowed CMHNs to be seen and helped them to discover how they could collaborate with primary care colleagues. We learnt that we had to be there, to be seen, to discuss with colleagues how we could help, actually to do it and then to provide evidence that we had made a difference to patients and their carers. At surgeries where GPs have regular meetings, and mental health care is an agenda item, changes are beginning to occur:

- More patients are being referred earlier.
- Referrals are beginning to be more appropriate.
- It is beginning to be recognised that one mental health professional cannot provide the best service alone; others will need to be involved.
- GPs have a better understanding of what mental health services can actually do.
- Some practices are beginning to request details of what was done with patients and how it was done.
- Previously held myths and stereotypes of each other's services have begun to be broken down.

The increase in the 'appropriateness' of referrals is significant as it means that services are beginning to understand what everyone does. This type of awareness can only be achieved through face-to-face contact and an acknowledgement of each other's skills and knowledge. Our Trust has also recently developed the role of primary care liaison nurses to link in with the primary care services, to raise awareness further of the mental health needs of older people, and of the means to address them. Initially, these workers undertook training with practice staff and with community services, to increase the knowledge and skills needed in working with this client group. They have also undertaken assessments of clients with potential problems in the primary care setting, and filtered them on to the appro-priate service provider. Earlier diagnosis of mental health problems should allow for speedier and more appropriate treatment, and recovery. It is hoped that this service will identify clients with mental health problems sooner, thereby releasing some of the pressure on secondary and tertiary services. However, as with all new service initiatives, uptake has varied from practice to practice.

The more service personnel come together to explore common issues, the more productive collaboration will prove to be. Both sets of staff have a great deal to teach each other and sharing knowledge and skills can be effective in improving services. One way of improving services for people with mental health problems in primary care might be to have one point of contact to which GPs could refer; that person would negotiate and make decisions on how best to manage the situation.

We are now more convinced than ever that fostering links with primary care is the most effective way of improving services, especially for older adults and their carers. The main benefits of closer collaboration that we have perceived to date are:

- the ability to offer better services;
- greater understanding of roles, activities and expectations of others;
- greater emphasis on holistic and proactive care;
- continuous opportunities for professional development;
- more appropriate referrals; and
- a reduction in the number of letters that are sent to various colleagues.

We have also reflected on the ways in which we have collaborated with various individuals and as a consequence have identified different patterns of communication:

- regular meetings with all partners and key practice members, complemented by frequent telephone contact;
- irregular meetings, arranged on an ad hoc basis by the CMHN, with frequent telephone contact;
- meetings with individual GPs on a regular basis with frequent telephone contact;
- irregular meetings with individual GPs, arranged by the CMHN, with frequent telephone contact;
- no meetings but frequent telephone contact;
- infrequent contact by telephone, letters, or material that updates primary care teams on mental health issues; and
- contact at times of crisis only; this is the least common form of contact and the one that we least prefer.

The issue of definition is a particular problem. Dementia could be classified as a serious and enduring mental health problem, which would give it priority-funding status. Dementia is actually viewed by many GPs as a social problem (Wolff *et al.*, 1995). CMHNs are often asked to assess clients when a crisis has already occurred, and the client is well advanced into their illness. Gunstone (1999) suggests that the earlier nurses can be involved with patients, the more likely it is that crises will be averted. Even the simple conducting of assessments can have positive benefits for care-givers (Wright *et al.*, 1999), although a diagnosis of dementia raises issues that need to be addressed or acknowledged by the person diagnosed. Early intervention can reap untold benefits for carers, allowing for education and preparation, and helping to avert their depression, which is at a much higher level than in the general population (Bergman-Evans, 1994).

STANDARDS AND PROTOCOLS

Perhaps it is not surprising that services vary greatly. Until recently there were no national guidelines or policy initiatives relating to older people with mental health needs (Pickard, 1999), and services were left pretty much to individuals on the ground. In 2001, the publication of the *National Service Framework for Older People* (NSF-OP) (Department of Health, 2001) focused attention and resources on this very vulnerable group. The NSF-OP could well enhance the outcomes of people with dementia. Standard Seven (of eight) deals specifically with mental health:

> *Older people who have mental health problems should have access to integrated services, provided by the NHS and Councils to ensure effective diagnosis, treatment and support, for them and their carers.*

> (Department of Health, 2001)

Currently it is expected that practice nurses undertake all aspects of the over-75 health check, although they receive little or no formal training in mental health care. Gray *et al.* (1999) observed that, although practice nurses are regularly involved in mental health assessments, many conditions go unrecognised, raising the question of the value of these assessments. The major problem, as highlighted in the case of Edwina, is that detection of people with dementia is still patchy. With the advent of the NSF-OP, primary care organisations will be encouraged to utilise appropriate evidence-based uniform assessments and protocols for the early identification and management of dementia. The NSF-OP identifies the fact that

> *... early and accurate diagnosis of mental health problems enables older people and those caring for them to understand what is happening to them, to access appropriate help and to meet their care needs.*

> (Department of Health, 2001)

The Alzheimer's Disease Society (Keady, 1995) has highlighted the poor detection and treatment of dementia in primary care. Having personnel who can carry out physical and mental health assessments, better collaboration between CMHNs and practice nurses, alongside input from primary care liaison workers, would be a move towards addressing this problem. The NSF-OP suggests that mental health services for older people should be community-oriented and provide a seamless package of care and support for people and their carers. Although the majority of people with dementia will be cared for within primary care, a number will be referred on to secondary services, especially where the taking of the anti-dementia drugs (cholinesterase inhibitors) could be commenced. This may in time impact on an increasing number of referrals to the CMH teams.

A number of issues raised within our professional practice should be addressed by the NSF-OP.

- Nurses and other professionals are increasingly aware of diminishing resources.
- Some services and professionals are working in isolation.
- An increasing number of older people live alone without any close family or support to advocate on their behalf.
- There are still differences between social care and health care.
- Kitwood and Bredin (1992) have devised an approach that emphasises the importance of treating people with dementia as individuals, and retaining their abilities for as long as possible. This is not always feasible within current service constraints.
- Current team practices have encouraged links with primary care settings but there is still the tendency to be viewed as 'part of, but apart from' primary care.
- Although it has time implications, teambuilding exercises may be beneficial to enhance the exploration of others' roles and to negotiate care practices.
- Current methods of record-keeping (paper files on a number of sites), in conjunction with occasional professional reluctance, can inhibit the sharing of information and expertise.

CONCLUSION

The NSF-OP has identified good mental health services as comprehensive, multi-disciplinary, accessible, responsive, individualised, accountable and systematic. We would like to think that the service provided and the interventions undertaken with Edwina and her family fulfil this model. We do acknowledge, however, that current practice among the multiple disciplines involved resulted in some duplicity of assessment, which may have put added pressure upon the situation.

Alongside this, we are also aware that there needs to be an increased amount of attention paid to maximising primary community and secondary support for this vulnerable group. Collaboration must remain at the forefront of our practice and our service planning.

This chapter provides more evidence that collaboration between services greatly benefits clients and their carers. It strongly conveys the authors' compassion and their common-sense approach to care delivery. Older adults constitute a vulnerable group who derive most benefit from services if these are adjacent, and if service providers know each other and can request assistance from each other when the client is ready. The authors' genuine interest in Edwina, and their commitment to her receiving the best possible services, are impressive. The importance of involving the client in her own care and assessment is emphasised. It is misguided to think that assessments can be carried out quickly; ample time and patience are needed in order to complete a valid assessment that elicits the real needs and problems of the client. Care has to be taken not to over-assess a person – assessments should be carried out when the client is ready and when she can benefit most from them. Collaboration means knowing the other professionals who can contribute to the care and treatment of the client, and having quick and easy access to them. The relationship with the client is critical in ensuring her optimum welfare. (Editors' summary)

REFERENCES

Badger, F. and Nolan, P. (1999) General practitioners' perceptions of CMHNs in primary care, *Journal of Psychiatric and Mental Health Nursing*, **6**, 453–459

Bergman-Evans, B. (1994) Loneliness, depression and social support of spousal caregivers, *Journal of Gerontological Nursing, March*, 6–16

Burns, A. and Levy, R. (1994) *Dementia*, Chapman and Hall, London

Department of Health (2001) *National Service Framework for Older People*, Department of Health, London

Gray, R., Parr, A., Plummer, S. *et al.*, (1999) A National Survey of practice nurse involvement in mental health interventions, *Journal of Advanced Nursing*, 30(4), 901–906

Gunstone, S. (1999) Expert Practice: the interventions used by a community mental health nurse with the carers of dementia sufferers, *Journal of Psychiatric and Mental Health Nursing*, **6**, 21–27

Keady, J. (1995) Implications for nursing of the Alzheimer's Disease Society Report, *British Journal of Nursing*, 4(14), 812–813

Kitwood, T. and Bredin, K. (1992) Towards a theory of dementia care: personhood and well being, *Ageing and Society*, **12**, 269–287

McFayden, J. A. and Farrington, A. (1996) The failure of community care for the severely mentally ill, *British Journal of Nursing*, 5(15), 920–928

Pickard, S. (1999) Co-coordinated care for older people with dementia, *Journal of Interprofessional Care*, **13**, 345–354

Rees, L., Lipsedge, M. and Ball, C. (1997) *Textbook of Psychiatry*, Arnold, London

Roper, N., Logan, W. and Tierney, A. (1981) *Learning to Use the Process of Nursing*, Churchill Livingstone, Edinburgh

Roth, M., Tym, E. and Mountjoy, C. (1986) CAMDEX: A standardised instrument for the diagnosis of mental disorder in the elderly with specific references to the early detection of dementia, *British Journal of Psychiatry*, **149**, 698–709

Wolff, L.E., Woods, J. P. and Reid, J. (1995) Do general practitioners and old age psychiatrists differ in their attitudes to dementia? *International Journal of Geriatric Psychiatry*, **10**, 63–69

Wright, L.K, Hickey, J.V., Buckwater, K.C., Hendrix, S.A. and Kelechi, T. (1999) Emotional and physical health of spouse care-givers of persons with Alzheimer's Disease and strokes, *Journal of Advanced Nursing*, 29(3), 552–563

PART THREE

MENTAL HEALTH PROMOTION

15 MENTAL HEALTH PROMOTION

Jennifer Law and Tom Harrison

For many professionals, mental health promotion remains at best vague and unclear. At worst, it may be regarded as futile. It conjures up images of Saturday afternoons in the high street attempting to interest passers-by in reducing their alcohol intake, or trying to persuade reluctant schoolchildren to stop smoking. It seems a world away from the everyday practicalities of the crowded daily surgery. This chapter aims to demonstrate that what at first appears to be an idealistic and nebulous discipline can actually have a practical impact on public mental health. It argues that a strategic approach, working in co-ordination with a wide group of agencies and individuals, in particular environments, can enable members of the general population to change their behaviour for the better. It is not achieved quickly, or simply, but through an accumulation of actions. At first sight, it appears to be an anti-professional approach because it does not aim at those who are already ill, but at those who are at risk. In fact, it stands alongside the medical treatment model, and enhances it. Effective mental health promotion requires the input of those people at whom it is aimed; they need to share their views and become partners in the process. The process of developing alliances results in potential patients gaining skills and knowledge that protect them against a host of difficulties, not just specific disorders. This chapter also discusses the role that recent legislation has played, gives some evidence of the effectiveness of mental health promotion, and concludes with a synopsis of how PCTs might either become pioneers locally, or join in with other groups who are already active. (Editors' note)

INTRODUCTION

When Dr Manson and Dr Denny blew up the sewer – using dynamite in cocoa tins – in A.J. Cronin's 1937 novel *The Citadel*, they succeeded in ridding the town of enteric fever. Until then, they had been unable to focus attention on the cause of the epidemic in any other way. Their action demonstrates the power of practical health promotion.

There are no such dramatically simple solutions in mental health promotion, although imagination and innovation are still essential ingredients. The real battle has to be fought in concert with a wide group of agencies, of which primary care is only one. Health-service professionals need to work alongside staff in housing and education, the police, the media, ethnic groups and religious organisations, as well as with people who have experienced mental health problems themselves, and those who have cared for them. The challenge of mental health promotion is that the task is seemingly impossible, and hopelessly nebulous. The average general practitioner sees the idea of actively participating as both overwhelming and impractical.

The first requirement of success is a recognition that the assault on ignorance has to be carried out on a broad front, employing a variety of weapons, and forging a range of alliances. We advocate the use of a settings schema, which divides up the targets of promotion into neighbourhoods, schools, places of work, the health service, primary care and the media. In this way, various approaches may be used, taking into account the particular audiences, but working in parallel, and focusing individual effort. The individual GP is expected to work in partnership, rather than alone; for some, this may prove to be the most difficult barrier to overcome.

Mental health is a major concern for general practice as is amply demonstrated by epidemiological findings. In the UK, mental disorders account for almost a quarter of the total disease burden (Andrews, 1998). Between a quarter and one-third of all surgery attenders in the UK have significant psychiatric disorders (Goldberg and Huxley, 1980), but approximately half of these cases remain unrecognised by the GP, and the evidence indicates that those who remain untreated experience continuing difficulties.

These studies fail to assess the impact of mental ill health that does not reach clinical severity. Jenkins (1985), however, found that minor psychiatric morbidity was the cause of one-third of all loss of time from work through sickness. From these figures it has been calculated that 93 million productive days are lost each year, costing industry in the UK around £2.9 billion (Bosanquet and Bosanquet, 1998). The effects on family life are incalculable.

Perhaps these statistics begin to make the case for the serious consideration of how such disorders might be prevented, or at least minimised, by methods supplementary to medical treatment. Interestingly, the World Health Organisation definition of primary care involves the mobilisation of resources at community level in favour of actions that improve health and control. This clearly extends well beyond the confines of the patient-doctor relationship, to working with whole communities.

In this chapter we aim to introduce a strategy, and some practicable ideas, to achieve this end. It should be made clear at this point that there is a debate raging between those who advocate a risk reduction approach in vulnerable populations, often based on the medical model of care, and those who argue that interventions should be population-based. The former has been described as 'attempting to control icebergs by sending warships to shoot off their visible portions' (Rose, 1993). This chapter will argue that both strategies are relevant, but will concentrate on the second.

In order to illustrate how mental health promotion may be implemented, we will use examples of progress being made in the West Midlands. At present, these do not specifically include GPs, but they do illustrate the overall strategic approach, the practical implementation of evaluated methods, the search for common ground with a network of agencies, and working with those agencies, and the constructive use of serendipity.

WHAT IS MENTAL HEALTH PROMOTION?

Mental health promotion presents a huge agenda, engaging with many people, so it is important to clarify the basic concepts.

Meanings of mental health

The first conundrum concerns the term 'mental health'. Too often, it is used instead of 'mental ill health'; thus, 'mental health' trusts actually treat disorders, rather than promoting the sanity of ordinary people. There is a temptation to adopt a single definition, which tries to encompass everybody's various experiences and meanings. This is a major challenge, and probably impossible. A more flexible approach is to develop a shared understanding of different realities, rather than relying on one pre-defined agenda. This should include lay perspectives, finding out 'where people are at'. While this may not always sit comfortably with the professional view, it does contribute to an understanding of the ordinary person's views about what affects his or her mental and emotional health.

One effective way forward is to identify and get a general consensus on the elements that contribute to the shared understandings. For example, recognising those aspects of a particular environment that are conducive to mental health, such as neighbourly spirit, makes it easier for all participants to understand and to act. With the use of individually or collectively defined mental health concepts for different groups and settings, the resultant planning is more likely to be effective and sustainable.

Promotion or prevention?

Because mental health promotion may involve a large number of people and significant resources it is important that any effort expended should be carefully planned and evaluated. There is evidence, albeit poorly disseminated, of effective activity and this should form the basis for further work. This will avoid any increase in the number of poorly designed, often amateurish interventions.

Prevention in mental health has a long history. The alienists of the nineteenth century were ardent advocates of the early treatment of mental illness. Caplan (1961) was the first person to advocate a systematic approach, identifying three levels of intervention:

1 *Primary prevention* – preventing new cases of the disorder;
2 *Secondary prevention* – reducing prevalence by early and effective intervention;
3 *Tertiary prevention* – managing and reducing secondary disability incurred by the disorder.

The debate is between those who advocate a risk-reduction approach, and those who favour a broader health promotion. The former viewpoint has dominated the medical and psychiatric outlook, because clinicians tend to be nervous of the complexity of social issues in the causation of different disorders. Interventions involving large groups of people are expected to waste scarce resources, and suggest political idealism.

In the field of prevention, Caplan's original concept has been simplified into a risk-reduction approach, which is considered to be of more practical value as it tends to concentrate on single disorders. Interventions are concentrated at three different levels: universal, selected and indicated (Gordon, 1987).

At the broadest, universal level, interventions are targeted at the general public, or whole specific populations. An anti-smoking campaign aimed at children in schools in England and Wales would be one example. Such interventions are expected to be widely beneficial, with no significant adverse side-effects.

At the second level, selected interventions are aimed at high-risk groups where the benefits are estimated to outweigh the possible costs, effort and risks. One example of this is the health visitor programme in the UK, where every post-natal mother is visited for assessment and to be offered further assistance if required.

At the third level, indicated interventions focus on high-risk individuals who show minimal but definite symptoms of disorder. The resource implications are usually high, but the benefits are considered to outweigh them. In general practice, this would include screening for symptoms of depression, and rapid action based on this.

This approach is complementary to that of mental health promotion. After identifying the frequency of common disorders, it has been demonstrated that early detection of some mental disorders in general practice can be highly effective in reducing individual morbidity, particularly with regard to depression (Araya, 1999). However, certain suspicions remain; when minor mental ill health affects such a large percentage of the general population, an individually oriented treatment strategy is very costly, limited in efficacy and runs the risk of medical- ising conditions that could be managed differently. For example, nearly 40 per cent of adolescents registered with eight general practitioners in London were found to have had significant psychiatric disorder. This was found to be mainly emotional, but was associated with marked physical symptoms, and increased health risks such as suicidal behaviour, drug abuse and smoking (Kramer and Garralda, 1998). Another study found that nearly 10% of girls and 5% of boys suffer from social phobias (Wittchen et al., 1999). Strategies targeted at assisting these young people to cope with their environment, and find ways of supporting each other, may be healthier, and have longer-term benefits, than the use of medication.

Medical or political solutions?

The debate about promotion or prevention is reflected in the way in which measurements of the mental health of a population are interpreted. Most epidemi- ological studies, such as those quoted above, identify 'cases' – that is, those disorders that reach a previously determined level of severity, which is considered to be significant enough to require treatment, and would be recognisable to a clinician specialising in the particular field. This distinction – between those people considered to be healthy and those identified as ill – is too simplistic. As Pickering (1968) recognised in the case of hypertension, much ill health is distributed throughout a spectrum of severity. This is particularly true of alcohol use, anxiety and depression. Rose argues that the clinical approach emphasises causation in terms of individual pathology, rather than revealing underlying social and environmental trends. He points out that 'the baffling problems of widespread minor neurosis and depression' are ignored. He then elucidates the point that worries many doctors; that this 'may be society's problem rather than the psychiatrist's' (Rose, 1989). Certainly, there is evidence that supports his point of view. The two most consistently recognised risk factors for common mental disorders are poverty and female role.

Is a leaking sewer a social problem, or a clinical one? Is the solution medical or political? It goes without saying that poor housing conditions should be improved, but the process of making the necessary changes becomes political, and the benefits are not always straightforward. Are there other methods of achieving the same end?

It has long been recognised that the distinction between health promotion, prevention and treatment is not absolute. Rose (1993) argues for understanding and controlling underlying characteristics of the population, which are the real determinants of health and disease. While his focus is prevention, the underlying principles complement the work of those advocating a model that builds on people's strengths and enhances protective factors, rather than relying on risk-reduction activity (Antonovsky, 1996). This is compatible with the understanding that health prevention and promotion develop quality of life rather than merely prevent disorder. The social rewards of enhanced self-esteem and participation may be much more powerful, perhaps, than the estimated benefits of sport on physical health.

The health promotion movement has built on concepts that extend beyond the purely treatment-oriented model. The declaration of the first international conference on health promotion, the Ottawa Charter, formulated a definition that is still widely accepted:

> *The process of enabling people to increase control over, and to improve their health. (p. i)*
>
> (World Health Organisation, 1986)

While this definition has often been adapted to suit the diverse range of health promotion programmes, they nearly all include the notion of empowerment. Generally, activities have focused on individuals rather than environments, attempting to empower the former in order to mitigate the negative influences of the latter.

APPROPRIATE SETTINGS

MacDonald and O'Hara (1996) recommend that action should take place at three different levels: the micro, meso and macro. The first represents the individual, the second represents small groups such as families, workplace colleagues or community groups. The widest (macro) remit is government, health service or even international. All such programmes should integrate activity between each of the layers, where possible.

Antonovsky (1996) advocates a 'salutogenic orientation', which focuses on how people remain healthy. He identifies protective factors that can operate both at individual level and in a community. For example, at the micro level, general education has been demonstrated to increase the likelihood of individuals remaining healthy across the lifespan. However, the effect is limited, because of the unconscious cultural expectations that override people's rational understanding. Further, he advocates making small shifts in the overall health of a population, through aiming at specific groups of healthy people at risk, rather than those who have already developed symptoms of disorder.

Empirically it has been found that five conditions enhance mental health and a further five damage it (*see below*). This provides a pragmatic way of analysing the processes at work in affecting people's quality of life. In planning a strategy it is important both to strengthen the positive factors and to counteract those that are inhibitory (MacDonald and O'Hara, 1996).

Mental health promotion, viewed like this, has a huge agenda on which to deliver. Workers in the field have generally concentrated on an issue-driven approach, focusing, for example, on teenage pregnancy, smoking, drugs or alcohol. Less commonly, whole groups or populations of vulnerable persons, such as adolescents, the homeless or the elderly, are targeted. We propose instead a settings approach, identifying not people but specific social and geographical environments – such as schools, workplaces or neighbourhoods – which frame the context in which mental health may be influenced.

MacDonald and O'Hara (1996) have represented this schema in the form of a map (Figure 15.1). This framework can assist in establishing a shared understanding of mental health and mental health promotion. It also provides a basis to identify existing activity, and to establish need.

An implicit feature of this map is that focusing only on interventions in the semi-circle above the mid-line are likely to be of limited benefit if elements underneath are not also addressed. It also reinforces the idea that, while health promotion can help people collectively to change things that are beyond the control of individuals, it is important also to operate at a policy level, in order to affect the broader community. This may not be immediately achievable; it is more likely to be cumulative. It should be remembered that there is an overlap between all the elements and levels of activity, and that they have effects across the lifespan.

In Birmingham, for example, a few people suffering from mental health problems were upset by newspaper reports of mental illness. As a result, there was a determination to tackle the issue of discrimination against those with severe mental illness. Stepping back from this issue, and looking at the social attitudes that already existed, led to the adoption of another approach. It was clear that stigmatising attitudes evolve in childhood, so work was begun in schools. A number of individuals gave ad hoc lectures on mental illness to pupils. However, it was difficult to identify clearly any changes in attitude. Gradually, it became clear that the young people had their own problems, which distressed and isolated them. It was necessary to start from their viewpoint in order to become meaningful to them. A number of studies have looked at the mental health of young people, but

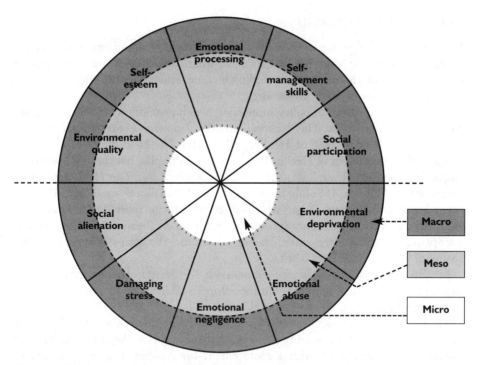

Figure 15.1 Map of mental health promotion: the integration of levels and elements. Adapted from MacDonald and O'Hara (1996)

only recently have they begun to look at their own perceptions. In order to address this neglect, as part of our study, we sought the views of 160 sixth-formers. This study found that they had difficulty in communicating about their distress, and seeking help for it (Health Education Unit, 1999).

The next step was to employ a theatre group, which initially presented everyday conflicts on stage. Following recognition by the social services department of their work, they subsequently engaged more actively with their audience, going into the schools and encouraging pupils to write and act out their own plays illustrating their problems. Mental distress became a focus for creativity, sharing and under-standing for the students. They started to form counselling services for those of their peers who were in distress. They had been able to acknowledge their own strengths and unhappiness, while learning new ways of coping. What is more, many of the skills developed – negotiating difficult situations, communicating emotions and asking for help – were generic. These are competencies that can be learned at any stage and applied to many situations.

Some of the inviduals involved in the study are currently in the process of devel-oping a specific strategy for mental health promotion in this area. It is planned that eventually this will be adopted throughout the city. This example demonstrates the often serendipitous nature of mental health promotion, and also how ever-widening circles of influence can begin to affect other levels and elements.

THE POLICY BACKGROUND

There are many different perceptions of what affects mental and emotional health. Ultimately, of course, everyone has to make their own choices, but a number of factors are outside their control, including income, education, housing, transport, and the distortions of mass advertising.

There is a groundswell of policy supporting health promotion, and mental health promotion in particular. The *National Service Framework for Mental Health*: Standard One (Department of Health, 1999), and *The New NHS: Modern and Dependable* (Department of Health, 1997) are two examples, but the first attempt in England to impose an overall strategy came with *Saving Lives: Our Healthier Nation* (Department of Health, 1996). In this publication, mental illness was identified as one of five key areas for action. Targets were first set for reducing morbidity and mortality, but the focus was on secondary (prompt detection and effective management) and tertiary (rehabilitation) prevention, failing to address the issues of improving the quality of life for whole populations.

In 1999, the *National Service Framework for Mental Health* gave specific guidance on primary prevention, but the effort to address whole populations and mental health gain was still too limited.

The structural changes in the NHS are primarily intended to address the inefficiencies in acute and community services. Central to this is the aim of enhancing community-led initiatives, with a requirement for combined, integrated action, achieved through partnerships. Primary Care Groups and Trusts could be pivotal in forging such community-defined and community-led alliances.

The New NHS (Department of Health, 1997) provides the structures to drive forward partnership working. The intention is to achieve this through the implementation of local health improvement plans, and the restructuring of services with the creation of PCG/Ts, health action zones and healthy living centres. Models of primary care delivery that incorporate multidisciplinary teams, and a joint budget, will maximise opportunities for preventive services.

The targets for health and social services, according to Standard One of the *National Service Framework*, are the following:

- to promote mental health for all, working with individuals and communities;
- to combat discrimination against individuals and groups with mental health problems; and
- to promote the social inclusion of those individuals and groups.

Part of the model of mental health promotion that we advocate here aims to identify barriers to progress. In this instance, despite the positive impact made by most of the legislation, two difficulties present themselves. First, the health authorities are given lead responsibility for implementation of mental health promotion. They have established few links between key areas locally, and other national programmes. As a result, they have no real system to deliver a broad public mental health agenda.

Second, lead officers, in different localities for implementation of the NSF, are preoccupied with Standards Two (primary care and access to mental health services) and Seven (preventing suicide). The inclusion of mental health promotion in Standard One does legitimate it in an important way; but successful implementation will still need the impetus of local champions. Unfortunately, the policy of a primary care-led NHS may lead to conflict with NSF key deliverables concerned with secondary care, while at the same time expecting a concentration on mild and moderate disorders and carers' issues.

There is a requirement to demonstrate linkage between policies. This will be measured through health improvement programmes (HImPs), in relation to specific identified settings and for specific groups of individuals: those at risk, vulnerable groups and those with mental health problems.

Working in partnership has many benefits, although a number of lessons need to be learned. A cohesive group of agencies, advocating a particular policy or approach, is likely to be far more effective than one organisation working on its own. The various channels of influence open to each become available to all. If social services, voluntary sector and primary care organisations can agree on an agenda for change, together they become a very powerful lobby. A major advantage for primary care lies in its capacity as a local partner in providing services, and in its role commissioning those services outside of the health service.

There is also evidence that if recipients participate in the planning of interventions, they clinically improve as a result of this involvement (Rainford *et al.*, 1998). It helps them overcome the alienation caused by the belief that they have no control over decisions, a feeling of isolation, and a lack of trust in other participants. A sense of ownership converts unwilling, passive, individuals into active and co-operative allies.

Making these links explicit puts mental health promotion on to other agendas. It also assists in securing a commitment at senior levels to integrated development of sustainable action.

THE EVIDENCE

There is now enough evidence to support a greater role for health promotion in reducing the social and economic cost of mental illness and improving the health of the general population. Mental health promotion is most effective when interventions are built on social networks, when it intervenes at a crucial point in people's lives, and when it uses a combination of methods to strengthen the resilience of individuals and communities. The benefits are many, and include the following:

- improvements in physical health and productivity, enabling people to enjoy life and survive difficulties by increasing emotional flexibility;
- an enhancement of citizenship, through giving people the skills and opportunities to adopt meaningful and effective roles in society; and
- the alleviation of mental disorder.

High-quality pre-school education and support visits for new parents can improve mental health, just as the learning of decision-making and problem-solving skills can improve social and emotional functioning, as well as employment outcomes (NHS Centre for Reviews and Dissemination, 1997).

Physical and mental health are inter-related, and each can impact upon the other. For example, depression has been found to increase the risk of heart disease, and there is also an association between physical inactivity and depression. Increased physical activity can help to improve communication skills, social networks and participation, and increase the likelihood of an individual seeking help when needed (Burbach, 1997).

These are just a few of the complex determinants of mental health, all of which have an accumulative impact, as described in the Black Report (Townsend and Davidson, 1982). However, it is unclear how they influence the causative pathway for a particular condition, and it is difficult to unravel the way they interact with each other. Friedli (2000) proposes one way around this, which involves the use of the following independent indicators, to assess effectiveness to focus activity and aid evaluation:

- partnership;
- regeneration;
- community involvement;
- social inclusion; and
- reduction of inequalities.

Social inclusion can be viewed as a feeling of being involved in a range of mutually beneficial relationships within an opportunistic and enhancing environment. This provides a strong basis for activities of mental health promotion. Low levels of trust are key indicators of the mental health of a community (Wilkinson, 1996). Similarly, a recent study examined the relationship between psychosocial work characteristics and changes in health related to quality of life in 21,000 nurses (Cheng *et al.*, 2000). This found that adverse work conditions, such as low job control, high job demand and low social support at work, were associated with a deterioration in health as significant as those associated with smoking and sedentary lifestyle.

While social class is an indicator of mental health or illness, the many protective factors such as employment, housing and economic status no longer appear to mark the division between those who are likely to suffer and those who will not. The Health of England Survey showed that self-reported health status was directly correlated with some of the indicators proposed by Friedli (Rainford *et al.*, 1998). People felt more stressed if they lacked control over decisions, had little trust of neighbours, and experienced restricted community involvement.

Primary care organisations in Birmingham are already supporting generic health initiatives in association with community bodies, the voluntary sector and informal care. These include school-based projects, mental health awareness programmes, and schemes for urban regeneration. An exciting opportunity has arisen with the appointment of primary care mental health workers, whose role could include linking mental health teams and primary care with the communities they work in. This is most effective when any innovation meshes in with pre-existing activities, and local circumstances.

A STRATEGIC APPROACH IN PRIMARY CARE

This section introduces some practical experience and ideas about how mental health promotion might be carried out by staff from primary care. It emphasises the need for a strategic approach rather than one-off exercises, which tend to be of little value, and may indeed even be counterproductive.

Another emphasis is lateral thinking. Even well-funded highly publicised campaigns can be unsuccessful if the approach is not holistic. Anti-smoking campaigns have proved ineffective in schools when they have relied entirely on educative approaches, using traditional teaching practice. Approaching the same children on the agenda of the way that tobacco companies are exploiting them and developing countries, has been much more promising, probably because it appeals to a rebellious streak.

Organisation

Primary care organisations (PCOs) have now become the central focus for public health strategies. Their primary remit is to improve the health of the local population, including the mental health. This presents both opportunities and challenges.

The first concern is the fact that mental health promotion has often been neglected by the existing health promotion services. In the West Midlands, a small number of health promotion workers have volunteered to work in the field of mental health with little, or no, support. Without resources or encouragement, they have struggled to make progress. The emphasis on mental health promotion in Standard One of the NSF is welcome, but it is not enough to reverse the trend on its own. Because of a lack of expertise in the field, workers may neglect mental health promotion in the face of the practical day-to-day demands of mental illness services. Local support, enthusiasm, and resources need to be mobilised to ensure success.

A second hurdle is the fragmented nature of primary care and relations with other agencies. There is likely to be considerable variation in the ability of providers of primary care to respond to the expanded role outlined by the government. The annual national evaluation survey of PCOs revealed that over one-third had identified mental health as a priority for improving the health of the local population. While it was recognised that the onus of responsibility lay with developments outside primary care, there is little commitment to building partnerships with community groups or voluntary organisations (Rogers *et al.*, 2000).

Furthermore, PCOs are likely to be too small to sustain a mental health promotion structure on their own. In order to maximise the few resources available, it might be preferable for a number of them to band together. The health authority might have a role in co-ordinating this, and in some areas this has come under the aegis of Public Health. In Birmingham, the health improvement programme has provided such a focus. Once the initial difficulties have been overcome, the strengths of PCOs can come into play. General practice is based in the community, and is central to the health care of a particular neighbourhood.

This gives the primary care team unrivalled access to the majority of the population, and also to groups of vulnerable people. Because most people with mental health problems seek help from this source at some point, members of the primary care team have a good idea of the environmental factors (such as unemployment or poor housing) that operate to cause distress. This enables a local strategy to concentrate on local conditions.

It is important to identify a particular person to co-ordinate and lead developments. If resources allow, this person may be supported by a team, with members responsible for the specific settings (*see above*). Training and education make a significant contribution to successful mental health promotion, and allow the conceptual shift to be addressed. Specialist expertise in population health gain will help the team to understand how to translate the determinants of health into common policy initiatives, in order to focus action.

Some areas appear to have started out already on the road of appointing a single individual to carry out the huge range of possible tasks, but this can cause problems. Advertisements for officers attached to single PCOs have been seen, but this may lead to different strategies within a district with overlapping boundaries, the pursuing of different agendas, repetition of similar mistakes, or the unnecessary replication of work. Other services, such as health trusts, social service departments, voluntary organisations, education departments, housing and the police, cover larger areas, and ensuring effective liaison is likely to need a wider remit. In the West Midlands region, Birmingham has appointed one full-time officer and this post is likely to be enhanced by workers taking responsibility for specific settings, such as young people and the media. This covers an area served by seven PCOs. Elsewhere in the region (for example, in Dudley, South Staffordshire, South Warwickshire and Worcester), effective strategies have been developed by individual health promotion officers, often working in their own time.

Strategy

Mental health promotion is about co-ordinating and developing a network of organisations, individuals and resources. This is a time-consuming process, and requires specific skills in bringing together people with diverse languages (technical and cultural) and agendas. It can be carried out before the appointment of a specific officer; but requires a lot of energy. If it is done successfully, it allows for clear job descriptions to be drawn up, which satisfy the needs of the likely key participants. In the West Midlands, a group of professionals met at a regional level for some 12 years, to work on a range of projects, before a specific mental health promotion worker was appointed. There were a few successes, but it provided impossible to sustain a complete programme. More recently, the task of clarifying strategy has become the responsibility of a much smaller group, which reports to a wider body.

More pragmatically, identifying and forging a network of interested parties is likely to be one of the first tasks facing the responsible individual.

It is important to define a strategy early on, which is acceptable to all participants, and should incorporate the following:

- a common understanding of what mental health promotion is;
- a laying out of aims and principles;
- a recognition of good practice that is already in place (both local and elsewhere); and
- an identification of particular groups to involve, and of the responsibilities of those groups.

The strategy should make connections between the many relevant national and local policies, relating to issues as widely diverse as housing policy, public health reports, and the local authority community plan. The document will inevitably require modification regularly as experience is gained, and as more partners join. It should not be set in stone. The framework it provides should also allow for diversity in practice. In Birmingham, a number of staff working in mental health services have been keen to provide education on mental illness in schools. This enthusiasm needs to be encouraged and channelled, rather than dragooned into a stereotyped response conforming to some previously laid out plan. Support can be given by providing information about past evaluated projects, previously prepared materials and, where necessary, training.

One further role of the mental health promotion team is the collection of information. It is important to know who are the interested people in the area being served, and to gather evidence of research and practice locally, in other regions and in other countries. Where possible, when projects are carried out, they should be evaluated against similar work done elsewhere.

SOME PRACTICAL STEPS

Perhaps the main lesson from all of this is that mental health promotion work is less likely to be successful if it is carried out in isolation. Putting up educational posters in the surgery is valuable – when it is backed up by other work. On their own, the posters are likely to be ignored. A talk about schizophrenia to a group of teenagers may enhance stigma rather than reduce discrimination, unless it is part of a package of education on mental distress, which is directly relevant to the teenagers' own experience of bullying, and stressful relationships or examinations. A single letter to a local radio station complaining about jokes aimed at those with mental illness will be forgotten. A campaign of correspondence and telephone calls from distressed listeners can lead to the offending broadcaster being taken off the air, as happened in the West Midlands.

Primary care teams and PCOs are in an ideal position to put mental health promotion on the agenda of a number of different organisations. This can be taken forward in three ways:

1 By communicating what mental health promotion is;
2 By having a realistic understanding of what can be achieved; and
3 By demonstrating how it interdigitates with other practice.

The health professionals' role may be one of advocacy and building capacity for self-help groups to operate independently. Self-help groups have been found to influence a wide range of factors; they have succeeded in reducing isolation and have improved social functioning, both at the individual and the community level. The primary care team can also take responsibility for identifying factors affecting mental illness, such as poor housing, poor social networks and isolation, but are not necessarily responsible for providing adequate housing or for introducing neighbours to one another. Orley (1998) details how health promotion principles can be applied by using a 'pyramid-selling' method. For example, mothers with good skills can be used as trainers of others, either as volunteers or for some kind of reward.

Much depends on what is already in place. Primary care workers joining an already active campaign would normally be welcomed as invaluable allies. This would be the case particularly if they are able to demonstrate that they have taken active steps in their own place of work to reduce discrimination, and have instituted new practices to reduce distress.

Mental ill health frightens people – both those who suffer from it, and those who come into contact with it in any way. Ensuring that the staff in primary care teams are understanding, and have overcome their own misconceptions, is perhaps the first step that needs to be taken in general practice. Even when most staff are sympathetic, others may act in a prejudicial manner. The consequences of failing to address these issues may be unforeseen. Team members themselves may have had mental ill health, or may be caring for someone who suffers from it. Discovering that their expertise in this area is valued, because they are able to explain what it is like to others, can help them to become more confident and feel less isolated. They may even volunteer to take responsibility for carrying out further work.

Many people with minor degrees of mental distress do not want formal psychotherapy or tablets; they would like someone to talk to. Self-help groups aimed at particularly vulnerable groups can help to reduce the risk of problems worsening. Vulnerable people might include children whose parents have separated, single parents, carers of people with physical illness, and individuals facing retirement. This approach can be enhanced by ensuring that information about counselling services is available; these services cover all sorts of issues, from bereavement and marital difficulties to excessive alcohol intake. The evidence clearly demonstrates that mental disorder is related to poverty. One way of helping to tackle this is by gaining the services of an advisory body, such as the Citizens Advice Bureau, in the surgery premises.

'Healthy living centres' have taken all this a few steps further. The Bromley-By-Bow Centre, created out of a decaying church in the East End of London, is now the admired model around the world for community regeneration and partnership. The process began by building relationships, giving one young woman a key for the building as a demonstration of trust. The underused building was offered to the community and some artists living locally gave art lessons in exchange for free rent. Then came the nursery centre, the community café selling healthy food at a reasonable price, sport and recreation facilities and the Bengali Outreach Project. A centre of this kind is currently developing in Newtown, Birmingham, and is expected to incorporate similar projects.

CONCLUSION

We have attempted to outline what mental health promotion is, its effectiveness, and how it can be implemented, but this is not an exhaustive account of the subject. It is clearly biased towards an approach based on partnership and practicality. Changing environments can significantly influence mental health, and at a political level this is important. At the level of general practice it is more pragmatic to reinforce people's own skills, so that they can make changes in their own life. Sometimes, this leads to local communities improving their neighbourhoods for themselves, as a number of action groups have done in the UK. The sense of mastery and success is fundamentally important in raising the morale of individuals, enabling them to withstand the stresses and strains of life more successfully.

In developing a nationwide acceptance of mental health promotion, the UK is still well behind such countries as Australia, Canada and New Zealand, which have been active in the field for 10 to 12 years. We believe that primary care teams in the UK are well placed to be leading players in improving the mental health of the nation. Within the West Midlands region, action has been taken to create an infrastructure that will support the development of Standard One of the NSF. General practice is seen as a key area of development. The opportunities are there. Now, can PCOs carry the torch for mental health promotion?

> *This chapter analyses the term 'mental health promotion' in various contexts, and provides sound advice on how to incorporate it into practice. The authors share insights accumulated over many years and are vigorous in their commitment to mental health promotion. Merely responding to individuals when they present in ill health, as the NHS has been doing for many years, does not assist society to create living conditions and health services that allow people to realise their maximum potential. In terms of mental health promotion the authors believe that mental health professionals, in collaboration with other health-service providers, have much to contribute in the areas of housing, education, the media and law enforcement. Mental health professionals cannot only identify the problems, but also offer solutions. They recommend that those involved in mental health care should consider using some of their time and skills to work with social organisations that have a direct impact on people's lives. In addition to having sound interpersonal skills, health professionals need inter-organisational skills, to enable them to work in and between organisations other than their own. (Editors' summary)*

REFERENCES

Andrews, G. (1998) Editorial review: The burden of anxiety and depressive disorders, *Current Opinion in Psychiatry*, 11, 121–123

Antonovsky, A. (1996) The salutogenic model as a theory to guide health promotion, *Health Promotion International*, 11, 11–18

Araya, R. (1999) The Management of Depression in Primary Health Care, *Current Opinion in Psychiatry*, **12**, 103–107

Bosanquet, N. and Bosanquet, A. (1998) Economic perspectives. In Jenkins, R. and Ustun, T.B. (eds.) *Preventing Mental Illness: Mental health promotion in primary care*, John Wiley, Chichester, pp. 131–139

Burbach, F.R. (1997) The efficacy of physical activity interventions within mental heath services: anxiety and depressive disorders, *Journal of Mental Health*, **6**, 543–566

Caplan, G. (1961) *An Approach to Community Mental Health*, Grune and Stratton, New York

Cheng, Y., Kawachi, I., Eugenie, H.C., Schwartz, J. and Colditz, G. (2000) Association between psychosocial work characteristics and health functioning in American women: prospective study, *British Medical Journal*, **320**, 1432–1436

Cronin, A.J. (1937) *The Citadel*, Victor Gollancz, London

Department of Health (1996) *Saving Lives: Our Healthier Nation*, The Stationery Office, London

Department of Health (1997) *The New NHS – Modern and Dependable*, The Stationery Office, London

Department of Health (1999) *National Service Framework for Mental Health*, Department of Health, London

Friedli, L. (2000) Mental health promotion: rethinking the evidence base, *The Mental Health Review*, **5**, 15–18

Goldberg, D. and Huxley, P. (1980) *Mental Illness in the Community: The pathway to psychiatric care*, Tavistock, London

Gordon, R.S. (1987) An operational classification of disease prevention. In Steinberg, J.A. and Silverman, M.M. (eds.) *Preventing Mental Disorders: A Research Perspective*, NIMH, Rockville, MD, pp. 20–26

Health Education Unit (1999) *Safe, Sorted but Sad?* Evaluation report on the second John Beasley Mental Health Promotion Day, supported by social services, Birmingham, 8 October 1999, Birmingham Health Education Unit

Jenkins, R. (1985) Minor psychiatric morbidity in employed young men and women, and its contribution to sickness absence, *British Journal of Industrial Medicine*, **42**, 147–154

Kramer, T. and Garralda, M.E. (1998) Psychiatric disorders in adolescents in primary care, *British Journal of Psychiatry*, 173, 508–513

MacDonald, G. and O'Hara, K. (1996) *Position Paper on Mental Health Promotion*, Society of Health Education and Promotion Specialists, London

NHS Centre for Reviews and Dissemination (1997) Mental Health promotion in high-risk groups *Effective Health Care 3*, 3, unpaged

Orley, J. (1998) Application of Promotion Principles. In Jenkins, R. and Bedirhan Ustun, T. (eds.) (1998) *Preventing Mental Illness: Mental health promotion in primary care*, John Wiley, Chichester

Pickering, G.W. (1968) *High Blood Pressure*, Churchill Livingstone, Edinburgh

Rainford, L., Mayson, V., Hickman, M. and Morgan, A. (1998) *Health in England*, The Stationery Office, London

Rogers, A., Gask, L. and Leese, B. (2000) Mental health: in the frame, *Health Service Journal*, 16 March, p. 30

Rose, G.W. (1989) The mental health of populations. In Cooper, B. and Eastwood, R. (eds.) *Primary Care and Psychiatric Epidemiology*, Routledge, London, pp. 77–85

Rose, G.W. (1993) Preventative strategy and general practice, *British Journal of General Practice*, **43**, 138–139

Townsend, P. and Davidson, N. (1982) *Inequalities in Health* [The Black Report], Penguin, Harmondsworth

Wittchen, H.-U., Stein, H.B. and Kessler, R.C. (1999) Social fears and social phobia in a community sample of adolescents and young adults: prevalence, risk factors and co-morbidity, *Psychological Medicine*, **29**, 309–323

World Health Organisation (WHO) (1986) *Ottawa Charter for Health Promotion*, First International Conference on Health Promotion, 17–21 November, Ottawa, Canada

Wilkinson, R.G. (1996) *Unhealthy Societies: Afflictions of inequality*, Routledge, London

16 WHAT HAVE WE LEARNED AND WHERE DO WE GO FROM HERE?

Frances Badger and Peter Nolan

BACKGROUND

Since its inception, the NHS has not been noted for communicating openly and clearly with the public about health issues, nor has it been particularly adept at involving service users in decision-making. It has appeared to presume that the support of medical advances is preferable to identifying and addressing the needs of local communities. Fifty years ago, the NHS aimed to take the worry out of paying for health care, and to fund itself through national insurance and taxes. Today, it costs about £40 billion annually, or nearly £1,000 per person every year. In 1942, William Beveridge wrote that improving the health of the nation involved much more than merely providing for the sick and infirm. He argued that services had to collaborate in order to fight what he referred to as the scourge of the 'five giants of poor health' – illness, ignorance, disease, squalor and want. Many who suffer from severe and enduring mental health problems, unemployment, poor education and hopelessness will readily recognise the social and psychological entrapments created by these 'giants'.

Collaboration and co-ordinated service planning and delivery of services are particularly important for users with mental health problems, who may require a broad range of professional and lay carers to address their needs. Complex problems need multiple solutions and collaboration is the underpinning driver that brings the conditions about where such complex problems can be dealt with and relieved.

Various drivers for change have existed in the past. Smith (1992) now finds the principal one to be the gap – which is widening – between what medicine could do given unlimited resources, and what can be afforded. More and more people are coming to realise that health is not necessarily the product of health services and that contact with health services may have only a modest impact on their health-related problems and their quality of life. Despite continuous innovations in medical technology and the ever-increasing demands for more and better health services, researchers are increasingly of the opinion that much of what health professionals do is based on the shakiest scientific evidence, and is of limited value only. Harvey and Wylie (1999) argue that, for services to become more effective, users must be informed, and encouraged to contribute to the design of services for local people. Having an informed and demanding public is a powerful lever for change and for bringing about better services. They point out that when people in the UK become ill, they know very little about what is available or what to expect.

Many take the health services for granted and assume that, because these services are provided by the state, they will automatically get the best if they become ill.

Collaborative service provision and work across agencies have long been recognised as prerequisites for the delivery of quality health services to users and carers. Few would disagree that they contribute to the effective use of scarce resources. The concept of partnership occupies a central place in New Labour's approach to a range of key policy areas, such as health, education, employment, crime and disorder and social inclusion. These are defined as 'cross-cutting issues', which means that they cannot be tackled by agencies operating autonomously; there is now a requirement for statutory and voluntary organisations and communities to work together to produce joined-up solutions for local problems (Charlesworth, 2001). However, partnership working is not necessarily easily or quickly implemented, no matter how urgently government policies require it. Almost three decades ago, a DHSS and Welsh Office Working Party examined collaboration between the reorganised NHS and local government. It had already been acknowledged that health services could not be developed or operated in isolation, and that they depended upon 'the humane planning and provision of a range of closely related services which [were] the responsibility of local government' (DHSS/Welsh Office, 1973). The Working Party report also affirmed that collaboration between health and social services must be firmly established to enable local communities to receive maximum benefit from the alliance.

However, the desired collaboration presupposes that the NHS is a cohesive entity, along with social services and the voluntary sector, with the constituent parts fully aware of the roles and functions, strengths and weaknesses of other parts of the organisation. Although different groups within different organisations may share the overarching aim of assisting people in need, there may be many subsidiary agendas directing how this might be achieved. The experiences of users, carers and service providers, and research, all suggest that the aspirations for collaboration between health and social services expressed in the 1973 report have been realised only in part. In the 1980s, policy dictated that competition would drive efficient and effective health and social services. Major restructuring of primary care health services, and, to a lesser extent, of social services, took the focus away from partnerships and joint working. The wheel has now come full circle and partnerships are once again seen as the solution to the delivery of health services.

It is often assumed that health-care providers share a common understanding of goals, agendas, roles and the definition of partnership. Given the location and structure of health services, Jefferys (1995) suggests that it is not surprising that teams and teamwork have generally been noticeable by their absence. Teamwork within primary health care starts from a more complex base than that found in local authorities, the NHS hospital sector or the private health care sector, where the majority of staff are employed by one organisation. GPs are not directly employed by the NHS, nor are they salaried employees; instead, they are contracted by health authorities. Within the same primary care team, there may be staff employed by NHS Trusts (health visitors, CMHNs, district nurses); some employed by the practice (reception staff, practice manager, nurses, salaried GPs); self-employed practitioners with a controlling interest in the practice (GPs); as well as self-employed practitioners who may rent rooms at the practice (chiropodists, counsellors, alternative practitioners). The construction of a team from such diverse disciplines is a challenge in itself, while the added complexities of employment contracts, professional codes of conduct, lines of management and pay scales all act as further confounding factors. Outside organisations that expect to collaborate with primary care 'teams' may find, as Ashburner (Chapter 3) amply illustrates, that there is confusion about who or what constitutes the team, and, indeed, whether there is a team at all. This is compounded where a group has different titles as in the case of CPNs and CMHNs. Some chapters make reference to both and in doing so may be referring to different groups or the same group.

Noting that the quality of services for people with complex needs, such as older adults and the mentally ill, had often been sacrificed to 'sterile arguments about boundaries', *Partnership in Action* (Department of Health, 1999a) focuses upon joint working at three levels:

1 *Strategic planning* – inter-agency planning for the medium term; sharing information about resources towards the achievement of common goals;
2 *Service commissioning* – agencies having a common understanding and a shared view of the needs of the community they are jointly meeting;
3 *Service provision* – regardless of how services are purchased or funded, the user must receive a coherent package of care.

This book is primarily about collaboration and partnership at the level of service provision, and aims to illustrate some of the ways in which seamless services can be provided, so that users and families do not have to 'navigate a labyrinthine bureaucracy' of services (Department of Health, 1999a). Under any circumstances, dealing with agencies or organisations with unclear structures can be a frustrating and time-consuming experience. And it must be even more exhausting for users with psychological and social debilities and their carers. *Partnership in Action* (Department of Health, 1999a) advocates innovative, interdisciplinary working, in order to:

• improve services for users and carers;
• avoid wasteful duplication and gaps in services;
• ensure public funds are used more efficiently and effectively.

While setting out frameworks for collaboration and identifying funding measures to support more flexibility, *Partnership in Action* (Department of Health, 1999a) recognised that there was no single, simple answer to partnership working between agencies and that solutions were not necessarily dependent upon structural changes.

Spurgeon and Field (Chapter 2) make it clear that there are sound reasons, now enshrined in national policy, for offering people with mental health needs the whole range of services they need within primary care. After all, the divide between emotional and physical wellbeing is artificial; physical health problems trigger emotional problems. People with severe mental illnesses are known to neglect their physical health, and this could be better addressed if they were in closer contact with primary care.

The *National Service Frameworks for Mental Health and Older People* (Department of Health 1999b, 2001), along with the *NHS Plan* (Department of Health, 2000) have clearly endorsed a variety of collaborations. Many ideas for promoting greater collaboration between the range of health-care organisations involved in the care of people with mental health problems have been put forward. These include shared pre- and post-registration courses; locating practitioners at the same base; liaison schemes; and CMHN attachment to primary care. The fact that health and social services personnel are beginning to share learning and educational programmes can only be regarded as a promising way forward as a means of breaking down professional and cultural barriers. Limitations of time and resources, the requirements of professional bodies, and widespread reluctance to make changes to existing professional training have resulted in initiatives being small in scale.

There *are* examples of current collaborative working in primary mental health care, but many of the partnerships are little more than 'fragile alliances'. Where they show signs of success, they must be supported and sustained to grow into true collaborations.

While 'interprofessionalism' or 'multidisciplinary working' are often seen as pre-requisites to improved health and social care across a range of settings, such approaches exclude many staff who do not possess professional qualifications. More importantly, they exclude users, carers and the voluntary sector. This book has accepted a broader definition of multidisciplinary collaboration because there is a growing realisation that collaboration is not solely about what providers can offer to users, and to each other. It is also about what users can offer, in terms of input into their own care, and into service planning and evaluation. Harvey (Chapter 4) speaks from a user perspective of the positive gains to be made from being able to offer something in return. The literature has repeatedly suggested that improving the health of the population is beyond the scope of professional bodies, especially those dominated by doctors (Gillam *et al.*, 2001). The King's Fund (Pratt *et al.*, 1998) found that lay members of Trusts and Primary Care Groups made a significant contri-bution to decisions about the types of services to be commissioned and also influ-enced the way in which decisions were made. Lay members forced other board members to revise their views on the benefits of lay participation. In time, they should be able to bring about wider public involvement in the planning and delivery of primary care services, provided that professionals can work collaboratively not only with each other, but also with service users and members of local communities.

All initiatives in collaboration are constrained by lack of resources, training and service accommodation. There are new monies available, but resources alone will not bring about the desired result. Personnel will need motivation, vision, a willingness to listen and share with each other, and above all a belief that services can actually be improved for service users and their carers. Attempts at collaboration require a robust determination. Success is not guaranteed and, sometimes, initiatives are unsuccessful.

EXTENDING COLLABORATION BEYOND THE HEALTH SERVICES – VOLUNTARY ORGANISATIONS AND USERS

Harvey's plea (Chapter 4) for service providers to utilise the voluntary sector, not only for what it can provide, but also for the opportunities it offers to users to reciprocate, is in keeping with government aspirations to harness the resources of this sector in a more systematic way (Department of Health 1999b). Yet the voluntary sector continues to be almost invisible to many service providers, or regarded as amateurish and as having few resources. While the voluntary sector is sometimes poorly funded (although this is not always the case), the information, support and insights it can offer have proved invaluable to many who have accessed it. Secondary health services have traditionally been reluctant to work with the voluntary sector, but this is not the case with primary care. Many GPs are seeing the benefits of working closely with voluntary organisations (Peters and Chaitow, 2001). When the Teaching Primary Care Trusts (TPCTs) are established – and it is anticipated that there will be 25 to 30 by April 2003 (Jackson, 2001) – they will bring together a wide range of health-care professionals, as well as complementary therapists, representatives of community organisations and voluntary organisations.

The National Service Frameworks for Mental Health and Older People (Department of Health, 1999b, 2001) suggest that the gains of working with the voluntary sector have yet to be realised. A national tracker survey of PCG/Ts (National Primary Care Research and Development Centre, 2001) reported that efforts have been made to involve key stakeholders, yet local communities and voluntary organisations are still under-represented. This is worrying when consideration is given to the fact that, as PCG/Ts increase in size and complexity, their capacity to be responsive to local needs may well be impaired rather than enhanced. Reconfiguring primary health care at the proposed speed also raises the possibility that some existing partnerships may be broken, while others may not have time to get started. It has been reported (National Primary Care Research and Development Centre, 2001) that three-quarters of PCG/Ts are developing integrated nursing teams, but only one-third are developing shared management for practice and community nurses. Only 12% of PCG/Ts say that they are working with no other local authority department apart from social services, but one PCG works with nine local authority departments. It remains to be seen whether the fully functional PCTs will impact on the number, structure and range of collaborations within primary care. PCG/T mergers necessitate major organisational and management change and may divert attention from their core function of developing services and improving health.

Dramatic changes have occurred over the years in the perception of the role of the 'patient', the 'client' and the 'user' in service delivery. From the silent and compliant 'patient', who did what the doctor told him or her, via the well-informed 'client' making decisions about his or her own care, there is a growing acceptance that 'users' are experts, both in their experiences of health and social services and in living with their illness. It is important to remember that, from the user's perspective, there are no distinctions between health, social services and the voluntary sector, or between qualified and unqualified staff. Expert care is expected from all. Users assume, not unreasonably, that service providers share information among themselves. A confusing array of service providers conducting similar assessments and requiring similar information therefore creates anxiety, irritation and bewilderment (Evers *et al.*, 1994).

User and public involvement should be systematically built into health services, with special attention given to involving rarely represented groups and communities. Service users should be invited to teach on basic training programmes, and to contribute to curriculum design and assessment of communication skills (Department of Health, 1999b).

DRIVING FORCES

The examples of collaboration given here were largely the result of individual efforts, and, with the exception of the child and adolescent mental health service cited in Chapter 10, were not underpinned to any degree by local structures or policy. Most were not the result of management-driven initiatives. Management that rarely meets with colleagues on the front line cannot assist collaboration. Social work teams within locality mental health teams who were drawn into collaboration were listened to and supported by managers they knew. Practitioners achieved greater job satisfaction, and enjoyed extending their roles and working with supportive colleagues (Chapters 6, 9, 13). Community mental health nurses for older people started working with primary care when they realised that some referrals were inappropriate, because local GPs were not fully aware of the nurses' service remit (Chapter 14). Outcomes of this collaboration have included improved understanding of the roles of CMHNs among primary care staff, better utilisation of telephone consultations with GPs, and, overall, a more responsive service for users. Other examples of collaboration (Chapters 5, 6, 7, 12) were driven by the conviction that people with serious mental illness were not being cared for holistically. Their physical and mental health needs were being addressed separately, and the former were often overlooked. Further chapters (including Chapter 13) show how lack of resources can sometimes be the driving force for collaboration between different services.

These drivers to collaboration are in line with the findings of the King's Fund (Pratt *et al.*, 1998), that solutions to problems of service delivery arise when people with different perspectives come together to work for a common cause. They are not necessarily dependent on external guidance, skills or money (Pratt *et al.*, 1998). This does not mean that best-practice lessons cannot be learned, but that the driving force for change is internal and locally specific. All of the practice-based chapters in this book feature 'ordinary' committed practitioners who decided to design and drive forward initiatives. Successful collaboration occurred when practitioners were not only able to identify problems, but also allowed the freedom and given the support to explore solutions.

COLLABORATION – A 'WIN–WIN' PROCESS?

Collaboration is the art of the possible. Efforts may not be perfect, or initiatives completed straight away, but skilled and committed service providers working within ordinary settings can achieve more together than on their own. To quote Harvey (Chapter 4), 'those who can measure up to the challenge have everything to gain and nothing to lose'.

Collaboration in primary mental health care has often been presumed to mean secondary services devolving their skills to primary practitioners. However, secondary mental health professionals may have insufficient understanding of the culture of primary care to enable them to work with personnel who are eagerly seeking a model of primary mental health care. As with all mergers and attempts at integration, there will be perceived winners and losers. The danger is that some groups may feel that they have been overlooked, not involved enough, or even deliberately left out, and this can lead to disenchantment, a feeling of being devalued and burn-out. To avoid this, a number of questions need to be asked.

- What are the limits to the capacity of primary care to deliver more services?
- Might expansion of services impede collaboration, because there are potentially more people and agencies with whom to collaborate?
- What are the gains of collaboration for secondary services? What can they learn from primary care?
- Overall, how can a 'win–win' situation be achieved? (Pratt *et al.*, 1998)

Success is dependent on appropriate development of the constituent parts without any damage to the environment of care. Arcelus *et al.* (Chapter 10) give a comprehensive account of the new role of the primary mental health worker and the gains for clients and for primary care. Secondary services' gain is an opportunity to focus their resources on users with major needs.

PRIORITISING MENTAL HEALTH

While almost 80% of PCG/Ts identify coronary heart disease as a priority, only 24% identify mental health in the same way (National Primary Care Research and Development Centre, 2001), despite the fact that the *National Service Framework for Mental Health* was the first to be published (Department of Health, 1999b). Much PCG activity has been about primary care practices sharing resources; little thought has been given to how primary and secondary services might collaborate and make better use of their combined resources. It may be the case that GPs are less familiar with the objectives of the NSF for Mental Health, than with the objectives of other NSFs. The NSF for Mental Health may appear somewhat utopian in its aspirations and perhaps threatening to primary care personnel. Other NSFs might be interpreted as being more measured in their presentation, and in their identification of specific markers to indicate that certain objectives have been achieved.

The challenge is for specialist mental health teams to find ways of working with primary care that ensure that clients with multiple and severe mental health problems do not lose out to those whose needs are perceived as less demanding, and who will recover faster. Where mental health services are located in primary care, there seems to be a tendency to focus on the largest presenting group, which comprises people with neurotic disorders (Burns and Bale, 1997). It is very difficult for mental health workers in primary care to manage clients with complex, enduring problems in 10 minutes and without the assistance of appropriately skilled personnel (Gask and Croft, 2000). Health-care personnel need time to develop relationships and carry out assessments, especially when clients have multiple problems, which need to be addressed sequentially rather than simultaneously. Rationing time with certain client groups has to be resisted, as it results over time in inevitable deterioration, increased suffering and more expense.

FRAMEWORKS FOR COLLABORATION

The need for collaboration is implicit in Standard Two of the *National Service Framework for Mental Health* (Department of Health, 1999b), as it is in the other six, but collaboration should not become ritualistic. It should be a carefully considered option, tailored to each user's needs. The user has a right to the best care available; this is enshrined within the Human Rights Act and the user should have a say in the nature and extent of the collaboration with other services. Practitioners' duty of care and professional responsibility demand that consideration is given to users' needs; this may not fall immediately within their own professional remit. Collaborative care should be considered when it is the most effective way to use resources.

Tensions and difficulties

There are acknowledged tensions in the world of primary mental health care. Primary care practitioners see large numbers of people with common mental health problems, and much smaller numbers of people with severe and enduring mental illnesses (SEMI). For primary care, the service priority has been the former group. Whereas secondary mental health services have always dealt with specific diagnostic categories, or people with complex problems, primary care has tended to deal with people with non-specific problems or problems that are sub-clinical. Suggestions of liaisons with secondary care may bring concerns that primary care is 'expected' to care for people with SEMI. Conversely, secondary care practitioners may fear that partnerships with primary care may lead to a diversion of their skills and expertise to the care of those who are perceived to have less severe and less enduring mental health problems. These fears can be dispelled, and collaborations can bring about gains for all practitioners whether they regard themselves as primary or secondary practitioners.

Practitioners have varied experiences of collaboration, and the uncertainties illustrated in Ashburner's Chapter 3 are evident to some degree in all. In some situations, collaboration may not be possible (Chapter 10), while partnerships with primary care are sometimes problematic (Chapter 5).

Factors that promote effective collaboration

Accounts of collaboration in the previous chapters reveal recurrent themes that assist in the identification of key factors. This can aid the development of a framework for collaboration within the context of primary mental health care.

The factors that promote effective collaboration can be classified into the following main themes:

- Foundations for collaboration;
- Essential elements of collaboration;
- Modes of collaboration;
- Outcomes of collaboration.

The various components of the themes that emerged from the chapters are listed below.

Foundations for collaboration

- Practitioners need to be committed to collaboration, and to believe that it is possible and an essential component of primary mental health care.
- It is important to realise that one discipline is unlikely to be able to deliver comprehensive care without the support or involvement of others, particularly in the case of someone with SEMI.
- Care for people with mental health problems can be improved if practitioners are realistic in assessing the amount and type of care they are able to provide, and well informed about the resources of colleagues, other statutory agencies and the voluntary sector.
- An awareness of private-sector resources may also prove to be increasingly important in the changing climate of health-care provision. These may be unknown to many NHS staff.
- Commitment to collaboration is essential. Practitioners had a strong belief that only by harnessing the skills of colleagues and other agencies could comprehensive care be delivered.
- Collaboration can be undertaken by individual practitioners, but gaining team commitment and support (or at least that of peers) is preferable. Sharing ideas about collaboration may reveal that special expertise and a sympathetic outlook are close at hand.
- Although collaboration between all those involved in mental health services is enshrined within government policy, the examples in the chapters did not appear to result directly from policy, nor from management directives, but were initiated by practitioners as a result of their own assessments of users' needs in relation to the services provided.
- Any team has a point at which, if it is overburdened, it collapses, and individuals resort to working independently.
- It is noticeable that little reference was made in the chapters to the need for education and training as a requirement for collaborative working.
- Practitioners need to be open to what other individuals and organisations can offer.

Essential elements of collaboration

- It is important that all practitioners within a team or group are involved in and supportive of collaboration. If this is not the case, and if the principal 'change agents' leave, collaboration may flounder, resulting in lost benefits; users, carers and practitioners may suffer as a result.
- Collaboration needs to be embedded within the culture of the respective organisations, extending to social events and educational activities, for example, and offering an openness to others.
- Collaboration is initiated by approaching others who might be open to partnership working.
- Attempts to engage the unwilling or the unenthusiastic as partners in collaboration offer few returns.
- Like all relationships, a collaborative relationship takes time to develop and for the full benefits to emerge. Indeed, much time can be spent endeavouring to collaborate with people who prove unhelpful. Initiating collaboration between practitioners of different disciplines is almost inevitably a slow process, particularly if there is a perceived difference in status and ideology.
- Collaboration involves recognising the limits to one's own practice. Collaboration is not an attempt to cover up for lack of professional knowledge or skills. However, fears that it may be interpreted as such by other practitioners can prevent it happening.

Modes of collaboration

- There are many different modes of collaboration in practice, and all may have the potential to be equally effective in producing positive gains for users and carers in the specific contexts in which they operate.
- Successful models are those that emerge as a result of the individuals involved, rather than those imposed as a result of policy initiatives.
- Patterns of collaboration are dependent upon a variety of factors, including the historical legacy of service configurations and resources, whether collaboration is built upon existing networks or developed as a result of new contacts, and the disciplines and individuals involved.
- Some practitioners collaborated and sustained collaboration by means of face-to-face contact; some encouraged users themselves to contact other organisations and did not necessarily know the outcomes of these contacts.
- Some practitioners collaborated with a few organisations or practitioners, while other practitioners collaborated with many. It is not clear whether multiple collaborations result in better outcomes for users, carers and practitioners.
- It is not certain whether practitioners collaborated with others whom they already knew, or with those they identified as best able to provide services for their clients. Some may have collaborated with professionals or agencies with which their organisation had a contract and not necessarily with those whom the individual health-care worker would have selected.
- There are many different points along the collaborative pathway. Some social services and nursing staff in community mental health teams had initially

embarked upon collaboration, but subsequently extended their roles to encompass what some might regard as the roles of other disciplines. This meant that vulnerable clients only had to establish a relationship with one practitioner.

Outcomes of collaboration

- Effective collaboration needs constant vigilance and must have progressed beyond being merely a 'fragile alliance'.
- The success of collaborative initiatives is not guaranteed. Constraints of time, difficulties in communication, resistance to partnership, or lack of personnel with whom to collaborate may mean that collaboration cannot take place.
- Collaboration is sustained by positive results and constructive feedback from collaborators. Some practitioners employed existing data to produce outcome measures to gauge the success of collaborations (such as users' attendance rates for primary care appointments).
- Apart from the example above, there is relatively little reference to the evaluation of the quality and outcomes of collaborations using a more empirical approach, and some authors acknowledge that there is much work to be addressed in this area. It is vital that outcome measures incorporate users' and carers' perspectives.
- Mental health is an area where the voluntary sector is vitally important, both for its range of services and expertise, and for the opportunity it provides for clients to gain support from people who have had similar experiences. Working in the voluntary sector gives users the opportunity to 'put something back' and may be an initial step towards returning to the workplace.
- Some secondary practitioners are concerned that closer contact with primary care may lead to their specialist skills not being available to people with serious or enduring mental illnesses, being diverted instead to those with more transient or less severe mental illnesses. As Chapter 7 demonstrates, this need not be the case and primary care is able to support people with SEMI.
- In some cases, expectations of what can be achieved through collaboration have been exceeded in terms of positive outcomes for users, a stronger and broader knowledge base for practitioners, and better understanding of the work of other practitioners.
- Collaboration with users, other than in their own care, appears to be limited. Also, little reference was made to the utilisation of ex-service users as potential collaborators. This may be because it is not high on the agenda of service providers. Additionally, users who recover from a mental illness may not wish to be identified by joining the user movement.

Taking the factors that have been derived from the chapters we now wish to suggest a model that encompasses the main components of productive collaboration. The factors that support collaboration in practice can be summarised under six main headings:

People-centred components

1 Service user focus;
2 Individual characteristics;
3 Professional competencies;

Organisation-centred components

4 Organisational climate;
5 Training and education;
6 Policy context.

These six areas and their constituent parts are summarised in Figure 16.1.

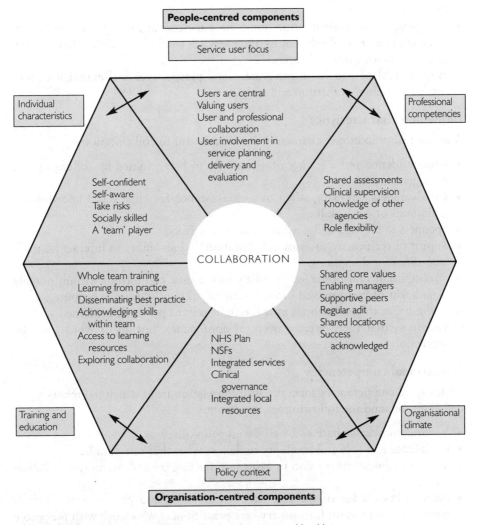

People-centred components

Service user focus

Individual characteristics

Professional competencies

Users are central
Valuing users
User and professional
   collaboration
User involvement in
   service planning,
   delivery and
   evaluation

Self-confident
Self-aware
Take risks
Socially skilled
A 'team' player

Shared assessments
Clinical supervision
Knowledge of other
   agencies
Role flexibility

COLLABORATION

Whole team training
Learning from practice
Disseminating best practice
Acknowledging skills
   within team
Access to learning
   resources
Exploring collaboration

NHS Plan
NSFs
Integrated services
Clinical
   governance
Integrated local
   resources

Shared core values
Enabling managers
Supportive peers
Regular adit
Shared locations
Success
   acknowledged

Training and education

Organisational climate

Policy context

Organisation-centred components

Figure 16.1 Components of collaboration in primary mental health care

Service user focus

- Users must be central to service provision and to the aims of collaboration. Each team should establish how this should be achieved.
- Users should be supported in establishing their own network of services. This may mean that service providers will have little knowledge of the involvement of other agencies, their assessments and their interventions, other than information that the user wishes to impart. The question of who should be the co-ordinating contact may need to be revisited as users' mental health and self-care abilities improve, and they are able to take increased responsibility for co-ordinating their own care. Service providers may find themselves in a supportive rather than a collaborative role as users undertake the role of key worker themselves.
- The benefits of collaboration must be balanced against the possibility of fragmented care. Will referrals to other services result in multiple, often similar, assessments for users and carers?
- Ways should be sought to integrate users' perspectives and experiences into service planning, evaluation and audit.

Individual characteristics

A number of practitioner characteristics are relevant to collaboration:

- self-confidence and a feeling of self-worth, of being valued by colleagues and management;
- self-awareness, knowing when to seek assistance for clients and knowing the limitations of one's skills;
- openness to change, and a willingness to take risks;
- a spirit of reciprocity to assist collaboration and an ability to interact honestly with different disciplines;
- a recognition that obstacles to collaboration may come from within, notably from a fear of being judged incompetent for seeking additional support;
- a firm belief that collaboration is the right way to proceed, combined with an awareness that there are a variety of approaches, not all of which may be successful.

Professional competencies

Professional competencies form the firm foundation from which to embark upon collaboration, and the following are important:

- a sound knowledge base and well-developed skills;
- confidence in a role and an ability to deliver what that role entails;
- access to clinical supervision to assist in reflecting on and promoting collaboration;
- detailed knowledge of the role of other agencies and professionals. This is particularly important for primary care practitioners who work with the whole range of physical, emotional and mental health problems. Users do not attend

primary care with their health needs compartmentalised and practitioners with a good knowledge of mental as well as physical health can offer a better service;
- role flexibility; willingness to accept agreed permeable professional boundaries if this improves services;
- willingness to share user assessments to avoid duplication of effort for both users and service providers;
- knowledge of local services, agencies, voluntary and self-help groups and of experts in other organisations.

Organisational climate

Individual service providers are enabled to collaborate when there is a supportive organisational climate. Collaboration may not be management-driven, but sympathetic management policy, attitudes and structures create an environment in which collaboration can flourish. In addition, organisations are supportive when:

- there are shared core values within teams;
- professional roles are extended as a result of team and peer debates about what is appropriate;
- services and the effectiveness of collaboration are looked at regularly, through formal audit, peer review, clinical supervision or reflective practice. Audit must take into account both users' and carers' evaluations;
- there is joint record-keeping;
- shared locations promote partnerships by facilitating informal contact between practitioners;
- individuals are permitted to take risks;
- there is an absence of 'blame culture' and 'finger-pointing';
- they create an atmosphere that is supportive and rewarding.

Training and education

Training and education are necessary to maximise practitioners' collaborative skills. Learning should be achieved through:

- whole team training for all staff who have contact with users, including reception staff;
- multidisciplinary, work-based learning, which supports partnership formation and networking;
- learning from examples of collaborative practice in primary mental health care;
- dissemination of best practice, both locally at PCG/T level, and nationally;
- access to resources at work (libraries, journals and the Internet);
- the establishment of an open-minded, enquiring environment, where individuals are able to share their knowledge and experience, and where they feel that they are being listened to.

Policy context

This context includes:

- the NHS Plan (Department of Health, 2000), which describes the post of primary mental health worker (PMHW), to be introduced in 2002. While this new post is welcome, its remit will need to be clearly stated to assist the process of collaboration;

- the National Service Frameworks for Mental Health and Older People (Department of Health, 1999b, 2001);
- clinical governance;
- integrated services;
- the role of PCG/Ts in promoting the mental health agenda. Working with user groups, PCG/Ts should seek to identify local examples of effective collaboration within mental health services and use them to promote best practice. Areas in which collaborative practice has either not been attempted, or not been successful, can then be examined in the context of local knowledge and resources. Providing a forum for networking and identification of local mental health resources are equally important functions of PCG/Ts.

THE CONTINUING AGENDA

A number of collaboration-related issues require further work. Practitioners may reflect intelligently on the outcomes of their collaborations, but there is also a need for more systematic evaluation. Findings can then be fed into training, education, and workforce planning. Informative evaluations and outcome measures are necessary, so that both successful and failed partnerships can be analysed, and the results incorporated into future service planning. Continuing audits of collaborations must integrate users', carers' and practitioners' perspectives and there is an urgent need to develop meaningful outcome measures.

CONCLUSION

Collaboration can be seen as a response to rationing and is often referred to as a means of resource management. It aims to improve services by maximising existing resources of personnel and expertise. It can be outstandingly successful in providing enhanced services, but it may also fail – as a result of changes of staff, resistant attitudes, disagreement about roles, lack of enthusiasm, or displacement by other pressing agendas or new initiatives, and the financial resources that accompany these. The outdated management system of control and command is not appropriate for the modern organisation. Systems that promote teambuilding, consensus working, open-mindedness and goal achievement are more likely to promote collaboration and partnership working.

Currently, there are many examples of fruitful collaboration within mental health care, initiated by social workers, nurses, consultant psychiatrists and community mental health nurses, among others. Collaborations tend not to be driven by management directives or policy statements. They are more likely to be the result of service providers identifying ways in which services could meet people's needs more sensitively, in a less stigmatising way, and closer to home. The role of management in the collaborative process is as enabler and facilitator. Practitioners must feel that their input is valued and that mutual respect is a core value of their organisation.

All collaborations require constant review and new partnerships need to be developed all the time. The time and skills invested in collaboration must show an ample return in terms of benefits to users, carers and practitioners. 'Standard' models of collaboration are probably unworkable because they fail to take into account existing cultures, structures and service configurations, as well as different population needs.

This book demonstrates the extent and quality of practitioner skills and resources in mental health services. Practitioners should be given credit for what has been achieved so far. Perhaps policy-makers should consider whether it is now appropriate to allow a respite from further new policies, to allow existing policies to become embedded in day-to-day practice. Perhaps the time has come to call a halt to policy-driven change in mental health services and to allow best practices in collaboration to be disseminated and adapted by innovative practitioners, who are able to respond to local circumstances and local need. If the only constant is change, how will we know what works in the long term?

REFERENCES

Burns, T. and Bale, R. (1997) Establishing a mental health liaison attachment with primary care, *Advances in Psychiatric Treatment*, 3, 2219–2224

Charlesworth, J. (2001) Negotiating and managing partnership in primary care, *Health and Social Care in the Community*, 9(5), 279–285

Department of Health (1999a) *Partnership in Action: New opportunities for joint working between health and social services*, The Stationery Office, London

Department of Health (1999b) *National Service Framework for Mental Health*, Department of Health, London

Department of Health (1999c) *Patient and Public Involvement in the New NHS*, Department of Health, London

Department of Health (2001) *National Service Framework for Older People*, Department of Health, London

Department of Health (2000) *The NHS Plan*, The Stationery Office, London

DHSS/Welsh Office (1973) *Working Party Report on Collaboration Between the NHS and Local Government on its Activities to the End of 1972*, HMSO, London

Evers, H., Badger, F. and Cameron, E. (1994) Inter-professional work with old and disabled people. In Leathard, A. (ed.) *Going Inter-professional: Working together for health and welfare*, Routledge, London

Gask, L. and Croft, J. (2000) Methods of working with primary care, *Advances in Psychiatric Treatment*, 6, 442–449

Gillam, S., Abbott, S. and Banks-Smith, J. (2001) Can primary care groups and trusts improve health? *British Medical Journal*, 323, 89–92

Harvey, S. and Wylie, I. (1999) *Patient power – Getting the Best From Your Health Care*, Simon and Schuster, London

Jackson, C. (2001) Teaching Primary Care Trusts – An important development for pharmacy in the future, *The Pharmaceutical Journal*, 206, 57–58

Jefferys, M. (1995) Primary mental health care. In Owens, P., Carrier, J. and Horder, J. (eds.) *Interprofessional Issues in Community and Primary Health Care*, Macmillan, Basingstoke

National Primary Care Research and Development Centre [NPCRDC] (2001) *National Tracker Survey of Primary Care Groups and Trusts 2000/2001: Modernising the NHS?* NPCRDC, Manchester

Peters, D. and Chaitow, L. (2001) Integrated medicine in primary care, *Holistic Health*, 69, 7–8

Pratt, J., Plamping, D. and Gordon, P. (1998) *Partnership: Fit for purpose?* King's Fund, London

Smith, R. (1992) Introduction. In: *The Future of Health Care*, a collection of articles published in the *British Medical Journal*, London

Appendix I Distinction between Severe Mental and Behavioural Disorders and Common Mental Health Problems

Severe Mental and Behavioural Disorders

Conditions that cause major disruption of social, occupational and/or domestic activities that are uncontained, or unstable or sustained for at least a few weeks.

- Acute or transient psychotic disorders [a]
- Recurrent depressive disorders (at least one episode having been severe) [b]
- Severe depressive episodes [b]
- Severe personality disorders
- Substance dependence syndromes [c]
- Substance induced psychotic disorders [c]
- Dementias [d]
- Obsessive-compulsive disorder
- Post-traumatic stress disorder [e]
- Prolonged depressive adjustment disorder
- Dissociative disorders
- Anorexia nervosa [f]

Severe Enduring Mental Illness

Conditions that cause major disruption of social, occupational and/or domestic activities and are chronic and recurrent unless adequately treated.

- Schizophrenia
- Delusional disorder
- Schizoaffective disorder
- Bi-polar affective disorders
- Recurrent affective disorders (at least one episode having been severe with psychotic symptoms)

Common Mental Health Problems

Conditions causing mild or moderate disruption of social, occupational and/or domestic activities that are contained, stable or time limited.

- Mild/moderate depressive episodes [b]
- Recurrent depressive disorders, episodes always having been mild or moderate [b]
- Dysthymia
- Harmful use of substances [c]

- Uncomplicated panic disorder
- Generalised anxiety disorders
- Phobic anxiety disorders – panic attacks
- Somatoform autonomic dysfunction
- Mixed anxiety and depressive disorders
- Adjustment disorders
- Somatisation disorders
- Hypochondriacal disorders
- Neurasthenia (post-viral fatigue/ME) [e]
- Bulimia nervosa [f]
- Binge eating disorder [f]

[a] subsuming puerperal psychosis.
[b] Subsuming special categories such as post-natal affective disorders and premenstrual dysphoric disorders.
[c] May appropriately be managed by community alcohol/drug teams – an addictive behaviours centre.
[d] May appropriately be managed by elderly mental illness services.
[e] May appropriately be managed by tertiary specialist psychotherapy services.
[f] May appropriately be managed by eating disorders services.

N.B. Common mental health problems may be 'complicated' by co-morbidity, active suicidal ideation, overwhelming psychosocial issues and/or treatment resistance, in any or all of which cases they may be viewed as severe and more appropriately managed within (or at least in consultation with) specialist mental health services.

APPENDIX II   THE EDINBURGH POST-NATAL DEPRESSION RATING SCALE (INCLUDING SCORES)

From Cox, J.L., Holden, J.M. and Sagovsky, R. (1987) Detection of post-natal depression: development of the 10-item Edinburgh Post-natal Depression Scale, *British Journal of Psychiatry*, **150**, 782–786

1. **I have always been able to laugh and see the funny side of things:**

As much as I always could	0
Not quite so much now	1
Definitely not so much now	2
Not at all	3

2. **I have looked forward to things with enjoyment:**

As much as I ever did	0
Rather less than I used to	1
Definitely less than I used to	2
Hardly at all	3

3. **I have blamed myself unnecessarily when things went wrong:**

Yes, most of the time	3
Yes, some of the time	2
Not very often	1
No, never	0

4. **I have felt worried and anxious for no very good reason:**

No, not at all	0
Hardly ever	1
Yes, sometimes	2
Yes, very often	3

5. **I have felt scared and panicky for no very good reason:**

Yes, quite a lot	3
Yes, sometimes	2
No, not much	1
No, not at all	0

6. **Things have been getting on top of me:**

Yes, most of the time I haven't been able to cope at all	3
Yes, sometimes I haven't been coping as well as usual	2

No, most of the time I have coped quite well	1
No, I have been coping as well as ever	0

7. I have been so unhappy I have had difficulty sleeping:

Yes, most of the time	3
Yes, some of the time	2
Not very often	1
No, not at all	0

8. I have felt sad or miserable:

Yes, most of the time	3
Yes, quite often	2
Not very often	1
No, not at all	0

9. I have been so unhappy that I have been crying:

Yes, most of the time	3
Yes, quite often	2
Only occasionally	1
No, never	0

10. The thought of harming myself has occurred to me:

Yes, quite often	3
Sometimes	2
Hardly ever	1
Never	0

Mothers are asked to indicate which answer comes closest to 'How you have felt in the past 7 days not just how you feel today'.

Mothers who score above a threshold of 12/13 are likely to be suffering from a depressive illness of varying severity; nevertheless, the EPDS score should not override clinical judgement.

APPENDIX III   MENTAL HEALTH SELF-HELP GROUPS AND VOLUNTARY ORGANISATIONS

Adapted from Appendix II of Gask, L., Rogers, A., Roland, M. and Morris, D. (2000) *Improving Quality in Primary Care: A practical guide to the National Service Framework for Mental Health*, published by The National Primary Care Research and Development Centre, University of Manchester.

This is not intended to be a comprehensive listing. NHS Direct (www.nhsdirect.uk) can provide additional information on self-help and voluntary organisations: Tel: 0845 4647.

Alcohol problems

Alcohol Concern (www.alcoholconcern.org.uk) puts people in touch with local alcohol advice and counselling services, and provides a range of leaflets. Waterbridge House, 32–36 Loman Street, London SE1 0EE. Tel: 020 7928 7377 (office), 24-hour helpline: 0800 917 8282, e-mail: AC@alccon.dircon.co.uk

Alzheimer's Disease

The Alzheimer's Society (www.alzheimers.org.uk) provides information and support for carers, a comprehensive range of leaflets and booklets, and campaigns for better services and increased public awareness of dementia. Gordon House, 10 Greencoat Place, London SW1P 1PH. Tel: 020 7306 0606, helpline: 0845-300 0336, e-mail: info@alzheimers.org.uk

Bereavement

CRUSE (www.crusebereavementcare.org.uk) is a national organisation offering free information and advice to anyone who has been affected by a death. Cruse House, 126 Sheen Road, Richmond, Surrey TW9 1UR. Tel: 020 8940 4818, e-mail: info@crusebereavementcare.org.uk

Bullying

The **Anti-Bullying Campaign** runs a helpline for parents whose children are victims of bullying at school. Parents' and schools' packs are available. 185 Tower Bridge Road, London SE1 2UF. Helpline: 020 7378 1446 (9.30am–5.00pm Mon–Fri).

Carers

The Carers National Association (www.carersuk.demon.co.uk) provides information and advice for carers and campaigns on their behalf. Ruth Pitter House, 20–25 Glasshouse Yard, London EC1 4JT. Tel: 020 7490 8818, Carersline 0808 808 7777 (Freephone 10.00am–12.00 and 2.00–4.00pm Mon–Fri).

The National Alliance of the Relatives of the Mentally Ill (NARMI) was formed by carers as a campaigning organisation. It now provides advocacy, medical information and information about government legislation. Members receive quarterly newsletters, updates on medication, the Mental Health Act and changes in housing and welfare benefits. Tydenhams Oaks, Tydenhams, Newbury, Berks RG14 6JT. Tel: 01635 551 923 (answerphone service – all calls returned same day).

Depression

The Depression Alliance (www.depressionalliance.org) is run by sufferers of depression. It provides an online chat room, electronic support, self-help resources and lists of groups. 35 Westminster Bridge Road, London SE1 7JB.

The Manic Depression Fellowship (www.mdf.org.uk) aims to enable people affected by manic depression (bi-polar) to take control of their lives. It offers a variety of services including self-help groups, information and employment advice. Castle Works, 21 St George's Road, London SE1 6ES. Tel: 020 7793 2600.

Eating disorders

The Eating Disorders Association (www.edauk.com) provides information and a nationwide network of self-help groups for people affected by eating disorders. Youth Helpline: 01603 621 414 (9.00am–6.30pm Mon–Fri).

www.serpell.com/eat.htm provides resources for people interested in finding out more about eating disorders.

Gay and lesbian

The Pink Practice provides resources relating to counselling and psychotherapy for people who describe themselves as lesbian, gay, bisexual or transgender. Tel: 0113-242 4884 (9.00am–7.00pm Mon–Thurs). They will usually respond within 48 hours to messages left on answerphone.

General

Contact (www.doh.gov.uk/mentalhealthcontact/index.htm) is a directory for mental health. This Department of Health publication, recently updated, provides a comprehensive listing of organisations working with a whole range of mental health problems. Print copies are available free from: PO Box 777, London SE1 6XH, e-mail: doh@prolog.uk.com

MIND (www.mind.org.uk) is a major charity that promotes the needs of people with mental health problems through campaigns, conferences, publications, and a wide network of local groups. MIND's information line is 0845 766 0163 outside London or 020 8522 1728 in London (9.15am–4.45pm Mon–Thurs, 11.45am–4.45pm Fri). As part of the Mindinfoline, a pharmacist from the United Kingdom Psychiatric Pharmacy Group's helpline takes calls on 020 8215 2274 (9.15am–11.45pm Thurs). MIND can be written to at Mind Information Service, 15–19 Broadway, London E15 4BQ.

The Mental Health Foundation (www.mentalhealth.org.uk) provides a wide variety of services for users and professionals, including courses and conferences, publications, leaflets, and links to other self-help groups. UK Office, 20/21 Cornwall Terrace, London NW1 4QL. Tel: 020 7535 7400, fax: 020 7535 7474, e-mail: mhf@mentalhealth.org.uk

The Mental Health Foundation, Scotland Office, 5th Floor, Merchants House, 30 George Square, Glasgow G2 1EG. Tel: 0141-572 0125, fax: 0141-572 0246.

At Ease (www.at-ease.nsf.org.uk) is a mental health resource for people under stress or worried about their thoughts and feelings.

Recovery (www.recovery-inc.com/intro) provides an online mental health self-help programme to help people regain and maintain their mental health for a range of problems. It focuses on techniques for dealing with the problems of everyday life.

The Greater London Mental Health Advocacy Network (www.comcom.org/ GLMHAN/index.htm) is an online directory of organisations for users, listed by agency name, borough, health authority and hospital.

The UK Advocacy Network provides a link to independent patient councils, advocacy projects and user forums for mental health service users. Volserve House, 14–18 Westbar Green, Sheffield S1 2DA. Tel: 0114-272 8171 (10.00am–4.00pm Mon–Fri).

The Advocacy and Community Online Resource Network (www.comcom.org/ acorn) has a menu of self-help organisations.

Patient UK Self Help (www.patient.co.uk/selfhelp) has a comprehensive listing of self-help resources, including those relating to mental health and behavioural problems. The Mental Health Foundation (www.mentalhealth.org.uk) also provides information on self-help resources.

Inter-cultural counselling

The **Nafsiyat Intercultural Therapy Centre** provides a psychotherapy and counselling centre for people from black and ethnic-minority groups catering for individuals, groups, families and couples. They have produced a video on mental health in Hindi, Urdu, Punjabi, Cantonese, Greek and English. 278 Seven Sisters Road, Finsbury Park, London N4 2HY. Tel: 020 7263 4130.

Parents/children/family problems

Compassionate Friends provides self-help and support to bereaved parents and their families, and supports telephone contact groups. 53 North Street, Bristol BS3 1EN. Tel: 0117-953 9639 (helpline 9.30am–10.30pm daily).

The Anna Freud Centre Family Support Service (www.annafreudcentre.org) provides a family support service for parents with children experiencing psychological and emotional problems. It also runs a helpline. 21 Maresfield Gardens, London NW3. Tel: 020 7794 2313.

Phobias

The National Phobics Society (www.phobics-society.org.uk) organises groups throughout the country for people experiencing anxiety. Zion Community Health Resource Centre, Hulme, Manchester M15 5FQ. Tel: 0870 7700 456.

First Steps to Freedom offers support to people with anxiety and obsessive-compulsive disorders. 7 Avon Court, School Lane, Warwickshire CV8 2GX. Tel: 01926 851 608.

Post-natal illness

The Association for Post-Natal Illness (www.apni.org) offers support and advice to mothers experiencing post-natal illness, including depression, and has a network of volunteers throughout the UK. 145 Dawes Rd, Fulham, London SW6 7EB. Tel: 0207 7386 0868 (10.00am–2.00pm Mon, Fri; 10.00–5.00pm Tue, Wed, Thurs), e-mail: info@apni.org

Post-traumatic stress

Trauma After Care Trust (TACT), Buttfields, The Farthings, Withington, Gloucestershire GL54 4DF. Helpline: 01242 890 306.

Psychiatric drug and tranquilliser problems

ADFAM National provides a helpline and guide to setting up a family support group. Waterbridge House, 32–36 Loman Street, London SE1 0EE. Tel: 020 7928 8900.

The Council for Involuntary Tranquilliser Addiction provides help for clients and professionals in the management of tranquilliser and antidepressant addiction. Leaflets available. Training offered to professionals. Cavendish House, Brighton Road, Waterloo, Liverpool L22 5NG. Helpline: 0151-949 0102 (10.00am–1.00pm Mon–Fri). Office: 0151-474 9626.

The UK Psychiatric Pharmacy group is based at the Maudsley Hospital in London and provides information on psychiatric drugs. Tel: 020 7919 2999 (11.00am–5.00pm).

Schizophrenia and psychoses

Hearing Voices is a user-led group helping people come to terms with their voices. It produces an information pack and a list of self-help groups around the UK. Hearing Voices Network, 91 Oldham Street, Manchester M4 1LW. Tel: 0161-834 5768 (9.00am–5.00pm Mon–Fri, answerphone all other times), e-mail: hearingvoices@care4free.net

The National Schizophrenia Fellowship (www.nsf.org.uk) provides support services and information aimed at helping people affected by schizophrenia and other major mental health problems. 30 Tabernacle Street, London EC2 4DD. Tel: 020 7330 9100, e-mail: info@nsf.org.uk

SANELINE is a helpline (0345-67 8000, 2.00pm–12 midnight, 365 days a year) for users affected by mental health problems, carers and professionals. It provides emotional support and information.

Sexual abuse

Abuse Recovery UK (www.abuse.recovery.uk.asarian-host.org) provides interactive support to survivors of sexual abuse either as a child or adult.

Suicidal thoughts

The Samaritans (www.samaritans.org.uk) provide confidential emotional support to any person who is suicidal or despairing. They aim to increase public awareness of issues around suicide and depression. The national phone number is 0345 90 90 90.

The Self-Harm Bristol Crisis Service for Woman (www.users.zetnet.co.uk/BCSW) provides a helpline, and runs and supports self-help groups. Tel: 0117-925 1119.

CALM (Campaign Against Living Miserably) Helpline: Freephone 0800 58 58 58 (5.00pm–3.00am daily). A special focus on helping young men who feel suicidal – free access by telephone to trained counsellors offering health advice and referrals to people in the north-west of England.

Young people

Young Minds (www.youngminds.org.uk) produces a range of leaflets, and runs a parent information service. 102–108 Clerkenwell Road, London EC1 M5SA. Tel: 020 7336 0445, e-mail: enquiries@youngminds.org.uk

Organisations cited in chapters

BRIB Working for Blind People, now known as Birmingham Focus for Blindness, 48–62 Woodville Road, Harborne, Birmingham B17 9AT. Tel: 0121 428 5000.

CRUSE Bereavement Care: 3rd Floor, Edward Building, 205 Corporation Street, Birmingham B4 4SE. Tel: 0121 687 8010.

INDEX